Horse and Stable Management

Horse and Stable Management

Fourth Edition

Jeremy Houghton Brown, Sarah Pilliner
and Zoe Davies

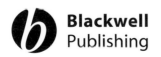

Blackwell
Publishing

© 2003 Jeremy Houghton Brown, Sarah Pilliner and Zoe Davies

Published by Blackwell Publishing Ltd
Editorial offices:
Blackwell Publishing Ltd, 9600 Garsington Road, Oxford OX4 2DQ, UK
    Tel: +44 (0)1865 776868
Blackwell Publishing Professional, 2121 State Avenue, Ames, Iowa 50014-8300, USA
    Tel: +1 515 292 0140
Blackwell Publishing Asia Pty Ltd, 550 Swanston Street, Carlton, Victoria 3053, Australia
    Tel: +61 (0)3 8359 1011

First published as *Horse and Stable Management* by Granada Publishing 1984
Second edition published by Blackwell Science 1994 and *Horse Care* published by Blackwell Science 1994
Third (omnibus) edition published 1997
Fourth edition published by Blackwell Publishing 2003
Reprinted 2004, 2005

Library of Congress Cataloging-in-Publication Data
Brown, Jeremy Houghton.
  Horse and stable management/Jeremy Houghton Brown, Sarah Pilliner, and Zoe Davies.—4th ed.
      p. cm.
Includes bibliographical references and index.
    ISBN 1-4051-0007-9 (Paperback : alk. paper)
    1. Horses. 2. Horses—Psychology. 3. Horses—Health. 4. Stables—Management. I. Pilliner, Sarah.
  II. Davies, Zoe. III. Title.
  SF285.3.B76 2003
  636.1′089–dc21   2003008648

ISBN-10: 1-4051-0007-9
ISBN-13: 978-1-4051-0007-6

A catalogue record for this title is available from the British Library

Set in 10/12.5pt Times and produced by Gray Publishing, Tunbridge Wells, Kent
Printed and bound in India by Replika Press Pvt. Ltd.

The publisher's policy is to use permanent paper from mills that operate a sustainable forestry policy, and
which has been manufactured from pulp processed using acid-free and elementary chlorine-free practices.
Furthermore, the publisher ensures that the text paper and cover board used have met acceptable
environmental accreditation standards.

For further information visit our website:
www.blackwellpublishing.com

Contents

Preface

Since the first edition was published in 1984, *Horse and Stable Management* has become the recognised source of reliable information on all aspects of the practical management of horses and ponies. It is now the established textbook for everyone who owns a horse or works with horses.

This fourth edition has been radically revised and re-organised to include the most up-to-date and accurate procedures and advice. With many new photographs, *Horse and Stable Management* includes chapters covering evolution and behaviour, conformation and action, routine preventive measures, nursing the sick horse, first aid, lameness and the management of breeding stock.

Horse and Stable Management is essential reading for those taking British Horse Society and Association of British Riding Schools examinations, as well as those taking college equine courses or National Vocational Qualifications in horse care and management.

This book was originally written to show sound modern practice and to answer the question 'Why care for the horse in this way?'. Only by empathy with the horse and appreciating how its systems work can we give appropriate care and management. Other books have since followed this approach, as have examinations and training. As befits the leader, this new edition stays true to this theme as it incorporates the latest research findings and experiences which guide best practice, also, it is more accessible for swift reference and sure guidance.

Good horse management means competently and pleasantly getting the best from a horse in all seasons and on all occasions, thus enhancing the pleasure for both horse and rider. To this end, quality care comes from understanding both the mind and the body of the horse and treating each horse accordingly.

The authors would like to thank Joanna Prestwich for providing the new photographs.

Part 1
The horse

Chapter 1
Horse care through understanding its origins

Horses and humans

An understanding between humans and the horses in their care is essential in the proper management of horses. An appreciation of the horse's evolution and natural instincts, structure and their basic requirements will help to ensure a good relationship between horses and their carers.

The most significant attribute arising from the horse's development is probably the ability to adapt. The horse has adapted first through changes in climate and vegetation and then to living with humans. The modern horse now relies on humans to meet its needs, and a consideration of the horse and its character provides for better understanding and care.

Evolution and domestication of the horse

Horses evolved over approximately 50 million years from fox-like creatures to the animals that we know today. Fossils found in North America and Europe give us a clear picture of the development of the modern-day horse from its prehistoric ancestors.

Ancestors

The horse's most distant ancestor was *Hyracotherium* (also known as eohippus or dawn horse), a specialised browsing herbivore, similar in size to a fox.

Hyracotherium had three toes on the hindfeet and four toes on the forefeet. Relatives of *Hyracotherium* lived from 50 to 38 million years ago and were swamp and forest dwelling. *Hyracotherium* first emerged in North America; however before the Baring Straits separated the two continents some animals migrated across the land bridges to Europe. *Hyracotherium* was a potential food source for large carnivores and therefore highly alert, with the ability to scurry away quickly from approaching predators; this is why horses have an inherent

nature of caution and alertness. Even the earliest ancestors of the horse had
acutely developed senses of sight, sound and smell to help them escape from
their predators.

Figure 1.1 outlines the evolutionary path of the modern horse.

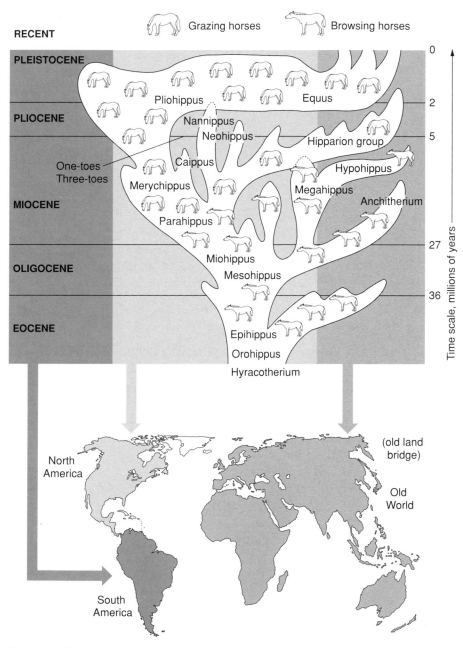

Figure 1.1. Summary of the evolutionary pathway of the horse.

Table 1.1. Some milestones in the evolution of horses

Horse ancestor	Millions of years ago	Notes	Geological period
Condylarth	65	End of dinosaurs	Palaeocene
Hyracotherium	54	Development of mammals	Eocene
Mesohippus	34	Modern mammals	Oligocene
Miohippus	24	Grassland hoofed animals	Miocene
Merychippus	17	Glaciers retreat	
Pliohippus	5	Human ancestors	Pliocene
Equus	2	Early humans	Pleistocene

The evolution of the horse was not a straight line of development, but a many branching tree, eventually producing *Equus*.

Survival of the fittest

Over the following millions of years, climate changes including ice ages with glaciations, led to the migration of huge numbers of animals to more temperate climates. Also, huge movements of landmasses effectively cut off migratory routes, thereby leaving some species stranded. Those unable to adapt to extreme weather conditions became extinct, whereas others slowly adapted to their new and different environments. Adaptation to new environments takes place through changes to the genetic makeup of the animal that are known as mutations. These changes take place over millions of years and result in a process of selection whereby those animals with genetic changes that result in increased ability to survive live on, while others become extinct. Many different types of animal that had mutated in this way succeeded *Hyracotherium*, some were highly successful whereas others were not and were lost.

The grazers

Climate changes led to changes in vegetation with new surroundings, such as cooler open plains and grasslands. Grasslands are by their nature open areas and the horses' ancestors no longer had the cover of bush and woodland. Two groups of three-toed horses were around at this time: the browsers and the grazers. The browsers eventually became extinct around 11 million years ago. The grazers adapted to their environment; they developed longer limbs specialised for speed to escape dangerous predators and the number of toes reduced from three to one to further support a speedy get away.

These grazing ancestors not only became taller and one toed, but at the same time further changed to suit their grazing way of life. Changes in the teeth and jaws enabled them to cut and chew large amounts of tough grass. Also, the size of the head changed to accommodate this battery of grinding teeth. The grazer's neck also became longer so that the taller animal could reach down to the grass to eat.

Grass is not as nutritious as the diet of the forest-browsing *Hyracotherium* and the horse's grazing ancestors had to consume much larger quantities of grass to support their increased size so they became trickle-feeding grazers, taking in large quantities of grass over long periods. This meant that changes to the animal's digestive tract had to take place and the gut adapted by increasing in size to digest large quantities of fibrous grass. This in turn resulted in the animals having longer and stronger backs from which to suspend the gut.

The grazing animals needed well-developed senses so that they could detect predators. They also developed the ability to sleep while standing to enable a quick get away. The horse gets up front feet first, after lying down, for a quick escape; whereas horned animals get up back end first in a defensive head down position.

The herd animal

At some point, the horse's ancestors developed an important social network for survival, living more safely and in harmony with others within their own herds. These one-toed horses belonged to the group *Equus* and these were the most recent ancestors of the modern horse, asses, zebras (Figure 1.2) and donkeys. For reasons that remain unclear, *Equus* became extinct in North America but several types of *Equus* survived in Europe and Asia. These evolved into different types, some were pony types whereas others were similar to small horses. These types gave rise to the many different breeds of modern horses.

Equus family

Table 1.2 lists some of the different species of *Equus* which live today.

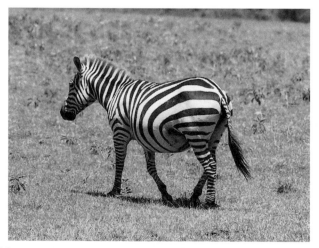

Figure 1.2. Zebra.

Table 1.2. Some present-day species of *Equus*

Common name	Scientific name
Domesticated horse	*Equus caballus*
Przewalski's horse	*Equus ferus przewalskii*
Persian wild ass (onager)	*Equus heminonus onager*
Domestic ass (donkey)	*Equus asinus*
African wild ass	*Equus africanus*
Burchell's zebra (plains or common zebra)	*Equus burchelli*
Mountain zebra	*Equus zebra*
Grevy's zebra	*Equus grevyi*

The horses and ponies of today have not changed greatly since *Equus* arrived roughly 5 million years ago. Their behavioural patterns are deeply rooted in their genetic makeup and must be considered and used during the training process.

Domestication

There is no doubt that mankind has contributed significantly to the success of the horse. Without human domestication there is reasonable argument to suggest that horses and ponies would have been greatly reduced in number, perhaps even becoming extinct. Humans would probably have simply hunted them for food, rather than using them in other ways. Before horses were domesticated for work, they were used as a food source. The horse's speed made it difficult at first for humans to keep up with them to kill them and the hunters had to become very inventive in their techniques. For example, evidence shows that some hunters used the technique of running horses off a cliff to kill them.

The first stage of domestication involved the nomadic tribes of central Asia keeping horses for their meat and mares for their milk production. The second phase of domestication took place with more placid types of horse, probably around 4000 BC. Farmers, when moving from area to area, used horses as pack animals to carry their goods. Sooner or later, a child or infirm person would also have been placed on this load. For bulkier loads the travois was devised with two poles crossed over the horse's withers and their butts trailing on the ground. Then came sledges and finally, with the advent of wheels, carts.

People began to ride horses, probably due to the need to herd animals. At about 1500 BC, a simple bone bit was devised. The horse became an integral part of human life and history.

Breeds and types

Horses were domesticated at different times and places throughout the world, leading to large varieties in breed and type. For example, in northwest Europe, with its wet climate, the native stock was akin to Exmoor ponies. In north Eurasia, with its colder climate, a heavier pony more akin to a Highland was domesticated. In western Asia, the fine-boned horses were Caspian's type and on the steppes of central Asia, the native horses were similar to the Akhal-Teke, which are still there today.

Modern horses and ponies can have their origins traced back to these four basic types. By breeding to meet human requirements the following now exist:

- hotbloods: Thoroughbreds and Arabs
- warmbloods: carriage and sports horses
- coldbloods: heavy draught horses
- ponies: with deep bodies and shorter legs.

These category names do not relate in any way to body temperature, in fact, they describe temperament and speed. The Thoroughbred tends to be more temperamental, faster, sharper and quick witted than the draught horse.

The larger and heavier horses are a comparatively modern feat of breeding as, in the 1500s, horses rarely exceeded 15 hands. The eighteenth century was the most notable for progress in selective breeding for specific purposes.

The horse in Europe and Asia

The Celts eventually arrived in Britain bringing their horses with them; these were crossed with indigenous types to produce the Celtic pony. The Celtic pony is the ancestor of many of the British native breeds, e.g. the Dales (Figure 1.3). The Romans and other invaders brought many different types with them to Britain.

From 6000 years ago, quieter horses were used to carry burdens and then ridden for herding purposes. The wheel was devised about 3500 BC and used for carts; later the spoked wheel led to chariots, which were pulled by onagers (Persian wild asses), which were larger than the horses of that time. Mounted soldiers were first seen in about 1000 BC and later mounted couriers provided swift communications. Light cavalry horses were critical to the Persian Empire (500–300 BC). Then Alexander the Great, riding his horse, Bucephalus, created the Greek empire. This was eventually over-run by Attila the Hun, who had the advantage of stirrups in 450 AD.

The horse collar provided more efficient pulling and so improved transport from about 500 AD. Heavier horses, still no more than 15 hands, allowed soldiers to wear more armour and the crusades between 1100 and 1200 provided a contrast between armoured knights and Arabs on faster more nimble horses.

In 1200 Genghis Khan from Mongolia used his soldiers on their small ponies, to capture much of Asia. They played polo for recreation.

The 'high school' style of riding began with the Renaissance in about 1500. Hunting on horseback started in the eleventh century and by the eighteenth

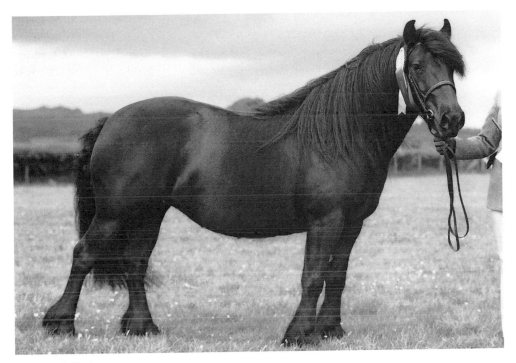

Figure 1.3. Dales pony.

century jumping was necessary due to the Enclosures Act. Racing was formalised in 1750, but the three great Arab sires, namely the Darley Arabian, Byerley Turk and the Godolphin Arabian, the foundation of all Thoroughbreds had already arrived. The Byerley Turk was put to stud in England in 1690. The Darley Arabian arrived in 1704 and was the great grand sire of Eclipse. The Godolphin Arabian arrived in 1728.

Cavalry were used in war until 1941 and the British army's pack mules were last used in 1975.

Horses were important in agriculture from the eighteenth century to the 1950s.

The horse in America

During the sixteenth century the Spanish Conquistadors arrived in North America by boat, bringing their horses with them. Thus horses were re-introduced to their native land where they had become extinct many years previously. These domesticated horses brought in by the Spanish became a major factor in the settlement of the continent; many escaped and became wild leading to the establishment of herds of wild horses in America. Many years later, the native North Americans and the gauchos of South America then tamed these wild horses.

The settlers in America used horses for exploration of the west. Horses were used to pull the famous wagon trains and to haul building materials as people moved in numbers across America. An important use of the horse was the Pony Express; riders carried mail in saddlebags on horseback, from Missouri to California, a distance of some 2000 miles covered by relays of horses and riders in about 8 days.

In America's Midwest, horses were used to work in the large fields being established by farmers. This involved the use of much bigger farm equipment and so larger and stronger horses were needed and farmers began to use larger draught horses brought in from Canada.

Natural behaviour of horses

The horse's main instincts are to survive and reproduce to ensure continuation of the species. The way in which horses evolved resulted in grazing animals that are regularly on the move and have great speed to escape predators (Figure 1.4). Horses are creatures of flight rather than fight and when threatened their natural reaction is to run away. However, if cornered a horse will kick or bite to defend itself. This means that horses are most relaxed in wide-open spaces within a herd environment as this provides safety and allows them to indulge in social behaviour such as grooming.

Modern management techniques have in many ways removed horses from this natural environment, often making them feel isolated. Horses are adaptable within reason, and with some forethought good stable management can fulfil many of the horse's natural behavioural patterns and requirements. This type of management will result in more contented, less stressed horses that are more able to cope with the demands of pleasure, performance and competition.

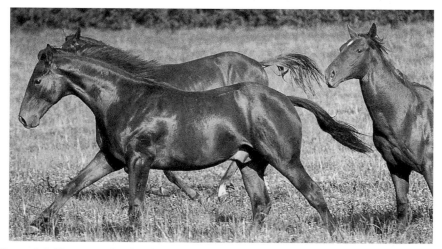

Figure 1.4. Horses evolved as free-ranging herbivores.

Natural management methods

Several aspects of stable management may be used to help fulfil the natural needs of the horse, including:

- water
- food
- shelter
- companionship
- space
- exercise
- understanding
- clean air.

Water

Clean fresh water should always be available. Dehydration and indigestion may lead to colic and can sometimes be the result of lack of water.

Food

As in nature, nutritious forage that provides a source of digestible fibre should be the basis of the feeding programme, keeping starch levels to a minimum. This allows horses to spend more time eating, keeping them occupied and less likely to develop stable vices or become bored. The proportion of concentrates must not exceed the forage part of the diet even in the peak fitness horse. Energy and protein sources should be matched to meet the horse's needs.

Shelter

In adverse conditions, horses need to have access to shelter. For horses at grass this may be a hedge, bank or built shelter, which allows horses to come and go at will. On the other hand, horses like to roam and play and should not be confined (unless due to injury or illness) for days at a time in a stable.

Companionship

Horses are naturally herd animals with a need for a social interaction (Figure 1.5). They like to be turned out with horses that they are known to get along with for several hours daily. Place grills in adjoining stables to allow horses to see, touch and smell each other. However, do make sure horses in neighbouring boxes are good companions.

Space

Horses generally prefer open aspects to their stables where they are free to observe their companions; however, as in nature, they may like some privacy when feeding.

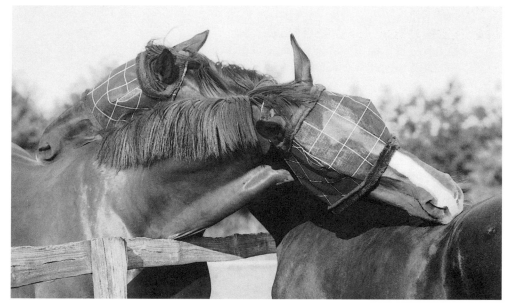

Figure 1.5. Horses enjoying a companionable scratch.

Exercise

Horses need exercise, after all they will move around a field grazing for as much as 16 hours a day if allowed. To confine horses to the unnatural environment of a stable for 22 hours per day (or even 24 hours per day on their rest day) is not recommended. Even some racehorse trainers with access to land now try and turn out fit racehorses daily to given them time to revert to their natural grazing and playful behaviour in open space.

Yards, horse walkers, play paddocks and other techniques can all help horses balance their performance lives with their natural needs.

Understanding

Over the past 5000 years a unique relationship has been established between humans and horses. It is the responsibility of the horse owner to provide the horse with the best possible environment and to ensure that stable management practices promote the mental and physical health and well-being of their horses.

Clean air

Horses need clean air. In the wild, horses rarely experience dust, but in a man-made environment, it is a major distraction to good health and performance. When any dusty operation is to be carried out, horses should be out of their stables. In stables the air should be gently moving through the stable and never stagnant.

Chapter 2
Describing the horse

The horse industry relies, to some extent, on a certain amount of specific, detailed terms relating to horses. The description of horses and ponies depends on identifying many features such as a sex, height, colour, markings, age and descriptions of type.

Sex

The following terms accurately describe the sex of a horse:

- a filly is a female less than 4 years old
- a mare is a female of 4 years old or more
- a colt is an uncastrated male of 3 years old or less
- a stallion is an uncastrated male of 4 years old or more
- a gelding is a castrated male
- a foal is a colt or filly less than 1 year old
- a rig is a male horse that has retained one testicle within the abdominal cavity.

Height

Horses are traditionally measured in hands, with a hand being equivalent to 4 inches (10.16 cm). All height measurements for competition horses and ponies are now given in centimetres (see Table 2.1). The measurement is taken with the horse standing squarely on a smooth level surface. The measurement is taken from the highest point of the withers using a measuring stick with a spirit level on the cross bar. For the purposes of the Joint Measurement Scheme the horse should be measured without shoes. For general purposes, 1 cm or 0.5 inch should be deducted for horses and ponies that are shod.

Many horses and ponies obtain life measurement certificates and these are taken by the panel of the Joint Measurement Scheme for horses over 6 years of age without shoes.

Correct height measurements are important for dividing horses into their correct height classes for show jumping, showing and other equestrian events. It also provides an accurate assessment of the horse when offered for sale.

Table 2.1 Horse measurement in hands and centimetres

Hands	Centimetres
11.0	111.8
11.2	116.8
12.0	121.9
12.2	127.0
13.0	132.0
13.2	137.0
14.0	142.2
14.2	147.2
15.0	152.4
15.2	157.5
16.0	162.6
16.2	167.6
17.0	172.7
17.2	177.8

Colour

Precise colour assessment is important when describing horses. Colour may change over the years. For example, foals are often born a different colour than that they will mature to; likewise grey horses become lighter, as they age. Also, some horses have different colour shades in the winter and summer. The points of the horse are used for more accurate assessment of colour, and these refer to:

- muzzle
- legs
- mane and tail
- eyelids
- tips of the ears.

The legs may be black or darker than the body or they may have white markings. A horse with no white markings at all is termed 'whole coloured'.

White patches caused by rubbing or excessive pressure such as girth galls and saddle sores are also used to help identify horses. White hair can also result from injuries such as cuts and are usually associated with some scarring. These acquired white patches should not be confused with natural areas of white hair in the identification of colour. Grey horses all become white with age, but are always described as grey and never as white.

- A bay horse is found in three different shades:
  - light bay: golden or reddish brown with black mane, tail and lower limbs
  - dark bay: rich, dark brown with black mane, tail and lower limbs
  - bright bay: horse chestnut colour with black mane, tail and lower limbs.
- A brown horse is darker brown almost black, with black mane, tail and limbs.
- A black horse is black with black mane, tail, limbs and muzzle.

- A chestnut is found in several shades:
  - liver chestnut: verging on brown with darkish (not black) mane, tail and limbs
  - light chestnut: paler shade and may have flaxen mane and tail
  - dark chestnut: rich red colour, sometimes with white limbs.
- A grey horse is found in several shades and has black skin:
  - iron grey: mainly black hairs and flecked with some white
  - light grey: mainly white
  - flea-bitten grey: dark hair growing in speckles through the white hair
  - dapple grey: white hair with circles of black hair over the body.
- A dun horse may be blue or yellow with a dark line or 'list' along the backbone:
  - blue dun: diluted black colour with black mane, tail and limbs
  - yellow dun: dark gold colour with black mane, tail and limbs.
- A palomino varies from gold to cream with similar coloured limbs and lighter or silvery coloured mane and tail.
- A piebald has large patches of black and white.
- A skewbald has large patches of white and any other colours.
- A spotted horse has pink or mottled skin and may have:
  - leopard spot: dark spots dispersed over a lighter background
    blanket markings: dark spots on the rump area of lighter colour
  - snowflake markings: white spots on a darker colour.
- An Appaloosa has a grey coat with darker coloured spots. Markings may be leopard, blanket or snowflake as above.
- A cremello horse has a light cream coat with white muzzle, mane, tail and limbs. The skin lacks pigment and the eyes may be blue or pink in colour.
- A roan is found in several shades with white hairs mixed evenly through the coat:
  - strawberry roan is red and white with similar mane, tail and limbs
  - blue roan is black and white (appearing blue) with black mane, tail and limbs
    chestnut roan or sorrel is white and light chestnut with matching mane, tail and limbs.

Markings

The horse's markings including scars, brands and acquired marks from injury or saddle sores, and so on are recorded on veterinary certificates and registration forms.

The head

- A star: is a white mark on the forehead. It may be further described as large, small, irregular or may even consist of a few white hairs (Figure 2.1).
- A stripe: is a narrow white mark down the face which may be a continuation of a star and may be further described as irregular, narrow, etc. (Figure 2.2).

- A blaze is a wide covering of white hair running down the face over the nose (Figure 2.3).
- A white face is an exaggerated blaze covering much of the horses face.
- A snip is a white mark between the nostrils (Figure 2.4).
- A white muzzle describes white skin covering both lips and the nostrils.
- White upper lip/under lip – white skin at the edge of the lips.
- A wall eye describes an eye that is grey-blue in colour, the sight is unaffected.

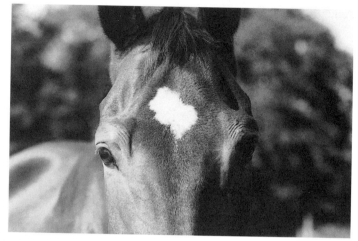

Figure 2.1. A star marking.

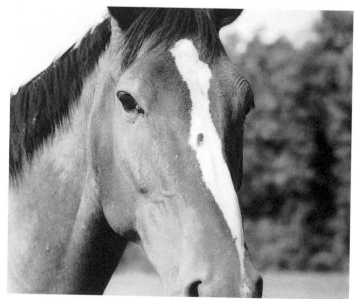

Figure 2.2. A stripe marking.

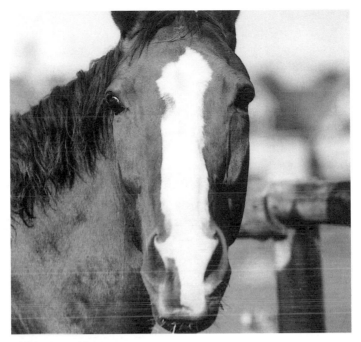

Figure 2.3. A blaze marking.

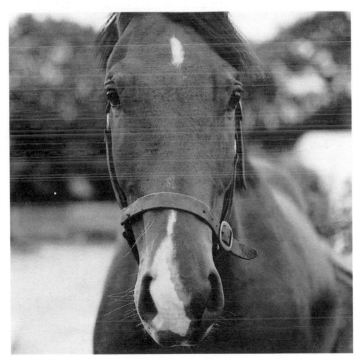

Figure 2.4. Horse with a star and large snip markings.

The body

- Dorsal stripe, list or ray – describes the dark line found along the backbone of dun horses and donkeys.
- Zebra marks – describe any stripes on the body.
- Whorls – small areas formed by changes in the direction of hair growth, occurring on the head, neck, body and upper limbs (Figure 2.5). Grey and whole coloured horses should have at least five whorl positions noted in their identification.
- Prophet's thumb mark – an obvious indentation in the muscle on the neck, shoulder or hindquarters said to be a sign of good luck and often seen in Thoroughbreds and Arabs (Figure 2.6).
- Flesh marks – patches of pink skin that grow white hair.

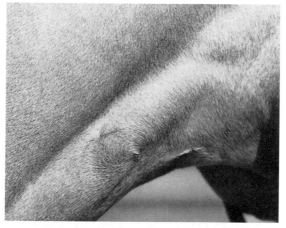

Figure 2.5. A circular whorl.

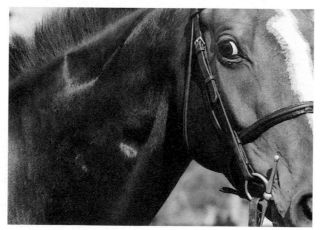

Figure 2.6. A prophet's thumb mark

Scars and/or brands may also mark the horse. Freeze brands resulting in white hair are a commonly used method of protecting horses against theft, each horse having its own unique number recorded on a national register. Brands indicate breed or country of origin and may be situated on the neck, shoulder or quarters. Identification brands may also be placed on the hooves (although these grow out and have to be remarked), or tattooed on the lips or gums. Some horses now have computer microchips of about the size of a grain of rice implanted into the superficial neck muscle.

The legs

White markings on the legs such as sock, stocking and leg are now only used for casual description and it is more correct to refer to the anatomy (Figure 2.7). Nowadays, the terms right and left are used instead 'off' and 'near', e.g. left leg to just below the knee instead of stocking.

Black spots on the white marks are called ermine marks. Any variation of the colour of hooves such as a white line down the hoof, should be noted. Hoof colour usually reflects the colour of the skin on the coronet.

Identification certificates

These are official certificates that must be completed by a veterinary surgeon, who will note down a description of all markings and colour on a sketch. The

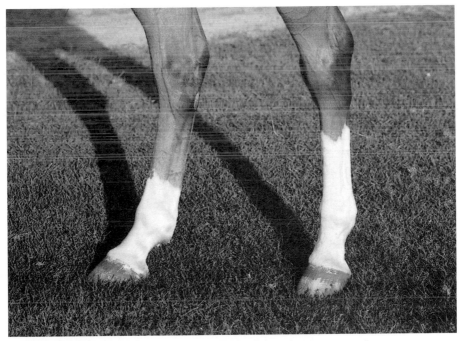

Figure 2.7. Left hind white to just below hock; right hind to lower cannon.

vet will also give a written description. White markings on the horse are outlined in red and filled with red diagonal lines, whorls are shown by an X in black, a tick in black shows scars.

The written description should be in black ink and should note the position of whorls and scars according to the sketch.

Age

A description of the horse is not complete without including its age. As the biting surfaces of the front incisor teeth wear away, the pattern on the tooth surface changes so that, with experience, the age of the horse can be estimated. This is described in more detail in Chapter 5.

Description of type

A brief description of the type or breed, if known, of the horse is helpful. For example, fine horses are described as lightweight; those with a little more substance and bone as middleweight and a substantial weight-carrying horse is known as a heavyweight. If the horse has characteristics of a certain breed, but the actual breed is unknown then it may be described as a 'Thoroughbred-type' (see below).

Types

Different horse types evolved to survive in different climates. Types that evolved in hot environments developed different physical and temperamental characteristics from those in colder environments. These are known as:

- hotbloods
- coldbloods
- warmbloods.

This does not in any way refer to body temperature.

Hotbloods

Sometimes referred to as blood horses, these types evolved in warm environments. Owing to high temperatures they developed fine skins and coats. Their heads are shorter and finer. Finer and longer legs helped to rid the body of excess heat. These types tend to be more sensitive and quick to react. Hotbloods tend to be more spirited and these include the Thoroughbred (Figure 2.8) and Arab.

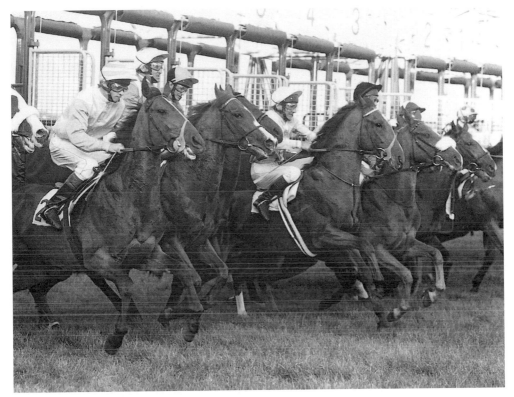

Figure 2.8. Thoroughbred horses.

Coldbloods

These include heavier breeds such as draught horses (Figure 2.9) and ponies. They are heavier and more thick set with deep wide bodies and shorter legs to maintain their body heat. They have thicker and longer coats with feathering around their lower legs to help keep them warm in the colder climates in which they evolved. The hair is thicker and coarser to trap air and provide increased insulation. Most coldbloods are efficient at maintaining condition, as food was less plentiful in colder climates and to this day they tend to be good doers.

Coldbloods tend to be more docile, preferring not to waste energy, and are tough.

Warmbloods

Warmbloods (Figure 2.10) have resulted from crossbreeding hotbloods and coldbloods. Breeders have attempted to match desired traits from both groups such as athleticism from hotbloods and the toughness and calmer temperament of the draught horse.

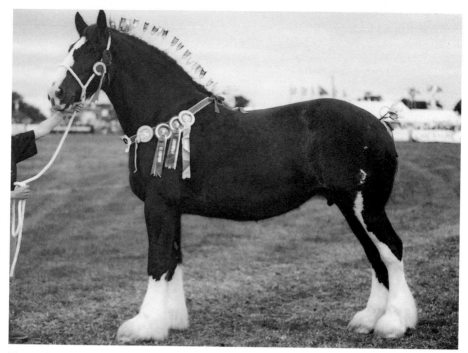

Figure 2.9. A draught horse (Shire)

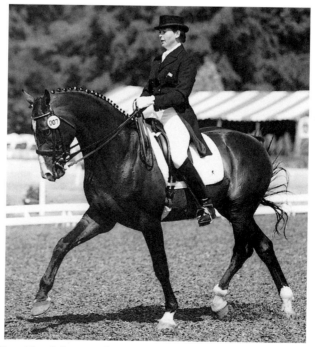

Figure 2.10. Warmblood dressage horse.

Breeds

From the time that horses were first domesticated, humans have bred and cross-bred different types to create useful breeds and types for certain desired traits. Many hundreds of breeds have been developed over the centuries, some of these have died out while others have lived on.

Horse breeds fall into one of the three types described above or ponies. Ponies are described as any animal under 14.2 hands.

A new breed is recognised by the production of a studbook.

Chapter 3
Conformation and action

Conformation refers to the horse's inherited structure. There is plenty of lively debate on this subject, but the physical shape and capability of horses are important to define. The conformation of a horse will affect its soundness and its ability to perform athletic manoeuvres throughout its lifetime.

Conformation has two main aspects:

- static conformation – the shape of the horse
- dynamic conformation – the way the horse moves.

A horse's actual performance in terms of speed, endurance and jumping are not included in conformation. Temperament may be taken into account when assessing dynamic conformation.

Static conformation

Head

The head should be lean and well set on the neck. It should be in proportion to the size of the horse. If it is too big, the horse will always tend to travel on the forehand. The lower and upper jaws should meet evenly at the front so the lips should be drawn back to check. If the upper jaw is longer than the lower, the horse is said to be 'parrot mouthed' or overshot. Conversely, if the upper jaw is shorter than the lower, the horse is said to be 'sow mouthed' or undershot.

There should be sufficient width between the branches of the lower jaw to allow plenty of room for the windpipe. There should be room between the wing of the top bone in the neck and the lower edge of the jawbone to allow the horse to flex its head. Ease of flexion will help the horse breathe when working hard.

The eyes should be well set, clear, large and prominent. The horse should not be fleshy round the jowl and there should be a fine nostril, not being too small.

Neck

The neck should be muscular with a length in proportion to the horse's body. The topline should appear rounded with an arch between the horse's poll and withers. Heavy crests, as seen in stallions and many Welsh ponies, are not desirable in mares and geldings. If the neck dips down in front of the withers it is said to be ewe-necked. This is often seen in severely underweight horses.

Withers

The withers should be of a good height, but not overly defined. There should be just enough room to allow for the attachment of the shoulder muscles. Withers that are too high make saddle fitting difficult, while low, thick withers are often associated with poor action and reduced mobility of the shoulder. This can also lead to problems with the saddle slipping forwards. In the adult horse the withers and croup should be of a similar height. If the withers are lower than the croup, the horse is termed 'croup high' and this can lead to these horses having a tendency to work on their forehand, however some racehorses and show jumpers do well with this conformation.

Shoulder

The shoulder starts at the withers with the cartilage extension of the shoulder blade, which runs forward to the point of the shoulder (see Figure 3.1 for the points of a horse). The line from the withers to the point of the shoulder is known as the slope of shoulder. The slope of the shoulder and the angle made by the pastern to the ground should be about the same. A horse with a slightly upright shoulder would therefore be expected to have slightly upright pasterns; this helps to distribute the forces through the limb evenly. An upright shoulder gives a shorter stride and the forelimbs are more likely to show wear and tear

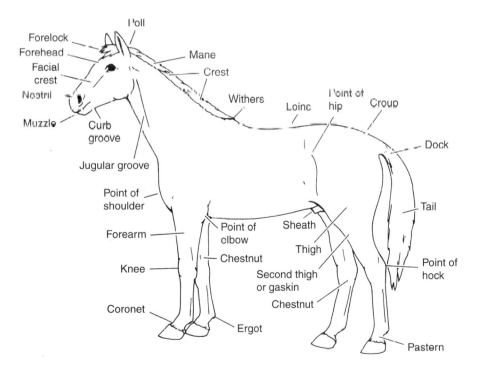

Figure 3.1. Points of the horse.

more quickly. However, the upright shoulder is often seen in harness horses as it provides better pulling power. A good sloping shoulder is preferred as this gives a longer, more flowing, stride.

Forelegs

The length of the humerus bone from the elbow to the point of shoulder affects the position of the forelegs. If this is slightly long, then the forelegs will be positioned too far back under the body, tie-ing in the elbow and restricting movement. The elbow should be placed well forward from the ribs. The forearm should be well muscled from the elbow and longer than the lower limb below the knee.

The foreleg should be straight down from the top of the limb to the foot (Figure 3.2). If viewed from the side it should run straight from the top of the leg to the front of the fetlock. If this does not run in a straight line, then the horse has poor conformation in this area and additional strain is placed on the tendons, joints and ligaments of the lower leg (Figure 3.3).

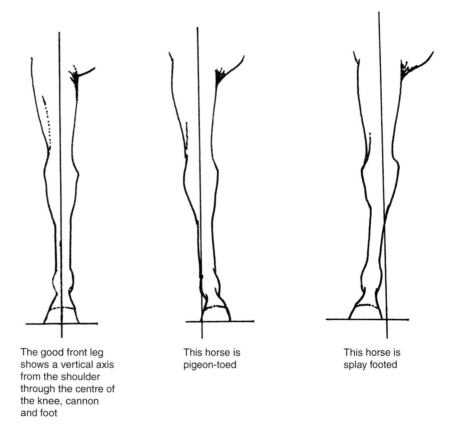

The good front leg shows a vertical axis from the shoulder through the centre of the knee, cannon and foot

This horse is pigeon-toed

This horse is splay footed

Figure 3.2. The front leg (front view) showing a good front leg, pigeon toes and splay footed. It should be noted that poor alignment and turning in or out are *not* the same; a horse's leg can have good alignment yet a toe turned in or out with the rotation starting at any joint.

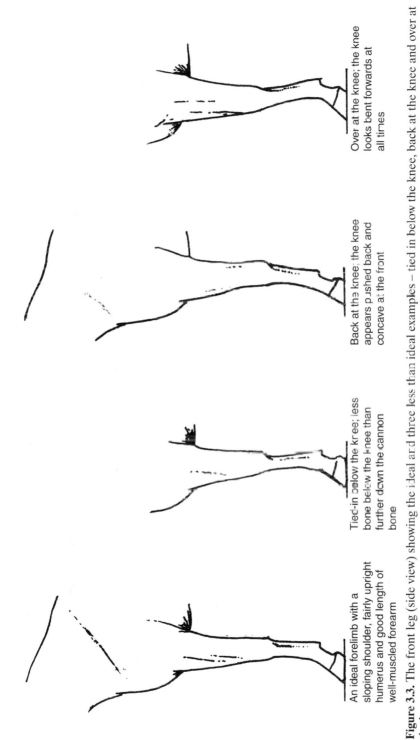

An ideal forelimb with a sloping shoulder, fairly upright humerus and good length of well-muscled forearm

Tied-in below the knee; less bone below the knee than further down the cannon bone

Back at the knee; the knee appears pushed back and concave at the front

Over at the knee; the knee looks bent forwards at all times

Figure 3.3. The front leg (side view) showing the ideal and three less than ideal examples – tied in below the knee, back at the knee and over at the knee.

Knees

The knee consists of a box of bones each separated by shock-absorbing cartilage. Knees should be broad, flat and deep to allow room for the attachment of tendons and ligaments (see Figures 3.2 and 3.3).

Horses are said to have 'calf knees' when they are back at the knee, i.e. concave when viewed from the side. These horses are not very suitable for fast work and/or jumping due to the added strain on tendons.

Horses are said to be 'over at the knee' when they appear to be forward from the elbow to the top of the pastern. This conformation is less likely to cause problems. The horse is described as 'tied in' below the knee if the cannon bone is narrower just below the knee than just above the fetlock.

The circumference of the leg just below the knee gives the measurement of 'bone'. This measurement actually including the tendons; heavier breeds of horses have more bone. As a rough guide, a horse of 16.2 hands should have over 20 cm (8 in) of bone for a lightweight and 23 cm (9 in) of bone for a heavyweight.

Cannon bones

These should be rather short straight and flat in front, with the tendons standing out cleanly at the back. This ensures the tendons are short and less liable to damage.

Fetlocks

These should not appear too round. Soft swellings on the sides of the fetlocks indicate wear and tear.

Pasterns

Pasterns should be of medium length, not too short or too long. Too much slope of the pastern puts greater strain on the tendons and, if they are too upright, excessive concussion may result in foot problems.

Feet

'No foot, no horse' an old adage, but based on fact. The shape and make-up of the feet are vital to long-term soundness.

Front and hind feet should be matching pairs, i.e. the front pair should be the same and also the hind pair. Any difference in these pairs may indicate problems, either previous or current. An exception to this rule would be the horse that has lost a shoe and therefore undergone excessive wear of that hoof in comparison to the shod foot.

The heels should be wide with a well-developed frog. The sole should be slightly concave and certainly not convex. Contracted heels may slightly restrict blood flow to this part of the foot increasing the risk of navicular syndrome.

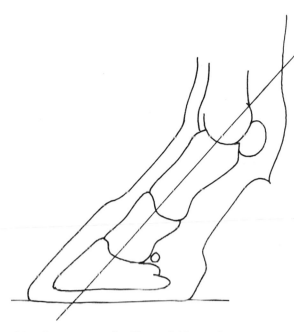

Figure 3.4. Good hoof–pastern angle. The pedal bone, long pastern and short pastern are correctly aligned and run parallel to the hoof wall and heel.

Large, flat feet may cause problems such as corns, whereas smaller feet have a greater tendency to develop unsoundness. Upright, boxy feet should also be avoided.

The hoof wall should be smooth and free from cracks, and it should not show too many rings as this may indicate chronic laminitis. Some rings are normal and often indicate a change in diet such as a change in pasture.

The quality of hoof horn is very important. Poor quality hoof horn leads to excessive wearing and difficulty in retaining shoes. Hoof horn seems to be of better quality on hardier native types and Arabs. Careful assessment of the diet may indicate the need for supplementation with biotin, zinc, methionine and calcium to help improve horn quality. Improvements will take at least 6 months.

Foot conformation should ideally be as follows:

- The front feet should slope at an angle of roughly 45° from the ground (Figure 3.4)
- The hoof wall should continue at the same angle as the pastern.
- The hind feet should have a more upright slope and should be narrower and longer than the front feet.
- All feet should point straight ahead. Forefeet toed in are known as pigeon toed: this is undesirable. Forefeet turned out are known as splay footed.

Chest and barrel

A deep, broad chest with 'well-sprung' ribs is essential to provide plenty of lung and heart room (see Figure 3.5). Horses that are shallow through the girth are described as 'showing too much daylight'. Horses that are too broad may produce a rolling action. The measurement from the lowest point of the girth to the withers should be approximately equal to that from the ground to the girth. Young horses often appear leggy but develop a deeper chest as they mature.

A horse with flat ribs is known as 'slab sided'. A horse of 16 hands or more should have a girth exceeding 1.83 m (6 ft). When viewed from the front the forelegs should have adequate space between them and not appear as if they have 'come out of the same hole'. They should drop straight down and not deviate at the knee or fetlock.

Good lung and heart room are essential. The first eight pairs of ribs are known as true ribs and are attached to the spinal vertebrae and sternum or chest bone. The next ten pairs of ribs are connected by long cartilage extensions to the breastbone and they are known as false ribs. Some horses have a nineteenth rib on one or both sides. The rearmost ribs should come close to the point of hip so that the horse is 'well ribbed up'. A wide distance between the last rib and the point of hip makes a horse appear long in the back and is often described as 'short of a rib'. A further weakness occurs when the underline of the belly slopes up excessively from front to back. This fault may cause the girth to slip back. The underline may also vary with diet and degree of fitness. Horses at grass

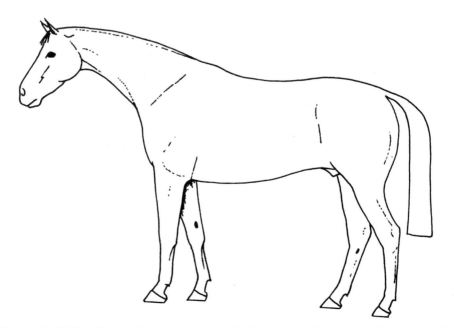

Figure 3.5. Well-defined withers and a strong back supported by a deep chest and well-sprung ribs.

often have a full gut and even appear pot-bellied, after stress of excessive work there may be a tightening of the abdominal muscles and the horse may appear 'tucked-up'. This is different from the overall leanness, which often accompanies hard trained horses on low forage rations.

Back

The back should be almost level and medium in length:

- short backs – strong but less comfortable for the rider
- long backs – gives a more comfortable ride, but are more liable to injury
- hollow backs – often seen in older horses as a sign of age, but may be a sign of weakness in young horses
- roach backs – arched upwards, these backs are uncomfortable for the rider even though they are strong. In older horses this may be a sign of arthritis.

Loins

Situated immediately behind the saddle area, loins should be broad, flat and well developed. A slack loin is often seen with a weak back and should be avoided.

Quarters

These provide the power for forward impulsion and should be muscular, rounded and a pair. Differences between the right and left side should be viewed with suspicion.

A horse is known as 'goose rumped' if the hindquarters slope excessively from croup to the tail and these horses tend to be lacking in speed (Figure 3.6). However, this conformation is often seen in successful show jumpers. A high croup is known as a 'jumping bump'.

Speed is expected in horses with plenty of length from point of hip to the hocks often referred to as 'well let down hocks'.

The tail should not be set on too low.

Hind legs

The horse should not appear split up the middle when viewed from behind, the muscles of the hind legs being well defined on both the inside and outside.

When the horse is standing square, the hind legs, viewed from behind, should show a straight line from the point of buttock through the point of hock down through the fetlock to the ground. Any deviations may indicate weakness placing additional strain on the important stifle and hock joints. The stifle and hock are very important joints working together to move the horse forward. The stifle should remain within the body and not be thrown outwards as the horse moves forward. The human knee is equivalent to the horse's stifle joint, both having a kneecap or patella.

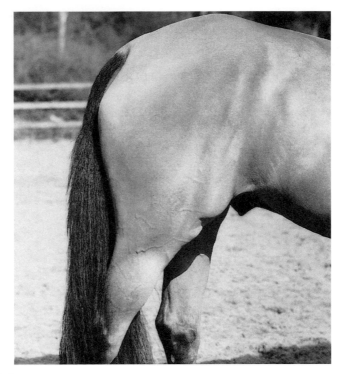

Figure 3.6. A goose rump.

There are a number of conformational faults associated with the hock:

- Cow hocks – feet turned out and point of hocks close together. These horses often brush (Figure 3.7).
- Bowed hocks – feet turned in and point of hocks wide apart (Figure 3.7).
- Sickle hocks – excessive angulation of the hock with feet placed more towards the forelimbs. More susceptible to curbs and wear and tear (Figure 3.8).
- Straight hocks – too little angulation of the hock, good for galloping, but less power for jumping (Figure 3.8).
- Hocks out behind – hocks stand out behind the horse, these horses jump well but do not tend to be good gallopers.

Dynamic conformation

Horses move according to their conformation and breed or type. Horses should move straight, particularly if destined for the show ring. Straight movers are less likely to suffer excessive strain and wear and tear of their legs. There should be slight knee action, but this should not be excessive unless required for the breed such as Welsh cobs.

Movement of the hind legs should indicate power and active hocks.

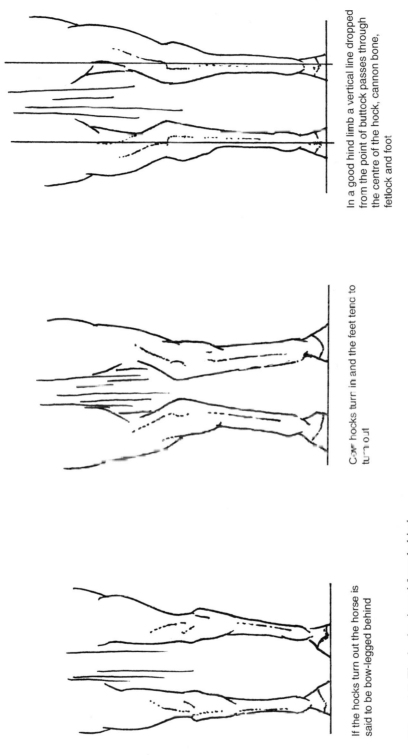

If the hocks turn out the horse is said to be bow-legged behind

Cow hocks turn in and the feet tend to turn out

In a good hind limb a vertical line dropped from the point of buttock passes through the centre of the hock, cannon bone, fetlock and foot

Figure 3.7. The hocks viewed from behind.

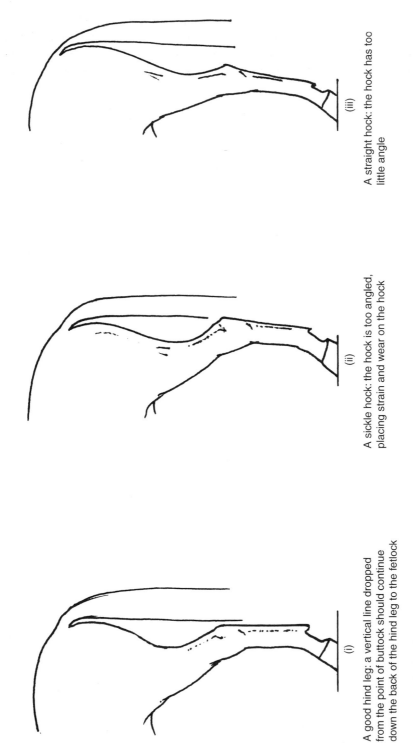

A good hind leg: a vertical line dropped from the point of buttock should continue down the back of the hind leg to the fetlock

(i)

A sickle hock: the hock is too angled, placing strain and wear on the hock

(ii)

A straight hock: the hock has too little angle

(iii)

Figure 3.8. The hindquarters viewed from the side. (i) A good hind leg. (ii) A sickle hock. (iii) A straight hock.

When assessing dynamic conformation, allowances should be made for small defects noticed in young horses as they have yet to strengthen up. However, serious conformational faults of youngstock are unlikely to resolve. Farriers may help to correct small deviations in youngstock through corrective trimming from foal through the yearling phase.

Walk

The walk is a symmetrical gait with a four-time beat (see Figure 3.9). The horse's feet follow one another in the following sequence:

- off hind
- off fore
- near hind
- near fore.

Regular steps of even length should be seen. Good walkers will place their hind feet in front of the hoof print left by their forefeet when walking up in hand. This is known as 'overtracking'. Good walkers are often good gallopers and this is a trait often searched for by prospective buyers at the yearling sales. Horses that place their hind feet in the hoof prints left by the forefeet are known as 'tracking up'.

Trot

The trot is a two-time gait with the legs moving in diagonal pairs:

- near hind
- off fore

and

- off hind
- near fore.

If the horse is extending at trot, there will be a moment of suspension between each beat (see Figure 3.10).

Viewed from the side, the strides of the left diagonal, near fore and off hind should be the same length as the right diagonal. A free moving shoulder with no sign of restricted movement is desirable as is a supple back, well-engaged hindquarters and freely, evenly flexing hocks.

The canter

This gait is three time, followed by a moment of suspension (Figure 3.11). If cantering to the right (or right-hand circle) then the sequence of footfalls is:

- left hind
- left fore and right hind together
- right fore.

Balance is achieved by the hind legs being placed well underneath the horse. The canter is the gait used to assess soundness in the wind.

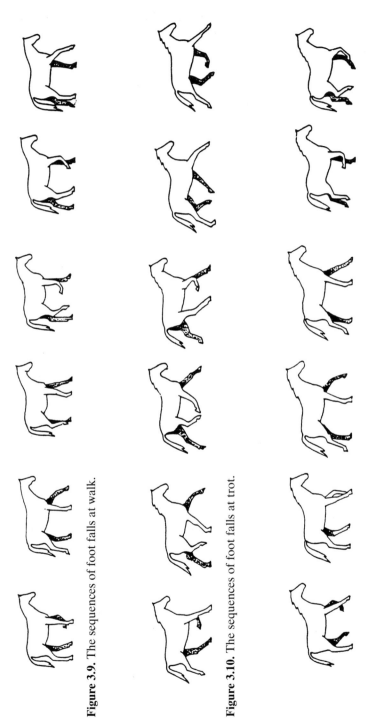

Figure 3.9. The sequences of foot falls at walk.

Figure 3.10. The sequences of foot falls at trot.

Figure 3.11. The sequences of foot fall at canter (left lead).

The gallop

The gallop should combine both speed and lightness with a good rhythm.

Faulty action

There are several different types of faulty action to look out for, most of these are observed at the trot. Although slight deviations are acceptable for normal use, they are frowned on in the show ring. Exaggerated movements may lead to unsoundness:

- dishing
- plaiting
- forging
- over reaching
- brushing/speedy cutting.

Dishing

Forefoot appears to be thrown out from below the knee, particularly at trot, but the actual fault lies in flexion of the elbow. It may occur in one or both forefeet. Severe dishing may lead to excessive wear and tear of the fetlock joints.

Plaiting

At walk and trot the horse places one foot in front of the other and is more often associated with narrow chest conformation. Excessive plaiting may lead to stumbling.

Forging

The hind shoe strikes the fore shoe and usually it may be corrected by good schooling to build up muscle. If the toes are too long the farrier may correct this.

Over reaching

The hind leg over extends and the toe cuts into the forelimb somewhere between the heel and knee. This often occurs when horses are jumping or galloping and may result in severe injury to the tendons of the foreleg. Horses known to over reach should wear protective boots.

Brushing/speedy cutting

The hind feet pass close by to one another and may brush against each other, if they come into contact higher up this is known as speedy cutting. This is often seen in horses that have toe out conformation in their front or hind feet. Affected horses will need to wear boots when ridden.

Assessment of conformation

Developing a 'good eye' for a horse comes with experience following close scrutiny of many different types of horses. Some breeds have particular conformational faults associated with them. For example, the draught horse is often goose rumped and straight in the shoulder, cow hocks are also often seen with these types. These horses were bred and used to pull loads; hence this conformation has developed over time. Assessing conformation of a horse should be undertaken in good light and with plenty of time allowed.

The most suitable horse or pony

After considering all aspects of conformation, both static and dynamic, all the factors should be taken into account and a judgement made depending on the intended use of the horse. A bomb proof, schoolmaster, child's pony will be preferred for its excellent nature and temperament, helping the child to develop riding skills. Minor conformational faults would be overlooked in favour of safety.

Perfect conformation is rare. Performance records of parents, grandparents and siblings should be inspected when purchasing youngstock.

Probably the most important factors when choosing a competition horse will be athleticism and good character. A horse with excellent conformation, but dubious temperament should be overlooked and left to professional riders.

Unsoundness

Unsoundness is a question of usefulness and not of disease. The position in English law was stated in the nineteenth-century case of *Coates* v. *Stephens* in the following way:

> *'The rule as to unsoundness is, if at the time of sale or examination, the horse has any disease, which either actually does diminish the natural usefulness of the animal, so as to make him less capable of work of any description, or which in its ordinary course will diminish its natural usefulness; or if that horse has, either from disease (whether such disease be congenital, or arising subsequently to birth) or from accident has undergone any alteration of structure that either does at the time or in its ordinary course will diminish the natural usefulness of the horse, such horse is unsound.'*

This is still the legal position today.

Veterinary surgeons now have a recommended form of examination of a horse for a prospective purchaser. After this examination the vet will conclude that the horse or pony is either suitable or not suitable for an intended purpose, for example, a child's pony, an eventer and so on. The vet's certificate is completed and given to the prospective purchaser who will then make a decision.

Five-stage vetting procedure

The aim of this examination of a horse or pony on behalf of the purchaser is to establish the facts about the horse and to conduct a five-stage examination looking for any abnormalities. This is a procedure that is carried out by the veterinary surgeon and the purchaser meets the costs. The purchaser is the client, not the vendor (seller). The vet will take down the details of the horse, name, breed or type, colour, sex, age by documentation and approximate age by the teeth.

The vetting is then carried out in five stages:

- the preliminary examination
- trotting up
- strenuous exercise
- period of rest
- second trot and foot examination.

Stage 1: the preliminary examination

The vet may stand and observe the horse at rest quietly in its environment, allowing heart and breathing rates to return to normal values after his or her arrival. Pointing of the toe, stiffness in turning or scuffing of the feet are noted. Evidence of crib biting, weaving or wood chewing is looked for. The handler then puts the head collar on the horse. If the horse is head shy, this will be noted. A stethoscope is then used to listen to the horse's heart on both sides of the chest. The horse is then taken out to the yard to look over in good light.

The horse is checked over for any unusual signs.

Stage 2: trotting up

The horse is trotted on a firm, flat surface. If adequate facilities are not available the vet may abandon the examination and arrangements made to have the horse taken to more suitable premises.

The horse should be walked away and walked back for about 20 m (66 ft). The horse is then trotted away and back for about 30–40 m (100–130 ft). The horse should have plenty of rope to allow free movement of the head and neck. The horse is then turned in a small circle around the handler doing two or three turns in both directions, before being backed up for a couple of metres.

Stage 3: strenuous exercise

The horse is exercised to the point of exertion, not exhaustion. This enables the heart to be listened to after exercise and any abnormal breathing noises detected. If the horse is fit to be ridden and there is suitable rider, then the horse should be ridden under saddle. If not, the horse is lunged. On reaching the area where the horse is to be exercised, the horse is trotted in a small safe circle around the vet on both reins. Then the horse is cantered in a larger circle on both reins, before an extended canter. Finally, the horse should be galloped passing close enough to the vet that he or she may hear any abnormal noises when breathing is synchronised with stride rate (see Chapter 13). The horse is pulled up and the heart listened to with the stethoscope.

Stage 4: period of rest

The horse is untacked and allowed to rest and stand quietly in the stable for 20–30 minutes. This allows time for any stiffness or stress associated with the exercise to become apparent. During this stage, the identification chart detailing the horse's markings and descriptions may be carried out (see Chapter 2).

The horse should not be taken out of the box during this time.

Stage 5: second trot and foot examination

The horse is brought out of the box and trotted away in hand and back for 40 m (132 ft) in both directions to detect signs of lameness. The horse is then turned round the handler in each direction as carried out in stage 2 and pushed back for a few steps.

Finally, the feet should be washed off and inspected, the vet is looking at the hoof/pastern axis, foot balance, uneven wear and state of the sole and frog. A hoof tester may also be used.

A blood test may be taken at the time of the vetting and for this the vendor will be required to sign a consent form. This may be stored for up to 6 months. The sampled blood may be used to test for various substances including phenylbutazone.

The vet may also recommend X-rays of the following: forelimb (knees, hocks, fetlocks, feet) and hindlimb (hock, stifle). Optional further examinations include: endoscope examination of the upper respiratory tract, tendon scan and an electrocardiogram (ECG).

The examination is complete. The vet will then gather the facts and assess the significance of any abnormalities in the light of the horse's future stresses or performance. The conclusions are then conveyed to the purchaser as fully and clearly as possible, often verbally before the final certificate is given.

The certificate states 'On the balance of probabilities, the conditions set out above are/are not (delete as appropriate) likely to prejudice this animals use for ...'. If necessary, further radiological examination or other specialised techniques may be undertaken by the vet after consultation with the purchaser.

Part 2
The horse in sickness and health

Chapter 4
The healthy horse

Health is not merely freedom from disease, but a state of well-being and vigour. Monitoring health and looking for early signs of problems are essential aspects of horse care. Watching patterns of individual horses and their behaviour are essential so that any difference from the horse's normal routine may be noted and if necessary acted on.

Signs of good health include the following:

- bright and alert attitude
- clear eyes, no discharge
- salmon-pink coloured membranes around the eyes and gums
- nostrils free from discharge
- mobile, alert ears
- shiny, smooth coat
- loose skin
- horse stands evenly, perhaps resting one hind foot
- no sign of sweating, unless hot weather conditions
- cool legs with no signs of heat or swelling
- droppings, green-brown colour (although this may vary with the diet) and free from unpleasant smell; should be passed eight to ten times a day
- urine, pale yellow to almost colourless, should be passed four to six times a day
- normal appetite and water intake.

Measurements such as those listed below, should be used frequently to monitor health.

These are collectively known as TPR (temperature–pulse–respiration rate) and the figures given below indicate normal values:

- temperature: 38°C (100.5°F)
- pulse: about 40 beats per minute
- respiration rate: 10–12 breaths per minute.

TPR of any new arrivals on the yard should be taken, and this procedure repeated at the same time of day for several days to ascertain the new horse's normal values.

Temperature

The horse's temperature is taken in the rectum with a clinical thermometer. The procedure is as follows:

- Shake the thermometer so that it reads several degrees lower than normal.
- Lubricate the bulb of the thermometer with petroleum jelly or saliva. Stand behind, but to one side, of the horse to avoid being kicked.
- Hold the horse's tail to one side and insert the bulb of the thermometer gently into the horse's anus, rotating it slightly as you do so. It should be inserted to half-way, at a slight angle to press the bulb against the side of the rectum.
- Leave in position for 1 minute.
- Withdraw and read the thermometer, taking care not to hold it at the bulb end. The mercury is most clearly seen if viewed through the apex that runs the full length of the thermometer.
- Clean and disinfect the thermometer before returning it to its case.

Many horses have a temperature that is normally 1°C lower than the value given and temperature may vary slightly throughout the day. The temperature should therefore be taken at the same time each day to establish a normal value for that horse.

In foals the normal value may be as high as 38.6°C.

Pulse

The pulse can be taken by pressing the fingers against an artery passing over a bone close to the surface, e.g. the facial artery on the inside edge of the lower jaw (see Figure 4.1) or on the radial artery inside the foreleg, level with the elbow. Some people like to take the pulse under the dock while taking the temperature. The simplest method of taking the pulse is to use a stethoscope just behind the horse's left elbow; after the horse has worked, even a flat hand lightly placed may be sufficient to feel the heart beat. The importance of monitoring pulse in such sports as long-distance riding has brought the use of the stethoscope into the range of the layman. The pulse rate of individual horses varies: a rate of between 35 and 45 beats per minute may be normal for a particular horse at rest, but a very fit horse may have a resting pulse rate that is considerably lower than this. A rate of 50–100 beats per minute is normal for a foal.

Respiration rate

To observe respiration, the horse must be standing still and undisturbed. The flanks should be watched from the side. Each complete rise and fall is counted

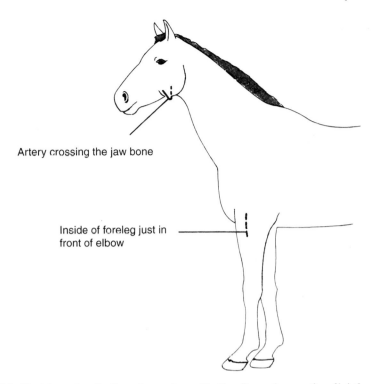

Artery crossing the jaw bone

Inside of foreleg just in front of elbow

Figure 4.1. Positions for feeling the pulse with the fingertips resting lightly on the artery.

as one breath. On a cold day, respiration may be observed by watching the nostrils as the warm air condenses as it meets the cold and breath can be seen. A range of 8–16 breaths per minute is acceptable in the adult horse at rest, 20–30 breaths per minute is acceptable in the foal.

Maintaining health

Current management practices have to some extent deprived horses of their natural environment. Key aspects to keeping horses should be managed to help maintain the horse's health and these include:

- fresh air
- exercise and rest
- protection
- mental health
- nutrition
- prevention.

Fresh air

Clean, circulating fresh air is vital for the respiratory health of horses. Horses should have plenty of access to fresh air outside of the stable by being given time out in the field.

For horses kept indoors for longer periods of time, research shows that all the air in a stable should be changed six to eight times each hour.

In particular, performance horses need a dust-free environment to maintain the health of their respiratory tract. Careful consideration should therefore be given to feed, forage and bedding, i.e. the general stable environment.

Exercise and rest

In the wild, horses exercise gently and steadily throughout the day, wandering and grazing. This process aids circulation and digestion. Ideally the stabled horse should have some access to a field every day.

Exercise should be built up slowly through a fittening programme and horses should not be left in the field or stable throughout the week and then be taken to a show on Saturday. Horses that are regularly exercised need time to rest and recover.

Protection

The wild horse has natural grease in its coat for protection. Excessive grooming and washing may remove many of these natural oils in the coat. Clipping also removes the protection of the coat from the weather. These horses need to be rugged up (see Figure 4.2) and offered protection in the field by artificial field shelters or natural hedges and trees. Clean, thick bedding should be provided to protect horses from injury and help keep them warm.

Mental health

The horse's natural mental health and well-being are important aspects of management. Horses that are mentally content are able to perform more consistently and tend to be more pliable than stressed horses. Some horses do become depressed if the stable environment is not suiting them and any signs of this should be acted on. Depressed and stressed horses have a reduced immune function leading to a higher risk of disease. Time out for these horses is vital.

Routine is important in the management of horses, they develop knowledge of feeding times and so on and these should be adhered to. They should be stabled next to horses they are known to get along with and turned out with good company to reduce risk of injury.

Nutrition

Horses must have access to clean fresh water at all times. A balanced diet should be provided, including plenty of forage to allow the horse to follow its

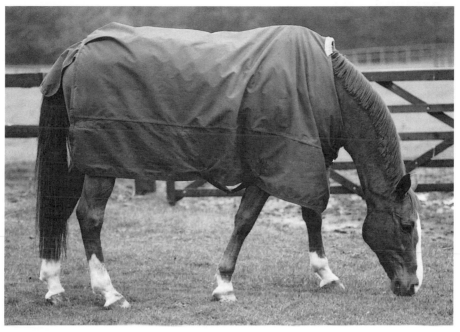

Figure 4.2. A horse in a turn-out rug.

natural feeding pattern of trickle feeding. The horse's digestive tract is ideally suited to eating fibrous food little and often. This is also important for mental health and reduces the risk of stable vices developing (see Chapters 16 and 17).

Prevention

The artificial lifestyle of modern horses exposes them to attack from parasites and infectious disease. Part of the management of horses is to keep them healthy and this must therefore include protection by following well-planned worming and vaccination programmes (see Chapter 5).

Chapter 5
Routine healthcare

Intensive management practices have contributed to high numbers of parasites, both internal and external, that live on horses. There are preventative measures which help to keep these parasites at bay in the equine population and should therefore be considered essential, as part of horse management. These programmes include vaccination and worming.

Another important aspect of routine healthcare of the horse is attention to the feet and teeth.

Worming

All horses carry internal parasites and most pasture is infected at some time if horses have been grazing it. As the level of the parasitic burden increases, extensive damage may be done to the digestive tract and other internal organs as worm larvae migrate through the body.

Internal parasites may cause severe health problems including:

- death
- colic
- loss of condition
- anaemia
- diarrhoea
- lethargy.

Horses may appear in good condition but still carry a significant worm burden; therefore it is important to treat all horses in the yard.

Control of internal parasites is based on breaking their life cycle through good pasture management and an effective worming programme.

Common internal parasites affecting horses include:

- large redworm (*Strongylus vulgaris*, *Strongylus edentatus*)
- small redworm (*Cyathostomes*)
- roundworm (*Parascaris equorum*)
- tapeworm (*Anoplocephala*)
- pinworm or seatworm (*Oxyuris equi*)
- threadworm (*Strongyloides westeri*)
- lungworm (*Dictyocaulus arnfieldi*)
- bots (*Gastrophilus*).

Internal parasites have a common life cycle, based on the egg, larvae and adult stages. Various species follow different migratory paths within the horse's body.

Parasite life cycle

If environmental conditions are favourable, eggs which may have lain dormant on pasture for as long as several years, hatch into larvae. These are known as first stage larvae (L1). These grow and moult into second stage larvae (L2) and then on to the third stage (L3). Eggs and L1 and L2 larvae cannot infect horses when ingested, they are digested in the horse's gut. L3 however is unable to feed and relies on being picked up by a horse within a couple of days. If not, it will die in the pasture. L3 larvae migrate up the blades of grass to increase their chance of being eaten. If conditions are moist, this is easier, if dry they are less able to migrate and often die.

Once eaten, L3 larvae burrow into the mucosal lining of the gut wall and moult into stage 4 larvae (L4). After a period of time L4 emerges, some complete their development in the gut, but others travel further to important organs such as the liver, heart and lungs. Larvae then return to the gut where they become adults before laying eggs that are passed out to the pasture.

Large redworm (*Strongylus vulgaris*)

Larvae migrate through important arteries to a position where the anterior mesenteric artery (supplying the gut) and aorta meet. They stay here for up to 3 months before returning via the blood vessels to the hindgut to become adults. Severe infestations may lead to weakening of the aorta, the largest artery in the body. Larvae may also cause blood clots (thrombi) cutting off the blood supply to parts of the gut. These parts may then die with resulting colic or even death.

The life cycle of *Strongylus vulgaris* is shown in Figure 5.1.

Small redworm (*Cyathostomes*)

There are approximately 40 different species of small redworm. Small redworm stay in the gut during their development, but burrow into the bowel wall where they become encysted, lying dormant, often for months. In the absence of a good worming programme these may build up in number often emerging *en masse* into the gut. This may cause severe irritation of the lining of the gut wall leading to acute enteritis and diarrhoea.

Roundworm (*Parascaris equorum*)

Common in youngstock, these worms live in the small intestine. They may be as thick as a pencil and up to 30 cm long. The female may lay eggs at the rate of 8000 per hour per worm. Eggs are highly resistant and may build up in the

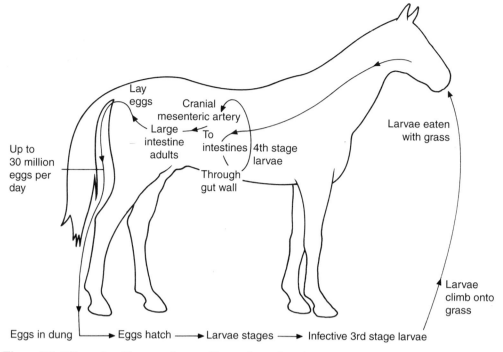

Figure 5.1. Life cycle of large redworm (*Strongylus vulgaris*): 200 days.

stable environment. Infective ingested larvae burrow through the gut wall and migrate via lymph vessels to the liver and heart and finally the lungs, where they are coughed up and swallowed. Once swallowed, they return to the small intestine.

Tapeworm (*Anoplocephala*)

Tapeworms may grow up to 80 cm long. They live in the small and large intestine. Their life cycle is different from other worms in that they require an intermediate host and this is a mite. There is some evidence that some horses can suffer from tapeworm infestation, but clinical symptoms such as colic and unthriftiness appear to be uncommon. The ivermectin group of wormers are not effective against tapeworm, and horses should therefore be treated with a double dose of pyrantel in the autumn.

Pinworm or seatworm (*Oxyuris equi*)

Eggs are laid at the horse's anus, from where they fall to the ground. The eggs contain larvae and the horse then eats these.

After hatching, the worms develop in the hindgut wall before returning to the hindgut lumen. The females laying their eggs may cause irritation making the horse rub its bottom and tail.

Threadworm (*Strongyloides westeri*)

These worms also live in the small intestine. They can survive in warm beds and may be particularly a problem of foals. Infection may occur through the dam's milk or via penetration through the skin. Foals with the infection may develop acute diarrhoea. The mare does not show symptoms and acts simply as a carrier.

Lungworm (*Dictyocaulus arnfieldi*)

These worms live in the horse's lungs. Donkeys are the major carriers of lungworm infection, but are often free from its symptoms. Infective larvae on pasture are ingested before migrating via the lymph and blood vessels to the lungs.

Adult worms produce larvae, which then travel to the throat before being swallowed. Horses develop a cough with lungworm infection whereas donkeys rarely do.

Bots (*Gastrophilus*)

These are the larvae of bot flies and not worms. Bots are the larval stage of the gadfly. The adult female lays yellow eggs on the hairs of the horse's forelegs from June to September. They irritate the horse causing it to lick them off. As the horse licks the larvae from the egg they attach to the horse's tongue. From here they migrate to the stomach and fix to the stomach wall. In spring they detach themselves and are passed out in the droppings. Ivermectin is useful against bots and should be used as a treatment in October/November.

Worm control

Worm control may be undertaken by anthelmintic (drug) treatment and pasture management.

Anthelmintic treatment (wormers)

Drugs for worming are known as anthelmintics. The use of drugs to treat horses for worms has played a major part in parasite control for many years. The theory behind their use is to kill the egg-laying adult worms and thereby reduce pasture contamination. Worming drugs may be used in two ways: interval dosing and target dosing.

Interval dosing

Interval dosing involves giving a specific drug at regular time intervals during the most high-risk time – spring and summer. Many horse owners continue to worm their horses through the lower-risk winter period or when stabled for most of the day. This may be expensive and often unnecessary. However, it is important to note that mild winters and an absence of frosts will lead to an increase in worm numbers. Worming drugs should be used at appropriate intervals, for example, a monthly use of ivermectin would be incorrect. The inappropriate or over-use of worming drugs increases the speed at which parasites develop resistance.

Target dosing

Faecal egg counts are performed prior to dosing. Treatment is then targeted at horses with significant (>200 eggs/gram) adult worm burdens. Larval parasites cannot be detected by faecal egg counts so such a routine should include larvicidal doses.

Methods of dosing include:

- power or granules added to the feed
- paste – given orally.

A worming programme should be decided on and routine worming of all horses (and donkeys) in a yard should be carried out. Most equine veterinary practices send out worming information and programmes to their clients and are happy to discuss the subject.

Worming is especially important in foals and youngstock.

Available drugs include:

- benzimidazole group
  - thiabendazole
  - mebendazole
  - oxfendazole
  - oxibendazole
  - fenbendazole
- ivermectin group
- pyrantel
- praziquantel.

Resistance has been shown to drugs from the benzimidazole group. Table 5.1 lists some commonly used equine wormers and their effects.

Ideally all horses sharing a field or a yard should be wormed with the same drug at the same time. Stabling for 24–48 hours following treatment does help to reduce the level of infection, but is often impractical particularly with horses kept at grass. New arrivals at a yard should be treated before turning out on the pasture, unless the previous worming history is known.

The correct dosage of wormer to give will depend on bodyweight. Manufacturer's instructions should be followed closely.

Foals should be wormed from 6 weeks of age, although many studs begin treatment from 2 weeks.

To determine the horse's bodyweight see Chapter 17.

Table 5.1. Commonly used equine wormers and their effects

Proprietary name	Drug	Worming frequency	Redworm small and large, ascarids, etc.	Tapeworm	Bots	Resistance known?
Equest	Moxidectin	13 weeks	Yes, includes encysted larvae	No	Yes	No
Eqvalan	Ivermectin	8–10 weeks	Yes, prevents build up of encysted larvae	No	Yes	No
Furexel	Ivermectin	8–10 weeks	Yes, prevents build up of encysted larvae	No	Yes	No
Strongid-P	Pyrantel	4–6 weeks	Yes	Yes, double dose only!	No	?
Equimax	Ivermectin, praziquantel	8–10 weeks	Yes	Yes	Yes	No
Eraquell	Ivermectin	8–10 weeks	Yes	No	Yes	No
Panacur	Fenbendazole	3 weeks	Panacur Guard 5 days for encysted larvae			Yes
Equitac	Oxibendazole	3 weeks	Yes	No	No	Yes
Telmin	Menbedazole	3 weeks	Yes	No	No	Yes

Pasture management

Keeping the pasture clean is a very effective method of reducing the worm burden. Removing droppings on a daily basis is ideal, if not once or twice per week. This is quite labour intensive, but worthwhile. Larger yards use vacuum equipment that is attached to a small tractor.

Rotating pastures with other livestock such as cattle and sheep also helps to break the life cycles and assists in 'cleaning' the pasture.

Vaccination

Vaccination provides protection against potentially serious or fatal diseases including:

- equine influenza
- tetanus
- equine herpes virus (EHV) – rhinopneumonitis
- equine viral arteritis (EVA)
- encephalitis.

Horses should be routinely immunised against those diseases from which they are most at risk in the country where they are kept.

Tetanus is given frequently in a joint vaccine with equine influenza with additional EHV and EVA given to breeding stock as appropriate.

Full certification of vaccination must be held by some performance horses, particularly under the British Jockey Club rules of racing and British Eventing or when competing at any event at any racecourse. Encephalitis, spread by biting insects, is a particular problem in North America.

Equine influenza

Effective vaccination against equine influenza helps to reduce the risk of outbreaks in competition horses, particularly racehorses and horses that travel regularly to compete. There are two distinct subtypes of this virus: A/equine/1 and A/equine/2.

All horses are susceptible, but infection is most common in young unvaccinated horses. Vaccinated horses may become infected, but show reduced symptoms. Equine influenza causes the following symptoms:

- coughing
- high temperature (42°C, 107°F)
- lethargy
- loss of appetite
- enlargement of the lymph glands under the jaw
- a watery discharge from both nostrils that often becomes thicker.

Outbreaks may affect whole stable yards and quarantine procedures should be put in place if a case is confirmed.

Tetanus

Vaccination against tetanus is an essential aspect of routine healthcare. The tetanus-causing bacterium, *Clostridium tetani*, lives in the soil. Spores of the bacteria are extremely resilient and may survive within the soil for many years.

Clostridium tetani attacks the horse's nervous system and most cases are fatal. Horses are particularly susceptible as the infection enters the body through small cuts and wounds. Newborn foals are at risk through infection entering the umbilicus.

Symptoms include:

- spasmodic tremors over the whole body
- stiffness
- third eyelid does not retract
- typical stance with head and neck thrust forwards and tail raised
- difficulty eating and drinking
- recumbency
- convulsions and death.

Prevention of this dreadful disease by vaccination is simple and effective.

EHV (equine herpes virus) – rhinopneumonitis

There are two herpes viruses associated with serious disease in horses: EHV 1 and EHV 4.

EHV 1

EHV 1 infection is associated mainly with respiratory disease, but may occasionally cause neurological symptoms, abortion and affect newborn foals. Respiratory disease is most common in young horses up to 3 years of age. Older horses may only show mild symptoms, if any, but may show exercise intolerance or low-grade airway disease. Unfortunately, immunity following vaccination or infection is short lived.

Symptoms include:

- high temperature (41.1°C, 106°F)
- a watery nasal discharge becoming thicker
- coughing
- depression
- enlargement of the lymph nodes under the jaw.

Abortion and disease of newborn foals and neurological symptoms are rare complications of EHV 1 infection.

EHV 4

This infection causes respiratory symptoms identical to EHV 1. It is not linked with neurological signs or disease in newborn foals, but, more importantly, EHV 4 is associated with sporadic cases of abortion. Vaccination of pregnant mares is therefore essential.

Guidelines for tetanus, equine influenza and EHV vaccination

Tetanus

- Initial course – two vaccinations 6 weeks apart.
- First booster – 1 year later.
- Successive booster – every other year.

Equine influenza

- Initial course – two vaccinations 21–92 days apart.
- First booster – 150–215 days after second vaccination (per initial course).
- Successive booster – every year, no more than 365 days following the last booster.

Equine herpes virus (EHV)

Pregnant mares should be vaccinated at 5, 7 and 9 months of gestation.

Routine care of the feet

The horse's foot is a highly specialised structure (see Chapter 10). The hind foot is longer than the front foot. Routine care is important to maintain the health of the feet and to prevent infections and injury. Regular and corrective trimming is important to maintain hoof angle, length and correct balance.

Care of the unshod foot:

- pick out feet daily
- assess condition, particularly of the frog and heel
- wash mud and dirt off the hoof wall and sole regularly
- use hoof oil sparingly, if at all, as oil products interfere with the natural hoof wall preventing absorption and evaporation of moisture
- check for cuts and puncture wounds to the sole and coronary band
- farrier to trim excess horn and tidy feet regularly.

Care of the shod foot:

- follow a regular shoeing programme every 4–6 weeks
- pick out feet daily, making sure to remove stones lodged under the shoe (see Figure 5.2)
- use hoof oil sparingly (see above)

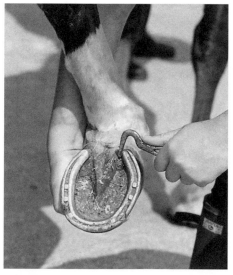

Figure 5.2. Picking out the shod foot.

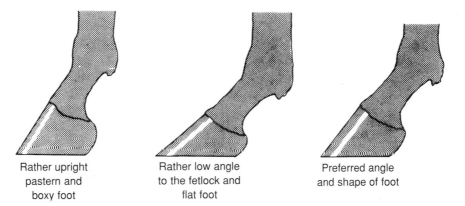

Rather upright
pastern and
boxy foot

Rather low angle
to the fetlock and
flat foot

Preferred angle
and shape of foot

Figure 5.3. Although not all ideal, these feet are all in balance, with an unbroken hoof–pastern angle.

- check for cuts and puncture wounds to the sole and coronary band
- check nails are tight and the clenches are still embedded neatly in the hoof wall
- check shoes are not loose and are still held firmly in position
- look for uneven wear of shoes and report to the farrier.

A list of what to look for in a well-shod foot is given below:

- The shoe should have been made to fit the foot, not the foot to fit the shoe.
- The type and weight of shoe should be suitable for the horse and the work required.
- The hoof–pastern angle should be maintained, as shown in Figures 5.3 and 5.4, and the foot trimmed evenly on the inside and the outside.
- The sole and frog should not be excessively trimmed.
- The frog should be in contact with the ground.
- Sufficient nails should have been used and they should be of the right size and well driven-home to fill the nail holes
- Clenches should be well formed, not too low and all in line.

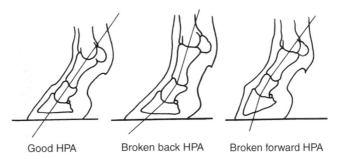

Good HPA

Broken back HPA

Broken forward HPA

Figure 5.4. The hoof–pastern angle (HPA) should be unbroken in the balanced foot.

- No daylight should show between the shoe and the foot, particularly at the heel.
- The heels of the shoe should not be short and put pressure on the seat of corn.
- The place for the clip should have been neatly cut and the clip well fitted.

The teeth

The horse has two basic types of teeth:

- molars – grinding teeth at the back
- incisors – cutting teeth at the front.

All male horses and some mares have four tushes or canine teeth situated between the incisors and the molars.

Horses, like humans, grow two sets of teeth: temporary milk teeth and permanent teeth. The milk teeth are small and white with a neck, whereas permanent teeth are much larger, pale brown or yellowy with no distinct neck.

The teeth provide a cutting and grinding system to help the horse eat.

The horse's tooth is well adapted to grinding the coarse, hard substances found in herbage.

The horse's tooth is made up of layers of three substances:

- dentine (centre of the tooth)
- enamel (thin layer, hardest substance in the body)
- cement.

The molars have big surfaces or 'tables' and the enamel is folded to make funnel-like depressions in the tooth that become filled with food and look black in colour. Inspection of the black infundibulum or 'cup' on the incisors is used to help determine the horse's age.

As the horse chews by moving its jaws from side to side, the molars grind the food; they also wear against each other. New permanent teeth have a large crown, much of which is below the level of the gum, so that in a 5-year-old horse most of the jaw is filled with teeth. The tooth wears down as it is used but that is compensated for as the growth of the tooth root forces the crown upwards. However, because the lower jaw is narrower than the upper, the wear on the tables is sometimes uneven. Small areas at the sides of the tables do not get worn down and they stick up as sharp edges. This may cause sores on the cheeks or the tongue. Potential areas of trouble are the inside edges on the lower jaw and the outside edges on the upper jaw. Rasping will deal with this problem (see below).

The teeth and ageing

As the biting surface of the incisor teeth wears away, the pattern on the surface of the tooth changes so that, with experience, the age of the horse can be estimated by examining its teeth. The first essential is to be able to distinguish the milk teeth from the permanent teeth; milk incisor teeth are small and white and appear to be pointed at the gum while the adult teeth are larger and yellower. The incisor teeth are called centrals (the pair top and bottom in the centre), laterals (the teeth next to the centrals) and the corners (see Figure 5.5). After a permanent tooth has erupted it takes 6 months to become 'in wear'.

Once the horse has a full mouth of permanent teeth, the age is estimated by the changing pattern on the tooth table, the angulation of the teeth which protrude more as the horse ages, and the shape of the tooth which changes from oval to triangular with age. As the horse gets older the 'cup' becomes shallower until it is known as the 'mark'. As the tooth wears down, the pulp cavity which carries nerves and blood vessels is exposed and, to avoid pain, secondary dentine is laid down to protect the pulp cavity. This gives rise to a raised 'dental star' on the tooth table. For a short time both the dental star and the mark are seen on the tooth table, but as the horse ages only the dental star is visible and it becomes increasingly central on the tooth table (see Figure 5.6).

The age of foals can be judged by looking at the growth of their tail and the stage of development, but generally the milk central incisors erupt by the time the foal is 4-weeks old and the laterals erupt between 1 and 3 months. By the time the foal is 1-year old it will have a full mouth of neat, white, temporary incisors but the edges of the corners will not meet.

The 2-year old will have a full mouth of temporary incisors that are all in wear. At about 2½ the temporary centrals will be replaced by permanent teeth so that the 3-year old will have permanent centrals that are in wear. At about 3½ the lateral incisors are replaced so that the 4-year old has four permanent teeth in wear. At about 4½ the corners are replaced so that the 5-year old has a full mouth of permanent teeth with the corners just in wear at the front edge. By then the tushes will have erupted in most geldings and some mares.

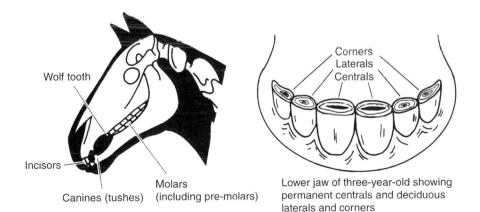

Wolf tooth

Incisors

Canines (tushes)   Molars (including pre-molars)

Corners
Laterals
Centrals

Lower jaw of three-year-old showing permanent centrals and deciduous laterals and corners

Figure 5.5. Teeth.

Four-year-old

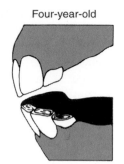

Milk teeth in corners
laterals just in wear

Five-year-old

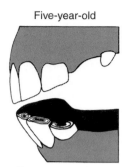

Permanent corners not
yet in wear

Six-year-old

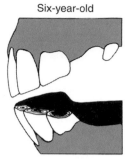

Corners still scroll shaped
but in wear with flat tables

Wear of central incisors

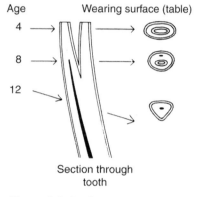

Age   Wearing surface (table)

Section through
tooth

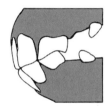

Seven-year-old

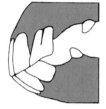

Fifteen-year-old

Figure 5.6. Ageing.

Table 5.2. Eruption of the horse's teeth

| Age of eruption | Incisors | | | Tushes | Premolars | Molars |
	Centrals	Laterals	Corners			
0–1 month	*					
1–3 months	*	*			***	
9 months	*	*	*		***	•
18 months	*	*	*		***	• •
2.5 years	•	*	*		• •*	• •
3.5 years	•	•	*		• • •	• •
4.5 years	•	•	•	◊	• • •	• • •

*Milk teeth.
•Permanent teeth.
◊Tushes.

The 6-year old will have a well-formed mouth with all the incisors in wear with level tables and obvious dark 'cups'. In the 7-year old the 'cup' in the centrals will have worn out, leaving the 'mark' that is not as dark. The top teeth may overlap the bottom ones so that there may be a little 'hook' on the back of the corner incisors.

By 8 years the cup will have worn out of the laterals, leaving a mark, and the centrals will have a dark line called the 'dental star' near the front of the tooth. The hook will have disappeared.

By 9 years the cup will have worn out of the corners, leaving a mark and the dental star will be apparent on the laterals. There may be a small hook and the centrals will have rounded off, giving a triangular shape. Galvayne's groove appears as a dark groove on the upper corner teeth at between 9 and 10 years.

The 10-year old will have stars and marks in all teeth, but the marks will be more indistinct and the stars will be clearer. The laterals will have rounded off to be more triangular. Galvayne's groove gradually grows down the tooth.

The 12-year old will only have dental stars in the centrals and the teeth are more triangular. The 15-year old will only have dental stars on the tooth tables and the teeth will have increased slope, while Galvayne's groove extends about halfway down the corner incisor.

Once the horse has a full mouth of permanent teeth, age determination can only be approximate as the type and level of nutrition of the horse can affect the changes outlined above.

Routine care of the teeth

The vet or horse dentist should regularly attend to teeth. Until the horse is 4 years old the teeth will need examining twice a year to make sure the milk teeth are not getting in the way of the permanent teeth.

After the age of 4 years, the teeth should be examined twice a year for sharp edges. These will then be rasped. Pain caused by sharp edges may also cause head shaking or lack of control from the bit. Older horses may need specialist care so as not to make worn or loose teeth worse.

Rasping needs two handlers. The horse, in a head collar is backed up into a corner facing the light and the assistant standing on the opposite side to the person doing the rasping, steadies the head and may be required to hold the tongue. The rasp must be dipped into water at regular intervals to keep the cutting edges clean.

Chapter 6
The sick horse

The horse will be challenged continuously by disease-causing organisms of one sort or another. These are the so-called invaders.

The invaders may be broadly categorised into one of two groups: microorganisms (Figure 6.1) and parasites (Figure 6.2). Parasites may live within the horse's body or on the surface.

Not all microorganisms are disease causing, some are able to live quite happily within the horse's body without causing any problems and others are essential for health, such as the beneficial hindgut microorganisms that digest plant fibre. Another example is the millions of bacteria which live naturally on the horse's skin without producing any disease.

An infection results from the establishment of colony disease-causing microorganisms such as bacteria, viruses or fungi. The disease-causing microorganisms are known as pathogens. These organisms actively reproduce and cause damage to cells.

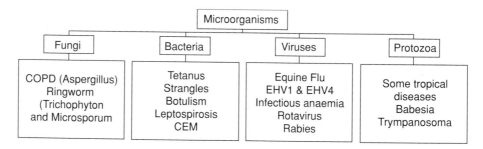

Figure 6.1. Microorganisms that invade the horse.

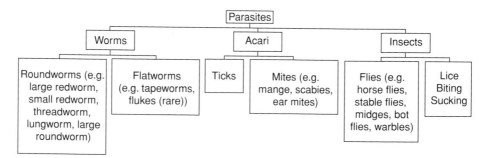

Figure 6.2. Parasites that invade the horse.

Infection should normally produce a response from the horse's immune system. In some cases, infection is spread throughout the horse's body and this is known as a systemic infection. Infection may also be localised within a particular area or tissue. The microorganisms vary in their ability to invade and multiply, and this capacity is known as virulence. Sometimes, organisms may spread from a part of the body where they are normally harmless to another part where they become harmful, for example, when there is leakage from the horse's gut into the surrounding abdominal space. This results in infection of the gut lining or peritoneum, known as peritonitis.

Entry of microorganisms from the soil into wounds or during surgery can introduce localised infection or the more serious systemic infection such as tetanus.

Disease-causing organisms include:

- bacteria
- viruses
- fungi.

All of the above are relatively simple organisms, which may multiply in the horse's tissues particularly when defences are low.

Other disease-causing organisms are parasites. These include single-celled parasites known as protozoa, worms (see Chapter 5), acari and insects. The horse's reaction to the presence of infection produces the symptoms of the disease. Blood tests often show that a bacterial infection will increase the number of white blood cells, whereas a viral infection tends to show a reduction in white cell count.

The symptoms of disease are therefore caused in part by microorganisms causing damage to cells and tissues, releasing toxins and drawing on the horse's nutrient supply. Symptoms are also caused by the horse's own defences using the immune system whose role is to destroy the offending microorganisms. The outcome will depend on whether the microorganisms or the horse's defence system gain the advantage. The strength of the horse's immune system, which is often a reflection of the general health and well-being of the horse, will strongly influence this outcome.

Apart from diseases in which the symptoms and signs are easily recognisable, such as tetanus or strangles, diagnosis will often rely on the isolation of the causative microorganism. Testing may involve microscopic examination of a specimen of infected tissue or body fluid by culture techniques or by detecting antibodies (proteins manufactured by the horse to defend against a particular organism) in a blood sample.

A problem in detecting infectious diseases is that there is always a time delay between the entry of microorganisms and the appearance of symptoms. This is known as the incubation period and may be as short as a few days or as long as several months. Furthermore, symptoms may never develop in some infected horses, but these horses nevertheless continue to carry the disease-causing organisms and unwittingly spread them to other horses. As a result of this spreading an epidemic can be well established before it is recognised and before control measures can be introduced.

Early recognition of symptoms is therefore important if treatment is going to be more effective.

Horses may be susceptible to some microorganisms, but not to others. This is because many of the microorganisms are species specific. For example, horses cannot catch influenza from humans.

Some microorganisms can cause severe reactions and symptoms, and these cause acute infections. Whereas others may produce a slow reaction of the horse's defence mechanisms and the horse is slow to overcome the disease. This results in a chronic infection.

Bacteria

Bacteria are a group of single-celled microorganisms which may cause disease. Bacteria have been recognised for over 100 years as a cause of disease. Some equine bacterial infectious diseases are listed in Table 6.1. Bacteria are naturally abundant in the air, soil and water, and most of these are harmless to horses. When they harm horses, they are called pathogenic. Pathogenic bacteria can be classified on the basis of their shape into three main groups:

- cocci (spherical)
- bacilli (rod-shaped)
- spirochaetes or spirilla (spiral shaped).

Disease caused by the cocci includes pneumonia and strangles. Bacilli cause tetanus and botulism.

The bacteria that invade the horse's body thrive in the warm, moist conditions. Some bacteria are aerobic which means that they require oxygen to grow and survive. They are therefore found in such places as the respiratory system or on the skin. Anaerobic bacteria, on the other hand, thrive in areas low in oxygen such as deep in wounds or tissues.

Table 6.1. Some equine bacterial infectious diseases

Disease	Bacterium
Tetanus	*Clostridium tetani*
Strangles	*Streptococcus equi*
Botulism	*Clostridium botulinum*
Rattles (summer pneumonia)	*Rhodococcus equi* (*Corynebacterium equi*)
Leptospirosis	*Leptospira interrogans* Serovars
Contagious equine metritis	*Taylorella equigenitalis*
Salmonellosis	*Salmonella* species

Many bacteria are naturally static and only move around the horse's body in currents of fluid or air. Others are very mobile and have filamentous tails to help them move. Bacteria are able to reproduce by simply dividing into two cells, these in turn divide again and so on. Under ideal conditions this can take place every 20 minutes. After only 6 hours a single bacterium cell can have multiplied to form a colony of over 250,000 bacteria. Luckily these ideal conditions rarely occur within the horse's body due to the action of the horse's own defence system in killing these bacteria.

As well as dividing, some bacteria can also produce spores. A spore is a single new bacterium, which is protected by an extremely tough outer coat that can survive high temperatures, dry conditions and a lack of nutrients. These spores can remain in this dormant state for many years. When conditions are correct they will 'hatch' and invade body tissues. Spore-producing bacteria include *Clostridia* responsible for tetanus and botulism. These spores are able to lie dormant within the soil for many years and are not susceptible to some strong disinfectants. When a horse has a wound (often very minor) the tetanus-causing bacteria (*Clostridium tetani*) can enter the body through this route. This is why it is so important to keep tetanus vaccinations up to date (see Chapter 5).

Treatment

The horse's body will attempt to fight invading bacteria, and sometimes this is successful without treatment. In many cases, though, treatment is necessary, this is usually in the form of antibiotics either given orally in the feed or by injection.

Superficial inflammation and minor infected wounds may be treated with antibiotic or antiseptic creams (see Chapter 8).

Viruses

Viruses are minute infectious agents, much smaller than bacteria, that have a very simple structure and a relatively uncomplicated method of multiplication.

Viral infections vary from relatively minor problems such as warts to extremely serious diseases such as rabies. It is thought that some virus infections also lead to cancer.

It is debatable whether a virus is a living organism as such or just a collection of nucleic material [deoxyribonucleic acid (DNA) or ribonucleic acid (RNA)] capable of replicating itself under specific, favourable conditions.

A virus' sole aim is to invade the cells of other organisms that they then instruct to make more copies of themselves. Outside of the living cell viruses are totally inactive. They are incapable of any of the activities, such as metabolism, that are normally associated with living organisms.

The number of different kinds of virus probably exceeds the number of types of all other organisms. Viruses are parasites and are known to be capable of parasitising all recognised life forms. They do not always cause disease however.

Replication

Technically, viruses do not reproduce, instead they undergo a process known as replication. Basically, the virus invades the host cell and begins the process of making copies of itself from materials within the host cell itself.

Viruses can gain entry to the horse's body through all possible entrance routes. They may be inhaled in droplets or swallowed in food or water. They may be passed into the body through the saliva of biting insects such as in equine infectious anaemia, or they may enter the horse's body during covering.

Once they have entered the host's body, many viruses will begin to replicate near the site of entry. Others may enter the lymph vessels and spread to the lymph nodes where many of them will be engulfed by white blood cells. Others may pass from the lymphatics to the blood from where they can invade every part of the horse. Viruses tend to have target organs such as the brain (as in rabies) or the respiratory tract (as in equine influenza).

Treatment

Fighting viral infections is very difficult because it is nearly impossible to manufacture drugs that will 'kill' viruses without affecting the host cell in which the virus is situated. Some antiviral agents have been produced in human medicine that prevent viruses from entering the host cells or by interfering with their replication within the cell. Immunisation can be a much more effective method of eradicating or reducing the effects of viruses. Vaccination programmes are used widely for the control of some viruses (see Chapter 5).

Fungi

Fungi are relatively simple parasites that include moulds, mildews, yeasts, mushrooms and toadstools. There are more than 100,000 species of fungi within the world. Most of these are harmless and may even be beneficial, for example, some moulds are used to make antibiotics. Fungi are larger than bacteria.

Some fungi occur as colonies of individual cells such as yeasts. Others form chains of tubes or filaments called hyphae, which are formed into a complex network known as a mycelium. Many fungi form millions of tiny spores which can be carried in the air and remain dormant until suitable conditions are available for them to grow. Fungal spores are mainly found in the soil.

Disease

Fungal spores can penetrate into the tissues of the host, such as with *Aspergillus* that can cause infection of the mucous membranes and guttural pouch. Some of the yeasts are present normally within the horse's gut where they may become a problem if the gut flora are upset or disrupted by the use of antibiotics. They can then overgrow the bacterial population because antibiotics are ineffective against fungi.

Probably the most common fungal infection of the horse is ringworm, which may be caused by either *Trichophyton* or *Microsporum*. Some spores of fungi particularly those found in mouldy hay may cause damage when inhaled by horses causing persistent allergic reactions in the lungs or chronic obstructive pulmonary disease (COPD).

Treatment

Fungal infections are treated with antifungal preparations.

The immune system

The immune system is a collection of cells and proteins that are able to protect the horse from potentially harmful infectious microorganisms such as those mentioned previously. The immune system is also responsible for allergic reactions and hypersensitivity in horses. Immunity may either be innate or acquired.

Innate immunity is present from birth and is the first line of defence against disease. Acquired immunity is the second line of defence and develops either through exposure of the horse to the infectious organism (after they have broken through the innate immune system) or through immunisation.

Chapter 7
Nursing the sick horse

Disease symptoms

A symptom is an indication that something is wrong with the horse and this requires prompt investigation.

The following should be monitored in horses:

- behaviour
- appetite
- action
- coat
- respiration/breathing
- temperature
- pulse
- dung and urine
- eyes
- lumps, bumps and swellings
- discharges.

Behaviour

The first sign of disease is often a change in behaviour – anything that is different to that horse's normal pattern. The person in charge of the horse must ask himself or herself the cause for the horse's change in behaviour. Is this attributable to external events, or to something in the horse's body or mind?

A mare about to foal or a horse with colic may display similar symptoms. Any abnormal activities should be noticed. The horse is normally alert and interested: any dullness or lack of zest should be regarded as a warning sign. It may be an indication of pain or of something else.

Appetite

A horse that does not hurry to the manger or finish a meal should always be regarded with suspicion. The horse may chew the food and let some slip back out, or it may have difficult in swallowing. The cause may be in the food or in the manger, but it may be in the horse's mouth or in its digestive system. A stabled horse that drinks more or less water than usual should be similarly regarded, although it is to be expected that a horse will be thirstier on hot days or after sweating.

Action

When the horse is free in the field or turning round in the stable, or being ridden or driven, telltale signs may become evident. For example, the ears may suddenly flick back or the tail may be clamped down. The horse may grunt when mounted or be unwilling to go forward. Its stride may be uneven or it may be lame. It may rest a leg when standing in the stable but this is only generally suspicious if it is a front leg.

When the horse resists going forward, it is one of the most difficult decisions that the rider has to make as to whether the animal is being stubborn or nappy, or whether it is in pain for some reason, or finds movement physically difficult or frightening. The great dilemma is to know when to be firm and when to be understanding.

Coat

A harsh, 'staring', dull, tight coat is unnatural and is usually a sign that something is wrong. The coat should be soft and move freely over the muscles. Except when the horse is cold, the hairs should lie flat and the coat should gleam. Rough or raised patches, rubbed hair or any local differences in one area should be watched out for. The horse should also be checked for cuts, wounds, splinters and bruises.

Respiration/breathing

Changes in respiration may be noticed in the stable or the field. The respiration rate will rise during fever and infection. Respiration type is also significant; shallow and rapid breathing is characteristic of infections of the respiratory tract. Respiration rate will be affected by the environment, rising in hotter and more humid conditions.

There may be a cough when the horse is feeding or working, and it is important that the circumstances and type of cough should be noted to assist in the diagnosis. The horse may make a noise when galloping. It is important to note if the noise is made by air going into or coming out of the lungs, as considered in Chapter 13.

Temperature

Whenever the horse is thought to be unwell its temperature should be taken. An above-normal temperature accompanies all cases of acute disease to a greater or lesser extent. It will also indicate fever, a local infection, such as an abscess or one caused by the presence of a thorn, and pain, whether acute or general.

A fall in temperature is characteristic of loss of blood, starvation, collapse, coma, hypothermia and some chronic diseases. An abnormal temperature indicates that the vet should be called.

Pulse

The pulse rate is a useful aid to diagnosis and to help determine fitness. The pulse rate at rest rises in cases of fever and acute pain; it falls in debilitating diseases.

Dung and urine

If the faeces are too hard, or too soft, strong smelling or slimy, all is not well within the digestive tract. Urine of unusual colour, cloudiness or smell may be a sign that problems are developing.

Eyes

A dull eye or one that is half closed is an indication that the horse may be feeling unwell. A special watch should be kept for damage to the eye. The inner side of the eyelid is a useful membrane to study, as it will change colour according to the condition of the blood. The gums may also be studied similarly. Healthy horses must be examined regularly so that any changes become apparent quickly. Care should be taken as there may be foreign bodies present.

Lumps, bumps and swellings

It is easy to find swellings on horses when grooming them; it is much harder to notice such things on animals in the field.

Swellings by the jawbone may indicate glandular problem. The inside of the mouth should be checked occasionally for ulcers and sores. When unaccustomed tack or clothing comes into use, particular care should be taken until the skin has hardened. A sore or rub is more easily dealt with if detected in the early stages. Where there is swelling, it should be checked for heat, and bruising, strains, thorns and infection should be considered.

A watchful eye should be kept on the legs; the tendons that go down the back of each lower leg should stand out clearly. Slight filling, or puffiness round the fetlock joint, is a danger sign that must not be ignored. The cause might be a knock the day before, a strain, exercise on hard ground or being shut in the stable too long.

Discharges

A runny nose is the common first symptom of a cough or cold but it may have other meanings, particularly if only one nostril is affected. Discharges may appear at any of the body's other orifices: eyes, ears, anus, vulva, sheath or teats. Each discharge will have its own particular significance.

Sick nursing

Care should be given to:

- stable – warm and clean with deep bed with banked up wall
- grooming – restricted, gentle
- feeding – high fibre, low concentrates with top quality forage
- water – clean and fresh, should be monitored
- TPR (temperature–pulse–respiration) – a chart should be made and completed for the vet
- hygiene (see below).

The horse must be comfortable and relaxed. If the horse is on box rest the diet must be adjusted. Fresh, cut grass may be given as an appetiser and plenty of hay. The vet will be able to give advice for post-surgical cases. Cereals should be avoided due to the high starch content.

The horse should be kept warm on deep bedding, leg bandages and rugs as and when necessary, with ample fresh air but no draughts. If the horse is sweating, it should be dried with a clean dry towel.

The horse's drinking should be monitored. The sick horse should be fed after any other horse in order to avoid the risk of spreading infection. The legs may also be massaged to prevent them filling. A very sick horse will not need thorough grooming, just a quick wipe over with a damp cloth, including nostrils, eyes and dock, but take care not to allow the horse to become chilled.

A TPR chart is useful and any instructions from the vet should be adhered to thoroughly.

Hygiene

Good hygiene for sick horses is even more important than usual. The grooming kit and feed containers must be kept spotlessly clean and disinfected before rinsing, if necessary. Before disinfecting the stable, it should be thoroughly cleaned out and then scrubbed with the warm disinfectant solution. There are also biological powder disinfectants now available. Allow a day after application of wet disinfectant before rinsing it off. A boot wash may be necessary where boots are dipped in disinfectant prior to and after visiting the horse. Hands should also be washed.

In cases of severely contagious disease, further protective wear will be required. The horse's grooming kit and stable utensils should not be used for any other horse.

Isolation

All diseases associated with microorganisms are infectious. The passage of the disease from one animal to the next can be made less likely by isolation procedures. There are two forms of isolation: within the yard for a contagious disease (one carried by contact), or outside the yard for airborne infection. The contact that spreads a contagious disease need not be direct. For example, a horse with a skin infection may be ridden under saddle, after which the saddle may be placed temporarily on a saddle horse. Later, another saddle rested on the same saddle horse may then pick up the germs and carry them on. Mildly contagious diseases can be kept under control by careful application of the principles outlined here.

Some diseases can be carried in the air. When a horse coughs, it releases germs that may float down wind. Birds and flies also carry germs. In the case of more highly infectious diseases, the ideal is an isolation box sited about 400 m (about a quarter of a mile) down wind of the stable yard. This gives a better chance of keeping a disease out of the yard itself. Such a box can also be used for visiting horses and, for the first fortnight, for new arrivals in a yard.

Giving medicine

Steaming the head

Where there is considerable discharge from the nostrils, the head may be steamed. To prepare for the treatment, a handful of hay is placed in a plastic bucket in the bottom of an old sack. This is then sprinkled with friar's balsam or oil of eucalyptus. Boiling water is poured over the hay so that it steams. The horse's head is put into the entrance of the sack and kept there for several minutes. More hot water is then poured over the hay and the procedure repeated. From time to time the horse will need a break. For heavy catarrh it may be necessary to steam the head twice daily.

In cases of pneumonia the sack should not be used as it limits fresh air. After the steaming process, the hay will be contaminated with nasal discharge and should be burned. The bucket and bag must be scalded to sterilise them.

Horses being steamed are best fed at ground level to encourage discharge. A little ointment containing menthol, oil of eucalyptus or something similar may be placed in the outer nostril. If the discharge tends to create a sore, the skin should be protected with petroleum jelly or nappy-rash cream.

Electuary

This old-fashioned paste still provides a useful aid to soothing a cough. It is usual to draw out the horse's tongue and, using the flat handle of a spatula, place the paste on the tongue. The treatment is repeated at least twice a day.

Drenching

Giving a horse liquid medicine can prove to be a difficult business. Some horses accept a drench quite easily, but others are not so co-operative, so it is wise to take precautions. The horse's head should be raised so that the liquid can be poured down its throat. This is not difficult with a small pony, but most people find their arms are too short to treat a horse this way. A rope should be attached to the middle front of the noseband of the head collar and the rope is passed over a beam. Additional height is gained by standing on a straw bale or two; this is essential if a beam is not available. An assistant can then control the horse and raise and lower its head as required. The drench is best placed in a plastic bottle. If a glass bottle is used, then the neck of the bottle must be bandaged in case the glass is broken by the horse's teeth. The animal's head is raised gently and the neck of the bottle is placed in the corner of the mouth. Gentle pouring may then commence. When one mouthful has been swallowed, another may be given. If the horse coughs, lower the head at once. If the medicine goes down 'the wrong way', it will end up in the lungs and may give the horse pneumonia. *Drenching should be done only by someone competent because of the risks involved.*

Other methods of giving medicines

Some powders and granules may be added to the food, but the horse has a sensitive nose and palate and may easily detect these additions and be put off. The meal should therefore be made particularly tempting by the addition of apples, carrots or beet pulp. If the horse fails to eat all of the prepared meal, the value of the medicine might be lost. Some medicines can be poured straight into the water bucket.

A useful way to ensure that the horse receives the appropriate medicine dosage is to make up a paste with icing sugar to which the medicine is added. Using a large syringe, without a needle, the mixture is squirted into the horse's mouth towards the back of the cheek. Some drugs are now supplied as a paste in a syringe for use in this way.

Some treatments require administration to the skin, and for some of these rubber gloves are required. In every case the great essential is to read the instructions or to follow the vet's directions.

Injections

It is now common for stockmen to inject certain classes of stock. The horse is not easy to inject as it has a tough hide and also sometimes produces a reaction to the injection. Furthermore, if the injection is not done smoothly and at the first attempt the horse is apt to become fractious and be difficult on the next occasion when injection is attempted.

Injections may be given intravenously (into the vein), and this is certainly a job for the vet. They may also be given intramuscularly. If the vet approves of an experienced person giving intramuscular injections, then he or she can demonstrate the proper technique.

Enemas and back-raking

It is sometimes helpful to the passage of faeces through the rectum to flush or lubricate this part of the bowel with fluids. There are several other reasons for giving an enema, and different fluids are used for different causes. The normal procedure is to lubricate the rounded end of a special tube and pass it through the anus into the rectum. Then, soapy warm water or liquid paraffin is passed down the tube. When dealing with a foal, gravity is often used, but in the case of a horse, a pump may help to pass the fluid along the tube. The giving of an enema is usually a task for the vet.

Back-raking is the removal of faeces, or of meconium in the case of newborn foals. In the horse or pony, a well-lubricated hand is used, but for a foal a small, smooth, well-lubricated finger is all that there is room for without causing inflammation. Generally, back-raking is best left to the vet.

Treatments using tubes

A stomach tube is used to place either a large quantity of fluid, or a small quantity without wastage, into the stomach. The tube is about 3 m (10 ft) long and about 12 mm (around half an inch) in diameter. It is passed up one nostril and goes down the gullet (oesophagus) towards the stomach. If the tube should accidentally go the wrong way at the pharynx, then it would pass into the trachea, and unless immediately remedied the fluid would pass into the lungs. *The stomach tube is only to be used by a vet.* Occasionally, there will be minimal bleeding at the nostril, but this is of little consequence.

Where it is necessary to empty the bladder, and the horse seems unable to oblige, the vet will pass a thin tube up the urethra into the bladder and thus allow the urine to escape. Such a tube is called a catheter.

Types of wound and wound healing

Wounds and wound healing are considered in Chapter 8.

Treatment of injury

There are several different therapies used to reduce inflammation and aid the healing of injuries and these include:

- cold hosing
- cold bandages, massage and astringents
- poulticing
- fomentations
- tubbing
- pressure bandages.

Cold hosing

Where there is any bruising or tearing of the tissues, cold applications will shrink the blood vessels. To control swelling after injury, cold and pressure may

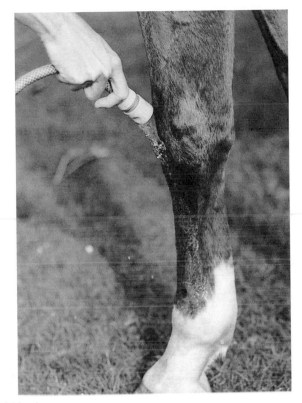

Figure 7.1. Cold hosing.

be needed for the first day, but then heat is required to aid healing. Cold is easily applied by running cold water. While an assistant holds the horse using a bridle, the hose should be run very gently, first on the ground and then on the foot; it is then worked gradually up the leg (see Figure 7.1). This should continue for 10 minutes, and several sessions per day are needed, using pressure bandages between sessions. If the horse can be stood in a suitable stall, such as in a horse-box or trailer, the horse can be allowed to eat from a hay net and the hose can be bandaged to its leg. Alternatives to cold hosing include standing or walking in the river or the sea.

Cold bandages, massage and astringents

An ice pack can be made by crushing some ice cubes in a cloth with a hammer or rolling pin, and then transferring this crushed ice to a polythene bag which may be bandaged to the leg over a thin layer of gamgee to prevent skin scald. Methods of bandaging are shown in Figure 7.2.

In addition to using cold bandages, some swellings – particularly those involving filling of the legs – respond well to massage. The legs should be rubbed upwards, towards the heart. To reduce friction, it may help to use soapy water,

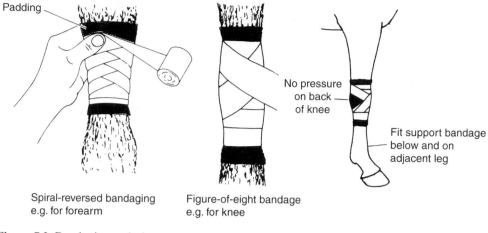

Padding

No pressure
on back
of knee

Fit support bandage
below and on
adjacent leg

Spiral-reversed bandaging
e.g. for forearm

Figure-of-eight bandage
e.g. for knee

Figure 7.2. Bandaging techniques.

baby lotion or oil. Alternating hot and cold applications also produces a massaging effect.

Some horses, particularly those that have to gallop or jump on hard ground, tend to get filled legs after work. This condition may be helped by using a cooling lotion after work, or by rubbing a diluted astringent into the lower leg in the evening. As a general rule, bandages should not be applied over these liniments or the skin may be blistered. As a preventative measure against legs filling, an astringent paste may be used. The hair is wetted, then the paste is applied, first against and then with the lie of the hair. The paste sets so the horse can be worked at home with the paste on. The paste can be washed off when the horse is required to be tidy.

Poulticing

Where there is damaged tissue, the application of heat will stimulate the blood supply to the area and this will help repair the damage. A poultice also has a drawing effect, which will help any pus form into an abscess. It is thus often useful for a wound, whereas an ice pack is useful for a bruise, and an astringent for reducing swelling.

Impregnated padding can be purchased ready for use, complete with instructions on the pack. Alternatively, a kaolin poultice may be used. The procedure is simple. The lid of the tin is loosened and the tin is then placed in a pan of boiling water for several minutes, until the paste is as hot as can be borne on the back of the hand. Paste is then put on a piece of lint, and covered with gauze, and is then applied. The poultice is then covered with a polythene sheet so that it draws from the wound and not from the air. The next cover is a piece of gamgee or similar padding, to retain the heat, and finally it is bandaged in place. The dressing is usually changed morning and evening. Alternatively, the cold paste can be applied to the lint and put in the microwave for 30 seconds. It is then covered with gauze, the temperature tested on the hand and the poultice applied.

If the wound or sore is in the sole of the foot, some people like to use a bran poultice. Boiling water is mixed with antiseptic and poured on to bran until a crumbly consistency is obtained: if the bran is squeezed, there should be no excess moisture. The mixture is allowed to cool until it can be tolerated by the palm of the hand and then it is placed in polythene inside sacking. The foot is stood in the bran and the wrapping secured around padding on the leg. It is tidier to finish off with a stable bandage. The poultice should be renewed at night and in the morning. The antiseptic will mask the smell of the bran so that the horse will not try to eat it.

A puncture wound is sometimes poulticed with a mixture of Epsom salts (magnesium sulphate) and glycerine. This has the advantage of not being edible and not making the sole hard as does kaolin.

Irrespective of the type of poultice in use, there is one situation that demands particular care. If an open wound lies over a joint, there is a possibility that the joint capsule may be damaged and a poultice could draw out the joint oil. A poultice should never be used in such cases.

Where the horse is taking more weight on the sound leg than on the injured one, this should be bandaged for support.

Fomentations

Fomentations are a useful way of applying heat to an area that is not easily poulticed. They should be repeated several times a day and continued for about 20 minutes on each occasion. A bucket and a container of hot water should be taken to the horse. Hot and cold water should then be mixed to a temperature that can just be tolerated by the human elbow. A double handful of Epsom salts may be added. A cloth, such as an old towel, is then soaked in the water, wrung out and applied to the area for a couple of minutes. This procedure is repeated, keeping the water as hot as can be tolerated.

Tubbing

Open wounds in the foot may call for regular applications of heat; this can be achieved by tubbing. The preparations are similar to fomentations but a non-metal bucket or tub is used. Some antiseptic may be added to the water and as much Epsom salts as will dissolve, thus making a saturated solution. The horse's foot is placed firmly in the tub or bucket (see Figure 7.3). The water may be hotter if the water level does not come above the top of the hoof. Generally, however, it is easier to have the water hand-hot. If the horse is reluctant to immerse its foot, hot water should be splashed gently over the leg until the horse is willing to lower it into the bucket. Tubbing should last about 20 minutes and should be repeated at least twice a day.

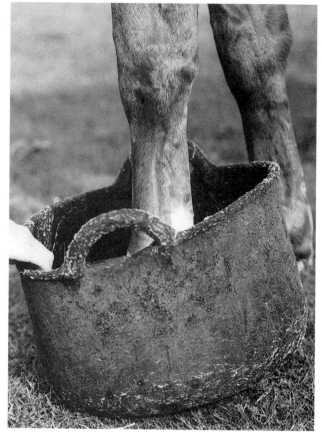

Figure 7.3. Tubbing.

Pressure bandages

A pressure bandage may be applied, for example, after a suspected tendon injury. This helps to limit the swelling that may interfere with the healing process if excessive. A crêpe bandage is applied over a thick layer of gamgee; care must be taken not to apply it too tightly. It should be removed twice per day and the leg massaged gently.

Feeding the sick horse

Providing the sick horse with balanced rations plays an important role in the horse's ability to fight disease. Correct nutrition provides one of the body's defence mechanisms. Proper feeding of the sick horse should always be considered as an integral part of the sick nursing and therapeutic regime.

Feeding may be difficult in that the horse's appetite may be depressed and swallowing may be difficult. The function of the gut may also be disturbed and this can lead to dehydration and an upset in the electrolyte balance. Weight loss often accompanies illness and injury.

Diet for the sick horse

The sick horse's diet should:

- be palatable
- contain good quality protein
- contain quality digestible fibre
- contain good levels of vitamins and minerals.
- be low in starch if the horse is on box rest.

Some specific nutritional management examples are given below.

Diarrhoea

This is often a result of large bowel disease in adult horses. The size of meals should be reduced and, for persistent diarrhoea, a vitamin B supplement and electrolytes given. Preprobiotics or probiotics may be useful.

Feeding free-choice roughage, salt and water is recommended, especially if the diarrhoea is due to starch overload or antibiotic therapy.

Avoid high starch rations and provide the horse with digestible fibre and oil to increase energy density.

Liver disease

The liver is the primary site of glucose production, and storage of vitamins A, D and E. The liver also functions to detoxify the body.

Horses with liver disease should be given a diet that does not overload the liver. Energy and protein can be provided in forms that do not rely on liver metabolism. Supplement the diet with vitamins A, D, E and K, as these are usually released by the liver into the bloodstream.

Diets for horses with liver disease should have relatively high levels of soluble carbohydrates and low protein. Alfalfa and clover should be avoided. Feed small amounts often.

Renal disease (or kidney disease)

Horses suffering from these problems will have similar requirements to those suffering from liver problems.

A low protein (but a high quality) diet should be fed. The kidney is the primary site of calcium excretion. High calcium feeds, such as alfalfa, may result in the excretion of high levels of calcium crystals in the urine. In horses with renal disease, these crystals accumulate in the kidneys, and could result in kidney stones. Bran and alfalfa should be avoided.

Pituitary dysfunction (Cushing's syndrome)

This is a common problem in older horses. This condition may reduce the horse's tolerance for calcium, glucose and fibre, while the requirements for protein, phosphorus, vitamin C and B vitamins are increased. Compound feeds formulated for older horses should contain 12–20% crude fibre so they can be used as a complete feed, reducing the need for hay.

Starvation

This is not a disease in itself, but this may cause many problems. It may result from dental problems, parasitic infection, reduced intestinal absorption, inappetance or lack of food. This will compromise immune function and wound healing.

Long-term starvation can cause a decrease in muscle mass, including the cardiac muscle.

Horses that have been starved, should have feed slowly reintroduced.

High-quality feed and forage with quality protein and some carbohydrates should be fed. Cereal feeds should be introduced slowly to ease the increase of the metabolic rate and the use of oil will help to increase energy density.

High levels of carbohydrates may cause stress to the weakened cardiac muscle.

Colic

If the colic is severe the horse may require surgery. After surgery, top-quality hay should be introduced together with a good vitamin and mineral supplement. This will help to stimulate gut motility, which can be compromised after the operation. After a horse is completely recovered from surgery, feed a diet high in quality fibre and water content.

If a portion of the large intestine is removed, or ressected, there is an increased requirement for protein, phosphorus and B vitamins, and a reduced capacity for fibre digestion.

Concentrates should be slowly introduced, at no more than 2 kg per meal. Fats are useful to increase energy density.

If the small intestine has been ressected, then the emphasis must be placed on the large intestine when it comes to the diet. This means that large amounts of cereals should be avoided, as the main site of digestion of carbohydrates is in the small intestine. Alfalfa and sugar beet pulp are very useful in these cases.

Oil may be fed if the ileum (part of the small intestine, see Chapter 15) has not been affected. If the ileum has been ressected, the vet should inject vitamins A, E and K.

There will also be an increased requirement for calcium as this is a major site of calcium absorption.

Chapter 8
First aid

First aid is an important skill with which all horse owners should be familiar. Even the smallest of wounds should be given some attention. A first-aid kit is a must for any yard, as prompt attention will aid the healing process.

First-aid kit

Contents of a first-aid kit:

- curved scissors
- bandages – conforming ones which mould to the limb, e.g. tubigrip
- crêpe bandage
- adhesive bandages, e.g. Elastoplast, which keeps dressings in place
- antiseptic wash, e.g. hibitane, dermisol multicleanse
- dressings – non-stick, e.g. melolin, fucidin intertulle
- poultice dressing, e.g. animalintex
- thermometer
- antibacterial cleansing cream, e.g. dermisol
- antibacterial and anti-inflammatory ointment, e.g. dermobion
- sterile saline solution
- roll of gamgee (not cotton wool)
- petroleum jelly
- antibiotic spray
- clean bowl and towel.

Care should be taken if using gentian violet, as it stains the wound dark purple and makes it very difficult to see the wound. This can be very irritating for the veterinary surgeon if he or she has been called out to treat the wound.

The use of tourniquets to reduce excessive blood loss is now outdated and pressure on the area should be applied instead.

There are various types of wounds and these can be broadly categorised into two groups: open wounds and closed wounds.

Open wounds

Abrasions: these are superficial skin wounds caused by rubbing or scraping. Examples are girth galls and saddle sores caused by ill fitting tack and clothing.

Incised wounds: clean with straight edges, they bleed freely and have very little bruising. They heal quickly by first intention. Examples are surgical incisions and cuts from glass or cans.

Lacerations and tears (see Figure 8.1): these have torn edges and are usually irregular in shape. There is some bruising and variable bleeding. Often tags of flaps of skin are present, which have little or no blood supply, which leads to the death of the skin flap. Protruding nails, wire or posts often cause these wounds. Barbed wire is perhaps the most frequent cause of these wounds.

Puncture wounds: these are potentially serious and consist of small openings in the skin, penetrating the soft tissue beneath. They usually inject bacteria deep into the tissues. Punctures can result from the thorns, nails and pieces of wire. They can also penetrate into joints.

Penetrating wounds: these are very serious as they enter deep into the body cavity of the horse, for example, the chest or abdomen. Organs may be damaged and emergency treatment is required from a vet. The wound should be covered to prevent further damage or loss and to stop air being sucked into the body. These types of injuries can occur when a horse stakes itself on a fence or jump.

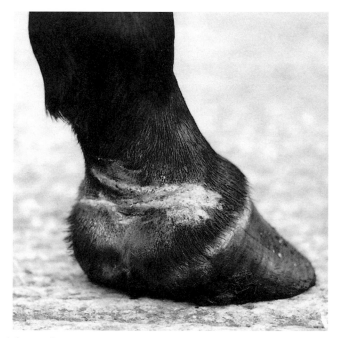

Figure 8.1. A laceration.

Closed wounds

Bruises: these are very common in horses and usually result from kicks. They should be treated with ice packs or cold hosed. The later application of heat will help to absorb excess fluid.

Contusions: caused by a blunt force inducing bleeding, bruising and swelling without breaking the skin surface. Blood-filled swellings may appear under the skin and these are known as haematomas. Large haematomas will need drainage after the bleeding has stopped. This should be done by the vet.

Sprains: this is damage to the ligaments that attach bone to bone around the joints.

Tendon strains or ruptures: these injuries are most common in the forelegs of the horse as they carry more of the body weight and are under more pressure, particularly when the horse is jumping at speed. The tendon may partially or fully rupture and there is considerable swelling and pain on palpation. The horse is usually lame.

Muscle tears or ruptures: this usually follows over-stretching of a fatigued muscle. There is variable lameness and inflammation.

Fractures: may be open or closed depending on whether bone fragments penetrate the skin. If a fracture is open, then the prognosis is guarded due to bone contamination and the greater risks of infection. Further damage to the fracture can be prevented by immediate immobilisation of the leg involved.

Wound healing

Healing

The healing process starts immediately after the injury has occurred; wounds can heal differently, depending on the site and the type of injury. Healing by first intention only occurs in non-contaminated incised wounds where the edges of the wound can be brought together and held closely with stitches, sutures or staples. The stitches usually stay in for a minimum of 10 days and should be protected with a bandage if possible.

Healing by second intention occurs in lacerated wounds and involves the wound contracting and the cells of the skin multiplying and migrating across the wound to form a scab and new tissue. Wounds on the body cause little scarring as the skin is loose and the wound can contract so that a minimum of new tissue has to be formed. The horse's limbs have little or no loose flesh and the new skin cells multiply excessively to form granulation tissue or proud flesh (Figure 8.2). This inhibits healing as the proud flesh prevents new skin from covering the wound. Proud flesh formation can be prevented by pressure bandaging and immobilising the wound as much as possible. Once proud flesh has formed it is removed by surgery or using caustic solutions.

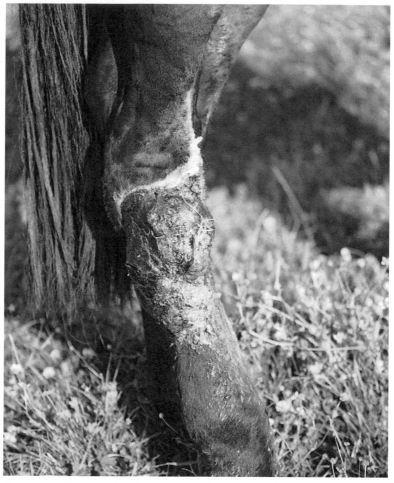

Figure 8.2. Wound healing showing proud flesh or granulation tissue.

Wound treatment

The immediate treatment of a wound or injury is extremely important as it can affect the long-term healing process. A first-aid programme is shown below.

- The bleeding should be stopped or controlled by the application of pressure.
- The vet should be called if the horse is shocked or in severe pain or if the wound is very dirty, bleeding profusely, contains a foreign body, requires stitching or if the horse's tetanus vaccinations are not up to date.
- The wound should be protected to prevent further damage.
- The wound must be cleaned using sterile instruments if at all possible. The hair around the wound can be cut away and then the wound should be bathed with cooled boiled water or sterile saline solution. Cold hosing is not recommended as low temperatures impair the healing process. It is better to use a

sterile syringe to wash deep wounds. If the wound is superficial, wash with an antibacterial solution and apply antibacterial ointment. Plain cotton wool may leave fibres within the wound which themselves become foreign bodies. If the wound is bleeding very heavily, apply pressure with a clean pad. The amount of pressure will depend on the amount of bleeding. If bright red arterial blood is spurting out, then apply heavy pressure with a gauze wad and then wrapping with vet wrap until veterinary assistance arrives. It is better not to wash away the blood so that the vet has some idea as to the extent of blood loss.

- Once clean, reassess the injury and call the veterinary surgeon if required. After application of a cleaning cream such as dermisol, cover with a new non-stick dressing such as fucidin intertulle and bandage if possible. Then apply gamgee and a conforming bandage. If the wound is quite deep or is a puncture wound, animalintex can be applied to help draw out any infection and this helps to keep the wound moist.
- To help reduce excessive swelling in skin injuries to the lower limbs walk horses out in hand.

The use of lasers in the treatment of wounds

Laser treatment stimulates the production of collagen and thus stimulates wound healing. Lasers have an antibacterial affect and they are becoming increasingly useful in the treatment of open wounds, but they should always be used alongside conventional methods of wound treatment. If treatment with laser is started within 24 hours of the injury occurring then the appearance of unwanted proud flesh can be halted. Wounds, which have been treated with lasers, tend to have little scarring and normal hair growth. This can be very important for horses where the cosmetic effects are important.

Laser treatment is thought to reduce inflammation and thereby reduce pain and infection. It should not be used on wounds which are already infected, or in conjunction with steroids, as it stimulates natural cortisone production.

Bone fractures

Fractures used to be untreatable and euthanasia was recommended in most cases. These days the prognosis depends on the position and type of fracture. New techniques mean that many fractures of the lower limb can be treated to a satisfactory degree, however, the materials, treatment and aftercare can be very expensive. Horse insurance for the payment of veterinary fees has supported the increasing incidence of fracture repair in the horse.

Fractures of the spine and upper limbs are much more difficult to treat in the older horse, whereas foals are often able to return to full use. Pelvic fractures are also very difficult to treat.

The first and most vital step in the treatment of fractures is immobilisation by the application of a splint. This will minimise further damage to the injured limb. Many horses with fractures are transported to veterinary clinics without adequate support. In these cases, fractures can become damaged further with the result that they become irreparable. If a fracture is suspected, then the limb must be immobilised properly. Horses that are in pain and distressed should be sedated and given analgesic drugs before the required manipulation of the limb and splinting are carried out. The horse can then be transported to the clinic for further investigation and treatment.

First-aid procedure

Safety

The horse must be controlled quietly but firmly. It is best to have it held by someone else, and if it becomes fractious a bridle should be fitted for greater control. A restraining influence may be obtained by holding up a front leg. When examining a hind leg, it sometimes helps to hold the horse's tail firmly downwards. A horse may also be restrained by grasping a fold of skin on its neck. There is no point in either the horse or a handler being hurt. If necessary a twitch should be used on the upper lip.

Simple methods of restraint are described in Chapter 18.

Calm

The attendants should talk reassuringly to the horse, pat and stroke it, and work without fuss or bother. This will maintain a calm atmosphere. Thoroughness is more important than speed.

Bleeding control

There are three types of bleeding or haemorrhage. First, there is the blood around a cut from the tiny capillaries in the flesh; this is not serious. The second type flows gently and is dark red; this comes from the veins and is called venous bleeding. The third type is bright red and comes from an artery; the blood runs freely and may spurt out under pressure from the heartbeat. An injury involving bleeding of the first type can wait for treatment until return to the horse transport or stable. However, an injury involving venous and arterial bleeding calls for immediate treatment.

Venous bleeding can be controlled with a clean pad such as a folded handkerchief placed on the wound, and then securing the pad firmly over the wound using a bandage, tie, stock or belt. Slight bleeding actually helps clean the wound and a little blood goes a long way, so try not to panic.

Where arterial bleeding is dominant, the blood flow is more difficult to stop and veterinary attention is needed. While you are waiting for the vet to arrive apply very firm pressure by pressing a clean dressing to the wound. If the wound is on the horse's leg put a pressure bandage on over several layers of gamgee but take care that the bandage does not act as a tourniquet and cut off the blood supply. The bandage should be removed as soon as the bleeding stops. If the wound is not on a leg, it may be necessary to hold the pressure pad in place until help can be obtained. The horse should be kept warm and quiet until it is taken home for treatment. If the need arises, help must be summoned or the horse led to the nearest house, where transport can be arranged. If any doubt exists the vet should be called as the wound may need suturing, and tetanus protection may be required.

Cleanliness

A dirty wound should first be washed under a cold, gentle hose, although care must be taken not to frighten the horse. Hair is then cut away from the region of the wound. A piece of cotton wool soaked in antiseptic solution is applied, taking care to wipe dirt out and not rub it in. Each swab should be used once only, and should not be put back into the disinfectant solution. When the wound is clear, it is dried with a dry piece of cotton wool. Wound powder is then lightly 'puffed on'. Antiseptic cream is useful for sores and grazes. Where a dressing is required to keep out dirt, the wound is covered with gauze, preferably medicated, and a cotton wool pad is bandaged gently in place.

Chapter 9
Lameness

Lameness is the most common cause for horses being off work. Lameness is an alteration of the horse's gait, usually as a result of pain or mechanical problems. Sometimes, horses are described as being 'unlevel' when their movement is uneven or there is an irregularity of rhythm. A horse that is persistently unlevel is probably suffering slight lameness and should be investigated further. Most lameness is caused by foot problems, but it may also be associated not just with the legs, but also with the back, for example.

The lame horse should be evaluated thoroughly so that the source or sources of pain may be found and treatment given.

Before looking at the horse, there are some points to be considered:

* age
* breed
* occupation (racing, hunting, jumping, dressage)
* fitness
* conformation
* shoeing
* gait abnormality – brushing, over-reaching
* recent history.

These points all give possible clues as to the cause of lameness. The examination should consist of two stages:

* observation at rest in the stable or field
* observation during exercise, either in hand or ridden.

Examination at rest

If possible, the horse should be observed while undisturbed and resting. This should include the position the horse finds most comfortable. It is normal for the horse to rest alternate hind legs intermittently, but it is unusual to rest a foreleg or point a toe. Some horses will rest a diagonal, i.e. a hind leg and the opposite foreleg, particularly when tired or having worked on hard ground. The horse should then be stood up on a square, flat, level surface and assessed for:

* conformation

- symmetry of bone structure and muscle development
- temperament, has the horse started to refuse?
- abnormal heat/swelling in legs or back
- size and shape of each foot
- each foot should be lifted, picked out looking for abnormal wear of shoes and/or feet
- hoof testers to apply gentle pressure
- tap the sole and hoof wall over each clench with a hammer.

This may be enough to locate the source of lameness, if not, the horse should be watched moving.

Examining the horse during movement

The horse must be properly restrained particularly if it has been on box rest for some time. A bridle or a cavesson and lunge line (see Figure 9.1) is more suitable than a headcollar when examining the horse during movement. The horse should be led along a hard, level, flat surface and the head and neck should be allowed to move freely.

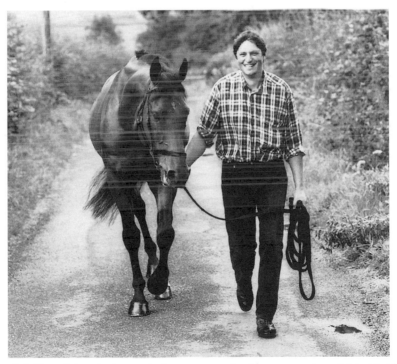

Figure 9.1. Examining the horse during movement using a properly restricted bridle (or cavesson) and lunge line.

First walk the horse away, towards and then past the observer, handlers should turn the horse away from themselves and the turns should be watched carefully for problems. This procedure can then be repeated at trot, although a severely lame horse may refuse and should not be made to trot.

In walk

Time should be spent watching the horse walk as it is easier because the legs are moving slowly.

- The way in which the horse places the feet on the ground is important. Is each foot placed squarely? Does one side land first? Does the toe land first?
- The flight of the leg through the air should be assessed. Does the horse lift each foot the same height off the ground? Do the feet swing in or out? Does the horse brush or forge? (see Chapter 3).
- Does each leg take the same length of stride? Is the stride length as would be expected for a horse of that type?
- Does each fetlock sink to the same degree as it takes the horse's weight?

In trot

Bearing in mind all the observations made in the stable and walk, the horse may now be examined at trot.

- The horse's head carriage should be watched carefully. The lame horse will nod as the sound leg hits the ground.
- The horse is said to be pottery if taking a shorter stride than normal with both forelimbs, indicating pain in both forelegs.
- If hind leg lameness is suspected, the horse should be watched from the side and from behind. The lame leg may take a shorter stride and this may be heard. If the lameness is in the hock or above, the horse may drag its toe, and the shoe may show signs of uneven wear. As it is impossible to flex the hock without flexing the stifle, and hip joints, it is hard to differentiate between these regions.
- The horse should be watched for uneven movement of the hindquarters with the quarter of the lame leg appearing to rise and fall more than the other side.
- The horse may nod as the foreleg on the same side as the lame hind leg hits the ground because the lame leg is not weight bearing. This may be confusing.

Small circles in walk

If the lameness has still not been pinpointed, the next step is to turn the horse in small circles. This assesses the flexibility of the horse's neck and back and its ability to move the outside legs away from the body and inside legs towards the body. It also puts added pressure on the inside legs as they have to carry more weight. Small circles will exaggerate any suspicion of lameness on the trotting-up turns. The horse should also be asked to move back to assess if it is a shiverer.

Large circles on the lunge

The horse can be lunged on hard ground to exaggerate foreleg lameness when the affected leg is on the inside. There are no rules for hind leg lameness.

Ridden exercise

Hind leg lameness may be exaggerated when the horse is ridden. This is sometimes most obvious when the rider is sitting on the diagonal of the affected leg. Some horses are 'bridle' lame and only show lameness when ridden.

Identifying the exact source of pain

After identifying the leg or legs affected, the veterinary surgeon will be able to locate the seat of lameness. Local anaesthetic may be used to block specific nerves supplying the lower leg. The idea is that if the pain originates in the desensitised area, then the horse should go sound

Vets also use other diagnostic procedures including:

* radiography (X-rays)
* ultrasound scanning of tendons and ligaments (see Figure 9.2)
* gamma scintigraphy
* blood tests
* surgical examination.

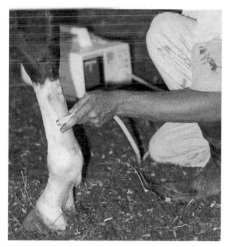

Figure 9.2. Ultrasound scanning of the tendons.

Exercise and the lame horse

When a vet has diagnosed lameness, the horse may be restricted on the amount of work or even placed on box rest. One of the following routines may be suggested:

- complete box rest – for very painful conditions, 24 hours a day
- stable rest – as the horse improves it may be led out for 5 minutes, twice per day, common with tendon injuries
- leading out only – longer periods of leading out
- walking out only – ridden again only at walk
- lungeing – horse is worked in circles on a lunge rein at walk, trot and canter
- light work – horse may be ridden lightly at walk and trot
- slow work – race horses may be given work at slow canter rather than fast canter or gallop.

Feeding the lame horse

If the horse's workload is reduced, so must the feeding of concentrates. Forage such as hay may be given *ad libitum* while the horse is on box rest. A cool cube, or low starch, high-digestible fibre compound feed may be fed, but not a high cereal performance feed. There are a few compound feeds available for ill or convalescing horses, otherwise feed a chaff base with a good-quality vitamin and mineral supplement and unmolassed beet pulp while the horse is off work. If the horse is being given medicine in the form of powders or granules the beet pulp will help to mix it in and disguise it. Clean fresh water must be available at all times.

Treatment for lameness

Lameness due to soft tissue damage may first be treated by the application of cold to reduce swelling, and later this may be interspersed with heat to draw blood to the area to aid healing. Heat may come from poultices, fomentations or ultrasonic therapy. Once the initial swelling has gone, it may be thought advisable to produce further inflammation by the use of counter-irritants. The simplest of these are known as 'blisters'. The first task is to clip the coat over the area. The blister is then applied according to the directions on the container. When blistering a tendon, the rear lower part of the leg should be covered with petroleum jelly or lard so that the blister does not run down the leg and inflame the heels. When blistering a joint, its inside angle should be avoided. The horse will need a cradle put on its neck so that it cannot nibble or lick the blister. Similarly, if the hocks are blistered, the tail must be kept bandaged up double so that it cannot swish over the blister and carry it to the flanks. The horse must be put on a forage-based diet before the operation and for a few days afterwards.

Less severe treatment is given by the use of 'working blisters'; these do not always need the hair to be clipped. Generally, they are rubbed in with a soft toothbrush each day until the skin becomes scaly. A working blister is normally to be found in most medicine chests, whereas the use of a full blister is a matter for the vet, who will advise on current thinking of its value.

The practice of 'firing' damaged tendons by applying electrically heated irons to the skin of the horse's legs is rarely carried out now. The technique of wounding tendons in a 'split tendon operation' to gain additional support tissue has also been criticised, but the use of carbon-fibre implants appears to be successful in some cases. The most popular treatment for tendon strain is box rest and cold treatment during the acute phase of the injury, followed by physiotherapy and controlled exercise until the horse is sound. Best results are obtained if the horse is then rested in the field to allow full recovery for as long as 12 months.

Whatever method is used to strengthen the legs, it is important to remember that the horse kept in the stable without exercise needs a forage-based diet, and that the sound leg, on the other side to the damaged one, will be taking additional weight and so will need support bandages. Eventually, and it may be after several months, the horse is turned out to grass. It may gallop about and could reinjure the damaged leg. The front shoes should be left on for a front-leg injury but the back shoes can be taken off and the feet cut back so that the horse is very footsore behind and thus not inclined even to trot. Drugs can provide an alternative restraint, which can be used for the first few days. It is essential that the horse be left out at grass for some months, as complete rest is the best cure for such injuries.

Physiotherapy

Today's horse must be fit enough to perform considerable feats and is thus exposed to the risk of injury. Physiotherapy is widely used during the training of human athletes, both to prevent injury and to aid recovery after it. These techniques are now being successfully adapted for use with the 'equine athlete' such as the hunter or competition horse. Obviously, it is more complicated to diagnose the exact site and type of pain in a horse and to gain its co-operation during treatment.

Traditionally, rest has been the treatment for the many athletic problems associated with horses. Now there are a number of techniques which, when used by competent people under veterinary supervision, lead to faster recovery, often of a more permanent nature.

A number of sophisticated medical appliances have been adapted to treat various equine athletic conditions. Some of these, such as faradism and ultrasound, work by applying energy sources directly to the horse.

Muscles give stability as well as function to joints. Deterioration of joint function can be the result of a previous slight injury that may not have been noticed. The horse cannot control or operate the joint as effectively as before, but is not lame. If not noticed, the next time the joint is stressed it may malfunction and sustain a serious injury. Permanent damage may perhaps result, or the horse may show poor form due to discomfort. This could be the start of a nappy horse.

Faradic

Faradic may be used for both diagnostic and therapeutic work. It consists of application of an intermittent alternating electric current, allowing the muscle in question to contract and relax, thus preventing atrophy.

The artificial stimulation applied by faradic current increases circulation to the injured parts without any damaging effects. Faradic can reduce adhesions and promote the interchange of fluids within the body with beneficial results. It may also help correct muscle imbalance and release long-term muscle tension.

Faradic is not tolerated by some horses and it has now been superseded by more effective techniques.

Ultrasound

This consists of high-frequency sound waves, well above the normal range of hearing.

Ultrasound can penetrate to a depth of between 5 and 10 cm (2–4 in) and affects the tissue in different ways. The resistance met in the tissues by the sound waves induces heat, a mechanical vibration is produced and the waves stimulate a chemical reaction. All three assist in the dissipation of swelling and inflammation, the removal of harmful breakdown products, the reduction of swollen tendons and the breakdown of adhesions.

Vibration and massage

The therapeutic value of massage and vibration has been known for many years. Their greatest value is in producing complete relaxation and dispersing muscle tension. Muscles cannot develop if they suffer from constant tension. Horses are generally exposed to unnatural ways of living and working, which can induce muscle tension. The temperament of the individual horse is of importance in its attitude to its work and to its owner/trainer. Muscle tension can prevent the horse from relaxing mentally and physically as muscles held in undue tension become exhausted. In this state they cannot develop and this may lead to muscle imbalance or incorrect development in shape or form. The elimination of undesirable muscle tension as soon as it is observed enables the trainer to progress with the horse's training programme and helps to maintain the animal's co-operation.

Remedial exercises

Injury can reduce the range of movement in joints, and by reduction of ligament suppleness or painful adhesions it can cause limitations.

Specific exercises can build up joint suppleness, help to break down adhesions slowly and to restore the horse's confidence in the use of the joint, and remedy muscle imbalance resulting from previous injury or use.

A combination of therapy and exercise is known as rehabilitation and the equine sports therapist will design a programme for an injured horse that aims to restore the horse to its full athletic potential.

Heat treatment

Heat in therapy can be used in three forms: radiant, conductive and conversive. The physiological effects of the three methods are basically the same and range from superficial to deep. Radiant heat is applied by means of infra-red light. Conductive heat is applied by hot-water bottles, electric heating pads, hot fomentations and poultices. Conversive heat is developed in the tissues by resistance to high-frequency electrical energy.

Heat promotes circulation in the area, which aids healing and also helps to alleviate pain; thus it relaxes and soothes the patient.

Generally speaking, cold therapy is used in the acute stages of an injury – applying heat to a new injury may be harmful. After the cold therapy has reduced the inflammation hot and cold may be alternated to great benefit.

Hydrotherapy

Generally, the application of water is a means of applying cold. However, equine swimming pools allow the heart and lungs to be kept fit without any weight on the legs. Remember that the swimming of horses should only be carried out by experienced professionals as poor swimming technique can be detrimental to a horse's development. Other forms of hydrotherapy include water treadmills and whirlpools.

Nursing

Care and attention to detail has a psychological as well as a physical benefit. As with people, horses respond in a happy, relaxed atmosphere with a positive attitude, gain confidence and becoming willing patients.

Part 3
The systems of the horse

Chapter 10
Systems of support and movement

The horse is a vertebrate: it belongs to the group of animals that have a backbone. The parts of the body are fixed to a frame, the skeleton, which is built from bone and cartilage for strength and to allow movement. The backbone and skull give strength and protection to the delicate brain and to the central nervous system. Joints are fixed together by ligaments and muscles attached to bones by tendons, allowing movement.

The most vulnerable part of the horse's skeleton is the lower leg and foot. The functions of these systems are:

- support
- protection
- locomotion.

Bones and cartilage

The skeleton of the horse is composed of over 200 bones. Weight for weight, bone is at least five times as strong as steel. Bones get their rigidity from hard deposits of minerals such as calcium and phosphorus, and they get their flexibility from tough, elastic fibres of collagen.

The hard outside of bone is known as compact bone. The inside is known as spongy bone and has a light honeycomb appearance. The core of the long bones contains bone marrow where all the blood cells, apart from some white cells, are made. There are two types of bone marrow:

- red marrow found in spongy bone – where the red cells and some white cells are made
- yellow marrow – a fat store found in some hollow areas in long bone shafts.

Yellow bone marrow may turn to red bone marrow when the horse is ill. The white cells formed in bone marrow play a key role in the horse's immune system.

The main functions of bone are:

- to provide support
- movement (when joints are brought in to play)
- to act as a reservoir for important minerals.

A thin layer of elastic connective tissue called the periosteum surrounds the bone. It contains cells, which make new bone.

The end surfaces where bones meet are called joints or articulatory surfaces. They are covered in cartilage.

Joints

Most of the horse's joints allow for bones to move, but different kinds of joints move in different ways:

- immovable or fixed joints (such as in the skull)
- slightly movable joints (such as the junction between the bones in the back)
- freely movable joints include:
  - hinge joints: let the bones swing to and fro like a door hinge, e.g. the fetlock
  - plane joints: joints that slide over each other, e.g. the knee
  - pivot joints: axis/atlas at the top of the neck
  - ball and socket joints: the hip.

Each freely movable joint is enclosed in a capsule, the lining of which is the synovial membrane. This secretes synovial fluid or 'joint oil', which acts as a lubricant. The outer cover of the capsule is fibrous and acts like a ligament, holding the joint together. There are similar capsules on prominent bone ends (such as the elbow), and these are called bursae (singular, bursa) (see Figure 10.1).

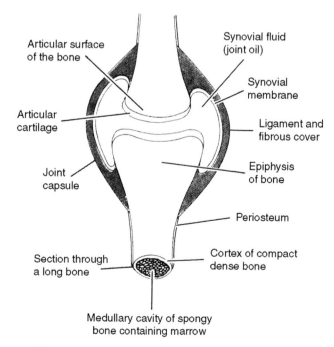

Figure 10.1. Bone and joint.

Ligaments are strong connective bands of tissue holding joints together. Some are within the joint capsule itself, but most are outside it, connecting the two bones on the sides, front and back of the joint.

Tendons and ligaments

Tendons are chord-like structures that attach muscle to bone or to another muscle. Ligaments attach bone to bone and are not as elastic as tendons. Each tendon is a continuation of the membrane around the muscle together with the outer membranes of its bundles of tendon fibres.

Tendons and ligaments are made up of long strands of collagen fibres aligned in parallel. There is very little blood supply to ligaments and tendons. Many tendons and ligaments are surrounded by an outer layer or sheath that protects them and provides oxygen and nutrients.

The tendon fibres have a crimped appearance, giving them a small degree of elasticity and a slight ability to lengthen.

Skeleton

The word skeleton comes from the ancient Greek word for 'dry'. The skeleton is made up of:

- bones
- cartilage
- joints
- ligaments.

The skeleton has two main parts: the axial and the appendicular skeleton.

The axial skeleton

The axial skeleton is shown in Figure 10.2. The skull consists of many small bones fused together to form protection for the brain, optic nerves, inner ears and nasal passages. One of the largest bones in the horse is the lower jawbone or mandible that is hinged between the eye and the base of the ear. The skull also contains the teeth. The back of the skull is formed by the occipital bone which has a junction with the top bones of the neck.

The neck contains the atlas, the axis and five other cervical vertebrae. The bones of the backbone or vertebral column are called vertebrae (singular, vertebra).

The chest part of the vertebral column contains 18 thoracic vertebrae to which are attached the 18 pairs of ribs. There are eight pairs of 'true' ribs attached directly to the breast bone or sternum. In addition, there are ten pairs of 'false' ribs, attached to the breast bone by long cartilage extensions. The horse has no collar bone.

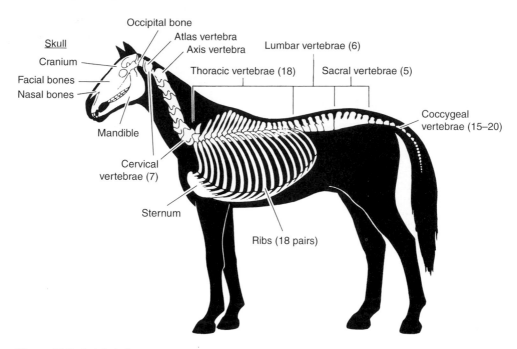

Figure 10.2. Axial skeleton.

The next part of the vertebral column consists of six lumbar vertebrae forming the loins. Behind the loins are the five sacral vertebrae fused together as a firm base for the pelvis and forming the croup. There are also some 15–20 bones called the coccygeal vertebrae that go down into the dock of the tail.

The neck and tail vertebrae are freely jointed to provide a wide range of movement, but little movement is possible through the thoracic and lumbar vertebrae. When we speak of a horse 'bending its back', most of the movement is in fact occurring in the neck. The apparent lateral bending is effectively a combination of neck, shoulder and limb alignment, the backbone remaining almost straight. The ribs limit movement through the barrel of the horse, and so any movement is confined to the region of the loins.

The vertebrae have vertical and transverse processes that aid muscle attachment. There is a canal or channel through the centre of the vertebrae housing the spinal cord. This is the continuation from the brain down the backbone. Occasionally, vertebrae seem to get slightly out of alignment and in some cases manipulation appears to help. Sometimes vertebrae will fuse together at their extremities. This can cause pain and reduced performance until the fusion is complete. Given time, however, the horse appears none the worse when the fusion is complete.

The appendicular skeleton

Figure 10.3 shows the bones that comprise the appendicular skeleton. The front legs are not joined by any bony attachment to the horse's axial skeleton. Thus, the weight of the horse is taken at the front by muscles, tendons and ligaments from the two front legs, so forming a sling in which the body is carried. This arrangement is part of the shock-absorbing mechanism built into the front legs. The other parts of this mechanism are the angles in the shoulders and fetlocks, the many bones of the knee and the design of the foot itself.

The foreleg starts with the scapula or shoulder blade, the top part of which consists of cartilage. The scapula forms the shoulder joint with the humerus or upper arm bone. The front of the humerus is known as the point of the shoulder. The rear or distal (lower) end of the humerus forms the elbow joint together with the radius and ulna, which are fused together to form the forearm. The radius is the main weight carrier of the two bones, and the ulna reaches up to form the point of the elbow (olecranon process). Below the forearm comes the knee or carpus, which is the equivalent of the human wrist. It is made up of two rows of small bones with a small additional bone at the back, called the accessory carpal or pisiform bone. This little bone makes the tendon pull at an angle to bend the knee.

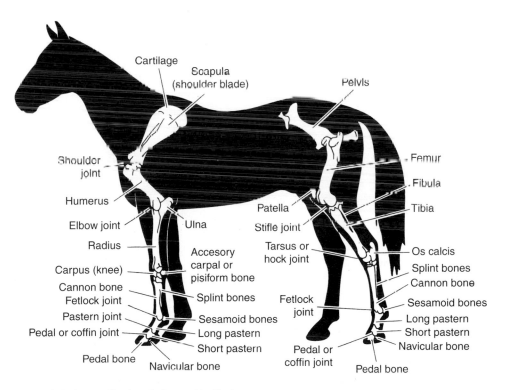

Figure 10.3. Appendicular skeleton: the limbs.

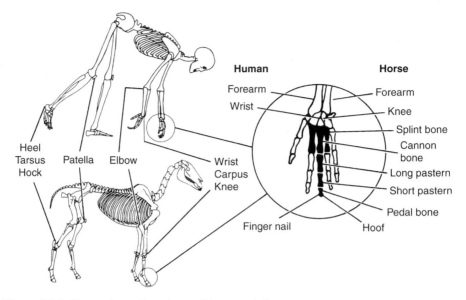

Human

Horse

Forearm

Forearm

Wrist

Knee

Splint bone

Heel

Cannon bone

Tarsus

Patella

Elbow

Wrist

Hock

Carpus

Long pastern

Knee

Short pastern

Pedal bone

Finger nail

Hoof

Figure 10.4. Comparison of equine and human skeletons.

Below the knee are the three metacarpal bones; the central large one is the cannon bone, and the two small bones on either side of it are the splint bones. The cannon and splint bones are the equivalent to the three bones running across the back of the human hand (see Figure 10.4). The bones equivalent to those of the little finger and thumb have disappeared during evolution.

The cannon bone meets the digit at the fetlock joint. This digit is equivalent to the human middle finger. It consists of three principal bones (the phalanges): the long pastern (first phalanx), the short pastern (second phalanx) and the coffin or pedal bone (third phalanx). The joint of the long and short pastern bones is the pastern joint. That between the short pastern bone and the pedal bone is the coffin joint.

At the back of the fetlock joint there are two small bones designed to gain mechanical advantage in bending the joint; these are the sesamoid bones (proximal sesamoids). At the back of the coffin joint is another sesamoid-type bone called the navicular bone (distal sesamoid).

The hind leg starts with the pelvic girdle (see Figure 10.5). This is made up from the fused sacral vertebrae and the two hip or pelvic bones (os coxae), which meet underneath at the symphysis. Each hip bone is formed from three bones fused together: the ilium, the ischium and the pubis. The ilium joins the sacrum on either side at the sacro-iliac joint. The front end of the ilium has the point of croup (tuber sacralae) near the sacrum and the point of hip (tuber coxae) on the outer side. The ilium unites with the ischium at the hip joint. The ischium has a rearward projection called the seatbone or point of buttock (tuber ischii). The pubis also meets at the hip joint, and the pubis, together with the

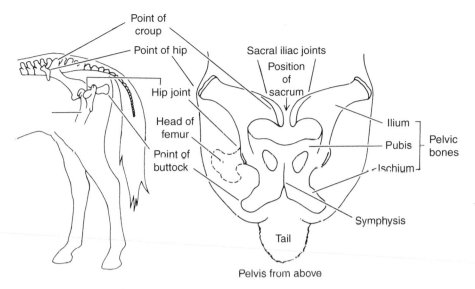

Figure 10.5. The pelvis.

lower part of the ischium, forms the floor of the pelvis. Thus, the pelvis forms a complete hoop of bones protecting the vital parts of the horse's body. A long flat pelvis is said to be best for high speeds.

The thigh bone (femur) comes from the hip joint and runs down to the stifle joint. At the stifle there is another sesamoid bone called the patella, which corresponds to the human kneecap. The femur meets the tibia, which is within the second thigh or gaskin. In humans, beside the tibia is the fibula; the fibula in the horse is only a vestigial remnant, sometimes no more than 10 cm (4 in) long. The tibia goes to the hock (tarsus), which, like the knee, consists of several small bones. The hock equates to the human ankle. At the back of the hock is a bone called the calcaneus or point of hock (fibular tarsal), which acts as a lever to extend the leg. It forms the heel in humans. Below the hock, the bones are similar to those below the knee.

Muscles

Muscles are special fibres that contract (tighten) and relax to move parts of the horse's body. They may be:

- voluntary muscles: muscles controlled by the will of the horse
- involuntary muscles: work automatically, such as the digestive tract wall
- cardiac muscle: heart.

Most voluntary muscles cover the skeleton and are therefore also called skeletal muscles. They may also be known as striped or striated, because there are dark bands on the bundles of fibre that form them.

Most involuntary muscles form sacs or tubes such as the digestive tract or blood vessels. These are known as smooth muscle because they lack the stripes or bands. Most muscles are arranged in pairs because, although they may shorten themselves (to contract), they cannot lengthen again by themselves. So a flexor muscle, which bends the joint, is paired with an extensor one that straightens it again.

Heart muscle is a unique combination of skeletal and smooth muscle. It has its own contraction rhythm to maintain the heartbeat.

A branch from a nerve controls each muscle fibre. These muscle fibres are arranged in bundles surrounded by connective tissue. When the nerve is stimulated the muscle contracts or shortens exerting a pull and the more muscle fibres involved, the stronger the pull.

Muscle fibres

These are made from hundreds or thousands of strands known as myofibrils, each marked with dark bands giving the muscle a stripy appearance. The stripes are alternate bands of filaments of two substances: actin (thin filaments) and myosin (thick filaments). Actin and myosin are able to interlock like the teeth of a zip.

Each fibre of a muscle is controlled by a branch from a nerve. These muscle fibres are arranged in bundles, as described above. Thus, for more strength the horse must build more muscle. Muscles are arranged in sheets and bands, and in herringbone and spindle-like groups according to their function.

Each muscle has an origin where it is attached to a stable part of the skeleton. At the other end it has an insertion into the part of the skeleton that it moves. Where the bone to be moved is distant from the muscle, there is a dense fibrous connection between them called a tendon. Tendons are usually cord or band shaped, but some are flat like sheets. They have little elasticity and are poorly supplied with blood. They also take considerable strain and, because of these factors, take a long time to heal when injured.

Just as a joint has a covering that supplies lubrication to help the moving parts, each tendon has a sheath where it passes over a joint, which protects and lubricates it. Similarly, just as a prominent bone end has a protective capsule (bursa), there are tendon bursae to help tendons pass over bones at a joint.

The muscles of the horse are complex. There are approximately 700 separate skeletal muscles in the horse. Some of the main muscles of interest to owners are considered below and shown in Figure 10.6.

Trapezius, the muscle on either side of the withers. It lies over the rhomboideus and splenius muscles. In some horses these muscles are poorly developed, which gives them prominent withers and 'ewe necks'.

Brachiocephalicus, the muscle that pulls the shoulder forward and is attached at its front end to the back of the head. This is why it is easier for a horse to jump well using its shoulders if it is given sufficient length of rein to extend the neck and head in flight. Similarly, at the collected paces where elevation of the steps is required, this muscle helps to carry the neck high and not stretched out, thus raising the shoulder.

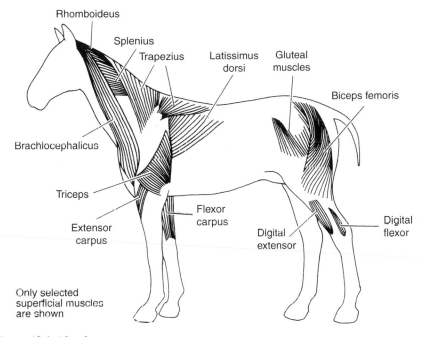

Figure 10.6. Muscles.

Latissimus dorsi, the muscles from the shoulder blade to the back. Those running along the back are the *longissimus dorsi*. These are the muscles on which the rider sits.

The elbow has extensor muscles called *triceps* and flexor muscles called *biceps*. The lower joints also have paired muscles, but in order to keep the lower leg light they are kept in the upper leg. This is advantageous for high speed. The extensor muscles acting on the hip are known as the hamstring muscles. These pass up the back of the hindquarters and attach to the croup. On fit horses these muscles clearly stand out with divisions between them.

By removing a minute portion of tissue (in a biopsy), laboratory analysis has shown fast-twitch and slow-twitch muscle fibres. The mixture of these in a racehorse has bearing on its sprinting or staying ability.

The lower leg and foot

A running man wearing heavy boots is slower than a man running in lightweight shoes. Evolution favours the fast-running horse to escape from its enemies, and similarly selects the horse with lightweight lower legs and feet. The remote ancestor of the horse had several toes; the modern horse has only one that takes all the strain and is sometimes the weakest link. This is particularly so in the front leg that takes all the strain on landing from a jump and which normally carries about two-thirds of the horse's weight.

The main strain is taken by the suspensory ligament (see Figure 10.7) coming from the back of the knee and running against the cannon bone down the back of the leg to the fetlock. Part of the suspensory ligament is then attached to the sesamoid bones and part divides into two and comes round the pastern from each side.

The two tendons running down the back of the lower leg are the superficial flexor tendon and under it is the deep flexor tendon, which has a check ligament. This takes some of the strain from the muscles situated above the knee in the forearm, or above the hock in the second thigh. The deep flexor tendon runs over the sesamoid bones down to the pastern, into the hoof and round the navicular bone. It is attached to the coffin or pedal bone. The superficial flexor tendon divides into two branches at the fetlock: these attach on both sides to both pastern bones.

The extensor tendons run down the front of the leg. As they take no weight, they are slim and generally trouble-free.

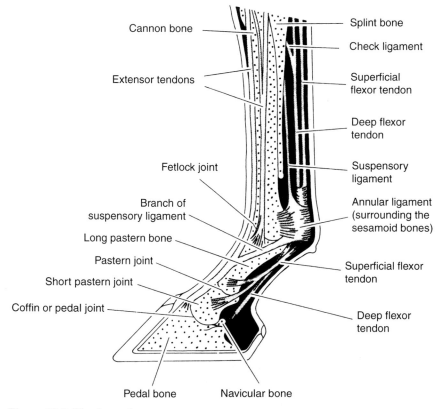

Figure 10.7. The lower leg.

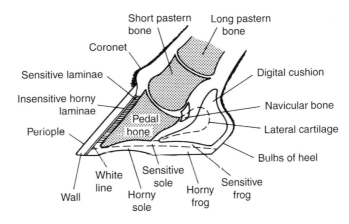

Figure 10.8. Foot structure.

There is a band of tissue at the coronet called the coronary band. This creates horn and so produces the hoof. The outer layer of the hoof, called the periople, serves to control the movement of moisture in and out of the hoof. There is next a horny layer and inside that the insensitive laminae. These mesh with the sensitive laminae that surround the pedal bone, and in this way the pedal bone is firmly held in the foot.

The lower surface of the foot is composed of the sole and the raised frog and bars that act like the treads on the wheels of a tractor, to help grip the ground. The shape of the underside of the foot is slightly concave, so aiding grip.

Under the back of the pedal bone is the pedal (plantar) cushion that takes and spreads some of the weight from the short pastern bone; it does this by pushing wide the lateral cartilages, two wings of cartilage attached to the pedal bone, so spreading the heel and pressing the frog against the ground. Much of the concussion of normal working is thus absorbed within the foot. The foot is well supplied with blood and the action of the pedal cushion being compressed at every step is like a small pump helping the circulation.

Figure 10.8 shows the structure of the foot.

Farriery

A normal hind foot is longer than the forefoot (Figure 10.9). When the horse is working under stress, it is important to keep the toe of the forefoot short, the frog in contact with the ground and the heels wide. This helps the foot to work most efficiently.

The rate of the growth of horn varies according to food, environment and exercise, and is greater at the front of the foot than at the heel. Wild ponies normally walk far enough and live in sufficiently rough conditions to keep their feet correctly worn. An unshod horse in a field may need its feet rasping every 6 weeks, as will a shod horse, although in the latter case wear of the shoe may dictate more frequent treatment.

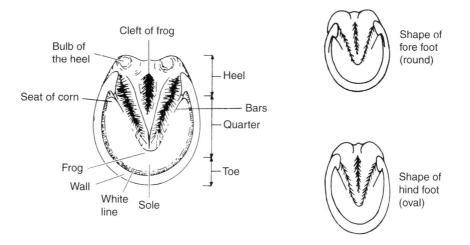

If the farrier is attempting to alter action by trimming the foot, this must be done only a little at a time, as it will alter the angle of wear on the joints. The foot is usually trimmed so that the angle of the pastern to the ground is the same as the angle of the foot. When rasping, it is harder work to take down the front of the foot and there is a tendency to take off too much at the heels or to reduce the bars, which may lead to contracted heels.

The preparation of the hoof for the reception of a shoe consists of removing loose particles of sole and tidying ragged pieces of frog. The bearing surface of the wall must be made level with the outer edge of the sole.

Although a shoe may not be worn out, it must be refitted every 4–6 weeks, otherwise it will be carried forwards by hoof growth. The weight of the horse borne by the shoe should not be far in front of the line down through the centre of the cannon bone, otherwise damage to hooves, joints and tendons will occur.

Muscle fibre types

There are several different fibre types within each muscle. Initially muscle fibre types are identified by colour, red muscle is associated with long-term or endurance work (e.g. chickens have dark meat in their legs as they use them for standing and moving all day).

The breast meat of chickens is white and this contains muscle fibre types for power.

The horse has three different type of muscle fibre:

- slow twitch – works steadily for long periods of time
- fast twitch – fast powerful muscles which may be: fast twitch high oxidative –

powerful and able to use oxygen for long periods of time: or fast twitch low oxidative – good for sudden bursts of power, but tend to tire quickly as oxygen quickly runs out.

Most of the horse's muscles consist of a mixture of the three types. During normal muscle contraction it is unlikely that the muscles need to exert their maximum strength, so not all the fibres are stimulated at once. There is an orderly selection of muscle fibres depending on the amounts of exertion, so for walking and standing only slow-twitch fibres are used.

The proportion of these muscle fibre types is largely genetic and often breed related. Even an unfit quarter horse (a sprinting specialist) will have more fast-twitch fibres than an Arab (endurance).

Fatigue

The aim of getting a horse fit is to be able to work it for longer before it gets tired, in other words to delay the onset of fatigue. A horse is said to be fatigued when it can no longer exercise at that level. If the horse is not allowed to slow down, exhaustion will set in.

There are four main factors, which contribute to fatigue:

- glycogen depletion (muscle sugar has run out)
- lactic acid build up
- dehydration and heat stress
- lameness.

Disorders of the skeletal, articular and muscular systems

Azoturia (Rhabdomyolysis)

Other names used for this poorly understood disease include Monday morning disease, tying up and set fast.

The disease results in muscle stiffness and pain of varying degrees. It may be mild or severe. Signs vary from slight hind leg stiffness to complete reluctance to move. Traditionally, the problem arose soon after onset of exercise, more commonly in fit horses on full rations and following a rest day. However, horses have been seen to develop symptoms at pasture, in the 10-minute box of a 3-day event or just while out hacking.

Some horses are prone to recurring attacks.

Whatever the cause, the result is muscle damage. This damage releases muscle enzymes [creatine phosphokinase (CPK) and aspartate aminotransferase (AST)] into the blood stream. A blood test taken by the vet will show the amount of these enzymes and therefore the amount of damage that has occurred.

Horses showing signs of the disease should not be moved if at all possible. If it occurs out on the roads, then the horse should be boxed home.

Treatment is rest and the vet will attempt to reduce inflammation and pain in the damaged muscles.

Electrolyte status has been implicated, as has a problem with storage of glycogen and these should be discussed with the vet. Some horses that frequently tie up have been moved to a low-starch, high-digestible fibre and oil diet, and have managed to compete successfully with no recurrence of the disease. Others have benefited from an assessment and correction of the electrolyte status. There is no scientific evidence as yet that selenium and vitamin E has any benefit for horses that tie up.

- Reduce concentrates if the horse has a rest day (or turn out to pasture for day).
- Warm up before and cool down after exercise properly.
- Pay attention to the electrolyte status of the horse (ask a nutritionist if necessary).
- Feed to match the level of work.
- Feed a low starch, high fibre feed. Use oil to supply calories if required.

Degenerative joint disease (DJD) (arthritis)

This is a disease of the cartilage within the horse's joints. Examples include ringbone and bone spavin. DJD may follow damage to the joint, sprain, fracture or infection. It may also result from poor conformation placing strains on the joints. Inflammation of the joint capsule leads to the production of enzymes, which break down the cartilage. Spurs of new bone may then develop around the joints. Eventually the joint space may become completely filled with new bone. Signs of DJD include:

- heat
- swelling of the joint
- lameness, may be gradual or sudden
- pain on flexion of the joint
- joint enlargement due to new bone and fibrous tissue
- reduced range of movement of the joint.

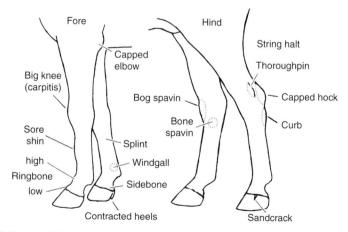

Figure 10.10. Leg problems.

There is no treatment for DJD. The aims of support are:

- pain relief
- reduce inflammation
- stop further cartilage break down
- encourage cartilage healing.

There are various drugs to help with DJD including phenylbutazone, flunixine meglumine, sodium hyaluronate injection and corticosteroids. All these should discussed with the vet. Glucosamine and chondroitin supplements may be helpful.

Bone spavin

This is DJD of the hock joint. It is a common cause of hind leg lameness.

Bone spavin is caused by wear and tear on the joints of the hock. Poor conformation such as cow or sickle hocks makes horses more susceptible to bone spavin. Clinical signs include:

- gradual onset of lameness that wears off with exercise
- change in hind leg action
- signs of pain when flexing the hock joint
- swelling.

Treatment

The horse should be kept in work if possible to encourage fusion of the hock joint involved. After the joint spaces have filled with new bone and fused, the horse may become sound, with some lack of flexibility of the affected joint. Pain-relieving drugs may be used.

Ringbone

This may be subdivided into one of four types:

- high articular (true) ringbone: DJD of the pastern joint
- high non-articular (false) ringbone: new bone grows on the lower end of the long pastern or upper end of the short pastern, does not involve the joint
- low articular ringbone: DJD of the coffin joint
- low non-articular ringbone: new bone grows on the lower end of the short pastern or the upper end of the pedal bone.

Causes include tearing of the periosteal attachments of various ligaments, direct injury to the bone, puncture wounds or wire cuts and poor conformation. Signs include some lameness and hard swelling in the pastern region. After X-ray diagnosis, some horses are able to continue work with pain relief. Fusion of the joint may occur.

Side bone

This describes ossification of the lateral cartilages that may cause lameness while the bone is forming. Side bones may be felt as hard areas in the bulb of the heel and forwards from that area.

Side bone is listed as hereditary and an unsoundness in English law within the Horse Breeding Act 1918, however ossification of this cartilage is normal. Treatment is limited to rest.

Splints

This is a bony enlargement of one or both of the splint bones. Each leg has a pair of splint bones attached to either side of the cannon bone by a strong ligament. This ligament is subject to tearing, particularly in young horses. This leads to new bone forming a splint. Splints tend to be found on the inside of the leg. There is heat, swelling and sometimes lameness. Causes include:

- working on hard ground
- direct injury such as a kick or a knock
- poor conformation.

Splints formed higher up may affect the knee joint.
Treatment includes:

- cold treatment and support bandages (see Chapter 7)
- anti-inflammatory drugs
- box rest
- topical application of dimethylsulphoxide (DMSO)
- surgery.

Bursitis

This results from inflammation of the bursa and often develops following trauma or infection.

This condition is known as synovitis if a tendon sheath in involved. Bursitis includes bog spavin, windgalls, thoroughpins (Figure 10.11) and carpitis. Causes include:

- a knock or kick
- too little bedding, capped elbow or hock (Figure 10.12)
- rearing over backwards
- strain or injury
- excessive concussion.

When the initial inflammation has subsided there is often a permanent swelling left. Treatment includes:

- rest
- cold therapy and support bandages (see Chapter 7)
- anti-inflammatory drugs.

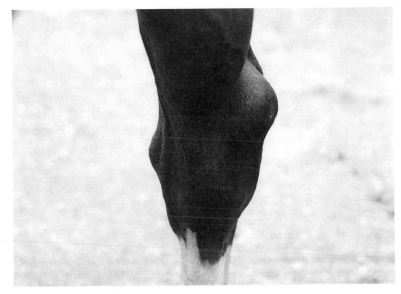

Figure 10.11. Thoroughpin.

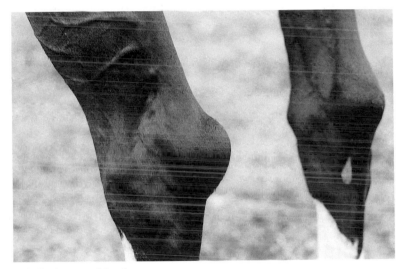

Figure 10.12. A capped hock.

Corns

This is a bruise that develops on the sole of the foot in an angle between the bars and the wall. Causes include:

- shoes that are too small
- shoes that are left on too long
- feet that are not properly balanced
- poor hoof conformation.

Lameness may be slight or severe and may be worse when turning the horse on a circle. The horse will react when hoof testers are applied to the affected area. The shoe should be removed and after slight paring back of the foot a red area of bruising can be seen.

The horse should have the foot tubbed and poulticed for a few days (see Chapter 7). Abcesses of the foot may follow bruising or develop from a penetrating wound or gravel, giving similar symptoms to a corn. Pus in the foot should be cut out and allowed to drain prior to tubbing and poulticing.

Navicular syndrome

This is a progressive, degenerative condition of the navicular bone, the navicular bursa and the deep digital flexor tendon. It may affect one or both front feet. It is seen in most types of horses but rarely in ponies. Symptoms may develop commonly in horses between the age of 6 and 12 years.

The cause is uncertain, but is seems to be associated with changes in blood flow in the foot and blood clots in the foot, impaired by such factors as poor foot conformation, enforced rest and irregular work. Other causes may be abnormal compression of the bone from the long toe's low heel conformation or excessive physical tension from the ligaments attaching the navicular bone to the long pastern.

Ulcers develop in the cartilage of navicular bone and this is then eroded. This results in injury to the deep digital flexor tendon, causing pain.

Signs include:

- shortening of the stride, pottery action
- lameness
- shifting weight from one foot to the other
- standing with one foot in front of the other, pointing the toe
- contraction of the heels leading to upright boxy hoof.

Diagnosis follows nerve blocks, X-rays and clinical signs.

Treatment

The earlier treatment is carried out the better the prognosis. Treatment includes:

- corrective shoeing
- exercise, to encourage normal blood flow through the foot
- isoxsuprine – improves blood flow through the foot
- warfarin – reduces the chances of blood clots forming in the hoof
- pain relief
- navicular suspensory desmotomy – surgical cutting of the ligaments joining the navicular bone to the long pastern
- neurectomy – desensiting the nerve supplying the back of the foot and navicular.

There is no cure for navicular and the prognosis is guarded.

Thrush

A smelly frog with moisture in the cleft, often black in appearance. This is caused by horses standing in dirty, wet bedding and the failure to pick out the feet regularly. Treatment involves cleaning the feet in disinfectant solution using a stiff brush. Treat the area with antiseptic dressing. Tubbing will also help, but make sure the frog is thoroughly dried. Keep both the feet and bedding clean.

Sprains and strains

Strains and sprains are synonymous terms and occur when a tendon or ligament is overstretched. They are far more common in the fore leg. Sudden stress on a tendon or ligament beyond its normal limits causes the fibres to tear.

Causative factors include:

- poor conformation such as upright pasterns or back at the knee
- fatigue
- fast work on uneven ground or in deep mud.

Strains may be mild or severe. A mild strain may still result in a moderate degree of damage to the tendon, without lameness. Signs include some heat and swelling around the tendon. Veterinary advice should be sought immediately to prevent further damage.

Severe strains result in a very lame horse and the tendon is hot and swollen. It is painful to the touch and the horse may be non-weight-bearing. If major disruption to the tendon has occurred the fetlock sinks.

An ultrasound scan will reveal the extent of the injury.

Treatment is aimed at:

- pain relief
- reduction of swelling
- providing support
- encouraging proper realignment of collagen fibres when healing.

Treatment includes box rest (with some walking out in hand) followed by controlled exercise, then an enforced rest at grass, of up to 1 year.

Tendon healing is slow process, but the following may be of some assistance in helping the tendon to repair:

- carbon fibre implants
- physiotherapy, laser, ultrasound or magnetic field therapy (see Chapter 9).

Firing and tendon splitting have shown no improvement in tendon healing when compared with rest, support and controlled exercise.

Chapter 11
Systems of information and control

Horses need to respond to their environment. They need fast and efficient internal communication systems in order to survive.

Horses have two co-ordinating systems: the nervous and endocrine (hormonal) systems that work together triggering responses to the environment. In horses, the flight or fight response to danger is brought about by both nervous and hormonal signals, however the nervous system is much faster in its reactions and is also responsible for the control of more delicate movements by the horse's body.

The endocrine system is involved with information transfer and consists of a series of ductless glands. It is much slower than the nervous system. The endocrine system works by controlling the horse's behavioural patterns by releasing hormones that are responsible for numerous body processes such as:

- growth
- metabolism
- sexual development and function.

The nervous system

The nervous system detects and interprets changes in conditions both inside and outside the horse's body and then responds to them. A change of stimulus produces a reaction. The stimulus is first received and then conducted to a central control system that interprets the message and causes an appropriate action to occur. The central nervous system consists of the brain and spinal cord.

The nervous system can be divided into two main parts:

- the central nervous system (CNS) that consists of the brain and spinal cord
- the peripheral nervous system (PNS), mostly communication nerves that carry signals out of the CNS.

Central nervous system

The CNS (Figure 11.1) consists of the brain and spinal cord that are protected by the skull and spinal column, respectively. The CNS receives inputs from the sense organs such as the skin, eyes, ears and so on, and sends signals to the muscles and glands via the PNS.

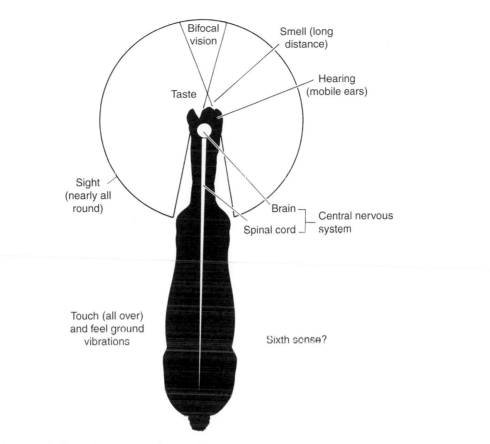

Figure 11.1. Central nervous system and senses.

Peripheral nervous system

The PNS consists of all the nerves that connect the brain and spinal cord to the rest of the horse's body. These include the cranial and spinal nerves. The nerves that carry signals to and from the brain are known as cranial nerves. Those that carry signals to and from the spinal cord are known as the spinal nerves. For example, the eyes, nose, tongue and ears are served by the cranial nerves, whereas the muscles and skin of the legs are served by the spinal nerves.

Hundreds of thousands of signals, both incoming and outgoing, pass each other within the same nerves simultaneously.

Autonomic nervous system

The autonomic nervous system consists of two sets of neurons with opposing effects on most of the internal organs. One set is known as the parasympathetic system and prepares the body for activities that gain and conserve energy such as the stimulation of the salivary glands and digestive juices, and the decrease of the heart and respiratory rates. The other set of neurons, known as the sympathetic system, tend to have opposite effects, preparing the body for energy-consuming activities such as flight or fight. The digestive organs are inhibited, the heart and respiratory rates are increased and the liver releases glucose into the blood, the adrenal glands secrete hormones.

Reflex actions

These are only a small part of the behaviour of horses.

A reflex is an action that occurs automatically and immediately, and, more importantly, predictably to a particular external stimulus. This reflex action is completely independent of the will of the horse.

Many reflexes are innate and examples include:

- shivering
- urination
- sneezing
- coughing
- swallowing
- blinking.

The horse is able to sleep standing up due to a postural reflex action.

Other reflexes are conditioned in that they are brought about by experiences of the horse through its lifetime. These experiences result in the formation of new pathways and junctions within the nervous system itself. The way in which these processes are acquired is known as conditioning. Learning is a type of conditioning in that once a response to a new situation has been repeated several times, then a response becomes automatically initiated next time that stimulus occurs. For example, a horse will learn to move away from the handler when a hand is placed against its side. Eventually, this will be done automatically and without conscious will.

Endocrine system (hormonal system)

The endocrine system is a much slower messenger system than the nervous system. This system controls the horse's behaviour patterns and it sends chemical messages in the form of hormones to specific organs in the horse's body (see Figure 11.2).

The word hormone is derived from the Greek *hormon* which means to arouse activity or stir up. Hormones are produced in special glands known as endocrine glands. The most important endocrine glands in the horse are:

- the ovaries
- the testes
- the adrenal glands

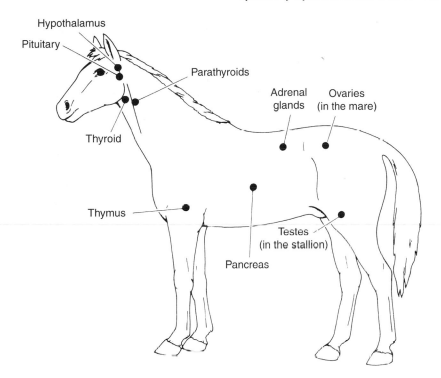

Figure 11.2. Ductless (endocrine) glands.

- the pancreas
- the pituitary gland
- the hypothalamus
- the pineal gland
- the thyroid
- the parathyroids
- the thymus.

Hormones are responsible for numerous body processes including metabolism, stress responses, growth, and sexual development and function.

The endocrine glands control many body processes including:

- puberty
- growth
- pregnancy and birth
- lactation
- aggression
- metabolism.

All endocrine glands have a good blood supply with capillaries running straight through them so that when the hormones are produced they can be released immediately into the bloodstream. Each hormone only affects certain target organs. Because hormones are carried in the blood, they are longer lasting than the quick, short-acting impulses carried by nerves. The main differences between the nervous and endocrine systems are:

- nervous messages are extremely rapid, hormonal messages are slow
- hormones reach all parts of the body via blood whereas the nerves go to specific points only
- nervous responses are mainly localised whereas a hormonal one may be widespread
- hormonal responses may continue for long periods, whereas nervous ones are short lived.

The endocrine glands

Hypothalamus

The hypothalamus is a nerve control centre at the base of the brain that is about the size of a cherry. The hypothalamus has indirect control over many of the endocrine glands including the thyroid gland, adrenal glands, the ovaries and testes. It is concerned with hunger, thirst and other autonomic functions.

Pituitary gland

The pituitary gland is sometimes referred to as the master gland as it is generally accepted to be the most important. The pituitary gland regulates and controls the operation of other endocrine glands and many of the important body processes of the horse.

The pituitary gland is about the size of a pea and hangs down from the base of the brain. It is attached to the hypothalamus by a stalk of nerve fibres. The pituitary gland consists of two lobes known as the anterior and posterior lobes. These two lobes produce a range of hormones:

The anterior pituitary produces six hormones:

- growth hormone – responsible for growth
- prolactin – stimulates milk production from the udder after birth
- adrenocorticotrophic hormone (ACTH) stimulates the adrenal glands
- thyroid-stimulating hormone (TSH) stimulates the thyroid gland
- follicle-stimulating hormone (FSH) stimulates the ovaries and testes
- luteinsing hormone (LH) stimulates the ovaries.

The posterior pituitary produces two hormones:

- antidiuretic hormone (ADH) increases resorption of water by the kidney and therefore reduces the volume of urine produced (see Chapter 10)
- oxytocin – produces contractions of the uterus during the birth of the foal and stimulates milk secretion from the udder in response to suckling from the foal.

Pituitary adenomas (tumours) otherwise known as Cushing's syndrome may be responsible for laminitis and cause a long and often curly coat even in the summer months.

Thyroid gland

This gland is situated on either side of the voice box or larynx. It consists of two lobes one on each side of the windpipe.

The thyroid is dependent on iodine. A shortage of iodine will therefore affect thyroid hormones. The thyroid gland controls metabolism and growth.

Parathyroids

These are a group of four small glands that lie behind the lobes of the thyroid gland in the horse's neck.

The parathyroids secrete parathyroid hormones that are released into the blood stream if the blood level of calcium decreases. This causes the bones to release more calcium into the blood, the gut (to absorb more calcium from food) and the kidneys to conserve calcium. These effects quickly restore the blood calcium level. If the blood calcium rises, the amount of parathyroid hormone secreted is reduced and the above effects are reversed, with the horse's body storing more calcium in bone and excreting more calcium in the urine.

Adrenal glands

These glands lie next to, and immediately above, the kidneys. Each adrenal gland is divided into two distinct regions, the adrenal cortex and the adrenal medulla. The adrenal glands produce two hormones: cortisol and adrenalin.

Cortisol helps to control inflammation and reduce the effects of shock. Adrenalin is a stimulant produced in response to stress; it increases the heart rate and blood pressure, preparing the body for fight or flight.

Pancreas

This is situated behind the horse's stomach in a loop of small intestine. The pancreas is an elongated triangular-shaped gland.

Part of the pancreas secretes the enzymes glucagon and insulin. Both insulin and glucagon are responsible for maintaining the blood glucose level within a normal range and diverting glucose to and from tissues. The pancreas also produces digestive enzymes. Horses rarely suffer from the common human condition of diabetes.

Thymus

The thymus is situated just behind the sternum between the horse's lungs. Again, it is made up of two lobes joined together in front of the windpipe.

The thymus plays a role in the immune system and it is particularly active in foals. The thymus gland is unusual in that it is active until puberty and then starts to lay down more fat and become relatively inactive. The thymus produces lymphocytes that are essential for the horse's defence system in resisting infections.

Ovaries

As well as producing eggs, the ovaries are glands and produce the female hormones progesterone and oestrogen. The oestrogens are responsible for the behavioural changes in the mare during her oestrus cycle.

Progesterone has a role in the oestrus cycle and is also responsible for maintaining pregnancy in the early days after conception.

Testes

The testes are responsible for producing the male hormone testosterone, which produces the characteristics of the male horse. Testosterone is responsible for the increased musculature of stallions because it has an anabolic effect.

Pineal gland

This is a tiny structure located within the brain itself. It is responsible for secretion of the hormone melatonin. The amount of hormone secreted varies depending on the day length as more is produced during darkness. The pineal gland is thought to affect mares in the spring: with increasing day length oestrus activity begins.

Disorders of the systems of information and control

Wobbler syndrome

This syndrome results from a narrowing of the cervical vertebrae in the horse's neck. This results in compression of the spinal cord and therefore loss of co-ordination and an abnormal gait. The horse seems to wobble and be unbalanced when walking. It is a progressive disease, but is most commonly seen in young growing Thoroughbreds, particularly colts. It can also occur in older horses of all types. It may appear suddenly, or it may become more noticeable progressively. Once symptoms occur the condition may remain static or it may deteriorate further.

This is an incurable disease and affected horses are not safe to ride.

Diagnosis is often confirmed by X-ray of the neck to see if a nerve is trapped. In the USA, surgery may be attempted to effect some improvement, but it will not cure the problem. It is thought that it may be due to nutritional imbalance in rapidly growing animals, but there may be also be a hereditary factor. Insurance companies now have a treatment protocol for wobblers that includes a drastic reduction of energy and some protein while maintaining mineral intake.

Shivering

This is a poorly understood disease, but an initial sign is that a horse will pick up a hind leg and hold it away from the body, with a slight flex.

The leg then starts to shake and normally both hind legs are affected (not simultaneously). The tail may also be held high and may quiver at the same time.

Symptoms are spasmodic and can be brought about by asking the horse to move backwards. It is commonly seen in the heavier breeds of horse, but the cause is unknown. It is a progressive condition with no known treatment.

Stringhalt

This condition is characterised by the horse hyperflexing one or both of the hocks. This is done when the horse walks and a goose-stepping action can be seen in the hind limbs. It may disappear altogether at the trot.

The condition may remain static or the horse may deteriorate further. The cause again is unknown, but horses in Australia have been found to develop stringhalt rapidly after the ingestion of plant toxins following periods of drought. These horses however usually make a full recovery.

Surgery may be attempted in some cases to remove a piece of the lateral digital extensor tendon, but in most cases the stringhalt returns. The affected horse is still able to carry on jumping, but dressage is not possible.

Laryngeal paralysis (hemiplegia)

This is more commonly referred to as roaring or whistling. This occurs as a result of damage to the nerve that supplies the muscles of the larynx on the left side. Affected horses make abnormal sounds when being exercised due to the muscle flapping within the respiratory airway. The nerve cannot be regenerated and so surgical intervention is required. This may be in the form of a hobday or tie-back operation or a tube may be inserted directly into the trachea thus bypassing the problem area. These tubes have to be kept very clean and often the surrounding tissue will reject the foreign body and another hole will have to be made. Some horses that have been tubed have gone on to perform extremely well (see page 155).

Stable vices

Stable vices are often referred to as nervous habits. The horse normally acquires them as a result of boredom or stress such as excessive confinement. It is thought that many vices such as crib-biting and windsucking have a strong hereditary factor. Weaving, crib-biting and windsucking are all vices that must be declared when a horse is for sale. It should be noted on the veterinary certificate as horses with these habits are classified as unsound.

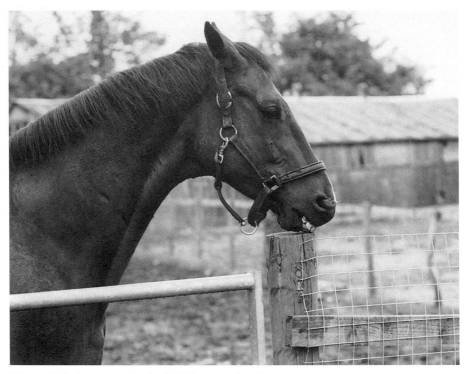

Figure 11.3. An example of crib-biting on a fencing post.

Crib-biting and windsucking

The actual causes of these problems are unknown. In crib-biting the horse grabs hold of any projecting edge, such as the stable door or fence post, with the teeth, arches the neck and gulps down air (see Figure 11.3). Wind sucking may follow on from crib-biting where the horse simply gulps down air without grabbing onto a surface.

Swallowing air leads to digestive problems and unthriftiness. Crib biters have worn front teeth or incisors. Many horses with these problems will continue even when out at grass. There are preventative collars (see Figure 11.4) that may be used with variable success, or foul-smelling substances that may be applied to surfaces to discourage the horse. A metal grille may be fixed to the door to prevent crib-biting. The most effective is probably judicious use of a muzzle and plenty of turn out in the field.

Weaving

This is often seen in racing stables where the horse swings its head from side to side over the stable door. In some cases the horse lifts each foot in turn as the forehand is thrown from the side to side, placing additional strain on the tendons and ligaments of the forelegs. Again, the exact cause is unknown, but it

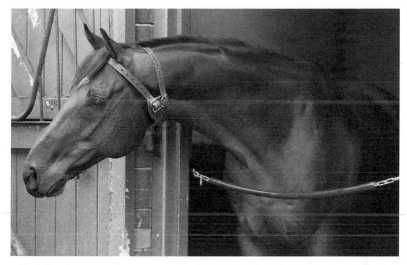

Figure 11.4. Equine mental stress may be detected by 'bad habits' such as crib-biting and windsucking.

is seen more frequently in stabled horses that are confined for long periods without turn out, such as in many racing stables.

An antiweaving grid is attached to the stable door.

The senses

It is impossible to known exactly what a horse feels, hears and sees or smells. Horses, like all mammals, have certain specialised structures that help to give them an awareness of their environment. These are essential for survival.

All mammals have sense organs responsible for sight, hearing (and balance), smell and taste. All these sense organs are extensions of the brain and are directly connected to it by nerves. These special sense organs all differ tremendously from each other in both structure and function.

The senses of the horse are:

- sight
- hearing
- taste
- smell
- touch.

Sight

The eye (see Figure 11.5) is probably the most highly developed of all the sense organs. The horse's eye is huge, one of the largest in the animal kingdom, even larger than that of the whale and the elephant. The eye of the horse also

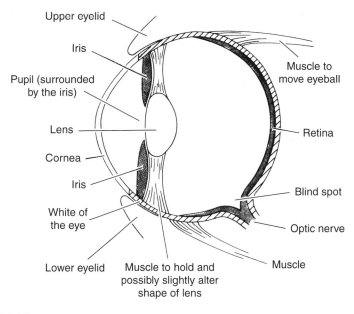

Upper eyelid

Iris

Pupil (surrounded by the iris)

Lens

Cornea

Iris

White of the eye

Lower eyelid

Muscle to hold and possibly slightly alter shape of lens

Muscle to move eyeball

Retina

Blind spot

Optic nerve

Muscle

Figure 11.5. The eye.

possesses a light-intensifying device known as the tapetum lucidum. This is a layer in the eye that reflects light back to the retina, enabling horses to see in dim light. This layer can be seen to glow in the dark (similar to cats' eyes). This points to the horse probably evolving as a nocturnal animal, being most active at dawn and dusk.

The horse has remarkable all-round vision. The eyes are set high up on the head towards the side rather than at the front. The eyes are in turn set on a long, flexible neck.

The horse's vision is mainly monocular (single eyed), seeing its surroundings as two pictures, from one each eye. It has some binocular vision directly in front of it.

The horse has two blind spots, just in front before the binocular vision starts and immediately behind its body. This is one reason why care should be taken when approaching horses from behind. Talk quietly so that the horse knows you are there.

It was previously thought that horses had a ramped retina, but now it is known that the central part of the retina gives the clearest picture. The horse moves its head in order to focus an image on this area and therefore needs to have some freedom of movement to do this when being ridden. If horses become alert to something in the distance they will stand with their heads held very high and their nose back, so that they can focus on the object of interest. Horses also have the added problem of their own muzzle obscuring the view. For this reason a horse's view is indistinct below eye level. By the time the horse is 1–1.5 metres

(4–5 ft) away from a fence it can no longer see it, most horses therefore are jumping blind from this point. Horses that race over fences are less likely to suffer from this problem because they have a longer take off distance and can see the fence before jumping.

The eyes are situated in bony sockets or orbits that are positioned in the skull for maximum protection. The orbit contains a large pad of fat that lies behind the eye and acts as a cushion if the eye should receive a blow. The horse has excellent reflexes, which is why they rarely injure their eyes.

It does take time for the eye to adapt when going from sun to shade and this may lead to nervousness when, for example, jumping into a wood.

Colour vision

Horses are not colour blind. Horses have specialised colour-detecting cells known as cones in the retinas. They seem to see yellow, orange and red best of all.

Ailments of the eye

The horse owner can easily see some conditions of the eye. However, some need specialist diagnosis from the veterinary surgeon.

Conjunctivitis. This is an inflammation of the conjunctiva. The membranes turn a deep red colour and become swollen. It is often quite painful for the horse and it may not open the affected eye fully. There is usually some yellow discharge from the eye. There are several causes of this condition including direct irritation from a foreign body such as a small piece of hay or straw, or infection. The foreign body must be removed and this can be done with the help of local anaesthetic drops that are placed in the eye. It may also be removed by washing the eye with warm saline solution (if the horse will let you).

Infections are treated with antibiotic drops or ointment. The ointment is preferred, because, although it is messier, it tends to stay in contact with the eye longer before the tears wash it away. Tears usually flush out liquid drops very quickly.

Cataract. The lens becomes less transparent and more opaque. Obviously, this affects the amount of light entering the eye that in turn affects the horse's ability to see. The degree of opacity will determine the degree of sight and some horses may become completely blind.

Cataracts may develop from birth, i.e. they are congenital. They may vary from small cloudy spots on the lens to complete opaqueness. These congenital cataracts rarely progress any further. Some horses, however, develop degenerative cataracts as a result of injury or disease. There is no effective treatment for cataracts.

Keratitis. This may develop from conjunctivitis or may result from a direct blow or injury to the cornea. The cornea contains nerve endings and is very sensitive. When an injury occurs to the cornea, the horse will usually not open the eye and tears will run down the horse's face. After the initial inflammation has subsided, a visible grey patch can be seen on the otherwise clear cornea. It is important that veterinary treatment is sought before an ulcer develops. If left the cornea may become perforated and the aqueous humour will leak from the eye causing the eventual collapse of the eyeball itself.

Hearing

Another equally important sense to the horse is that of hearing. Horses need their senses to help them survive in the wild. Being able to hear helps them to detect anyone or anything approaching.

Horses have a highly developed and sharp sense of hearing, and their sensitive ears can detect a wide range of sounds from a very low frequency to a very high one. A horse can hear sounds that are outside the human range, but, as with humans, their hearing begins to deteriorate with age.

The horse's excellent sense of hearing is helped by the highly mobile ears that can each rotate through 180° degrees and are controlled by no fewer than 16 muscles. The horse can also use its head to pinpoint the exact source of a sound.

Because the horse's sense of hearing is so acute they can become distressed when placed in a noisy environment. Horses, particularly youngstock, may become highly strung if they are kept near busy roads, railways, airports and so on.

It is well known among horse owners that windy days can turn their normally safe hack into a nightmare as the horse becomes much more nervous. This is because sounds are being carried by the wind, and the horse has far greater difficulty in pinpointing the source.

Horse owners should make as much use of the horse's excellent sense of hearing as possible, by talking quietly to them and using their voice as a training aid. Use softly spoken, simple words of command.

When moving around horses, particularly in the stable, talk to the horse so that it knows exactly where you are because, as previously mentioned, the horse has two blind spots one in front and one immediately behind the body.

Anatomy of the ear

The ear consists of three parts (see Figure 11.6):

- the outer ear
- the middle ear
- the inner ear.

The inner ear, in particular, is responsible for balance and informs the brain of the position of the head at all times.

The horse has large, mobile ears that can move independently from each other through a rotation of 180°. This enables the horse to pick up sounds from different directions without moving its body.

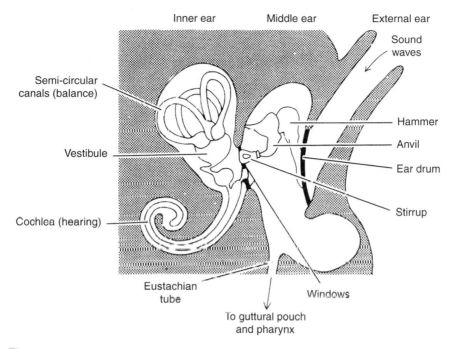

Figure 11.6. The ear.

Most horse owners are familiar with the outer ear or the visible part of the ear. The middle ear is separated from the outer ear by the tympanic membrane of eardrum, which is connected to three small bones with 'horsy' names, known (from outside in) as the malleus (hammer), incus (anvil) and stapes (stirrup). These little bones provide a mechanical link with the eardrum.

The horse is unique in that it has two large sacs connected to each of the two Eustachian tubes (one for each ear) and these are known as the guttural pouches. They are situated between the pharynx and the skull and have a capacity of about 300 ml. The guttural pouches lie very close to important nerves and arteries. There is a condition known as guttural pouch mycosis (caused by a fungus) that can be life-threatening if the vital nerves and blood vessels become affected.

The inner ear consists of a series of membranous tubes (labyrinth) that are filled with fluid. This performs two functions: that of hearing and that of balance and orientation.

Horses also use their ears to give visual signals to other horses and humans. The position of the ears can give us clues as to the mood of the horse. Pricked ears are typical of horses that are alert, interested or startled. If the ears are pinned flat back, then this is a threat signal. In the wild the pinning back of the ears was a protective measure in the case of attack by a predator. If the ears are pinned back they are less likely to be torn or damaged.

Ailments of the ear

Ear mites. Ear mites occur in horses and more often than not do not produce any clinical signs of infestation. However, in some horses these mites may be responsible for severe irritation that may cause head shaking. Ear mites may be removed by treating the horse with antiparasitic drugs.

Swollen parotid gland. The parotid gland is one of the salivary glands and is therefore responsible for the production of saliva. It is situated at the base of the outer ear (pinna) and it may become swollen. This particularly affects horses and ponies that are out at grass grazing. The cause of the swelling is not known, but it usually subsides by itself when the horse is taken off the grass.

Bleeding from the ear. This must be taken very seriously as it usually is the result of a skull fracture. It may also be caused by guttural pouch mycosis as discussed elsewhere.

Taste and smell

The senses of taste and smell are very closely linked in horses, so much so that they are often thought to be inseparable. Many horses are renowned for being fussy feeders.

Taste

Taste sensations are produced from minute raised areas on the tongue called papillae. The taste buds are situated on the surface of these papillae. The highest concentration of taste cells is situated at the back of the tongue.

Taste stimuli also increase gastric secretions in the stomach.

Taste is an important factor in the ability of horses to select their food, particularly if they are deficient in some nutrient. It has been proved scientifically in other animals that if they are mineral deficient, they will select foods high in that mineral (if it is available to them). This ability to correct dietary deficiencies is lost if the sensory nerves to the taste buds are cut. We know it is particularly true where salt is concerned, so a salt lick should always be made available to horses.

Although it is known that in humans that four specific tastes occur – sweet, salt, bitter and sour (acid) – there are considerable differences between species in tests. For example, it has been shown that while cats hate sugars and will avoid them, horses have shown a definite sweet tooth hence their preference for sweet feed or molassed mixtures. It has also been shown that horses cannot distinguish between pure water and highly concentrated sucrose (sugar) solutions.

Taste can vary considerably within a species, so different horses will show individual preferences to the same taste. It is thought that this has a genetic basis.

Smell

The sense of smell is commonly associated with seeking and selecting food and water, and is also a communication system within groups of horses.

Horses in the wild needed to be able to smell the presence of predators so they could make their escape.

The sense of smell is also important in horses for their reproductive patterns and social behaviour.

All horses have the ability to hold up their noses and curl the upper lip in a gesture, which is known as Flehmen. This is often seen when horses are presented with a strange or strong smell, but it is most often seen in stallions in their courtship activity with mares that are in oestrus.

Horses also use their sense of smell to smell droppings on the pasture or on a patch of grass that has been staled by another horse. Stallions or geldings showing stallion-like behaviour will then dung on top of these smells to mark the territory as their own.

When new horses are introduced to a group, they will blow air into the others' noses and a process of recognition or otherwise will be seen.

Mares rely on their sense of smell to bond with their foals. As soon as the foal is born the mare will lick and smell the foal. If she loses her foal and is given an orphan to foster then the orphan is usually covered in the dead foal's skin so that the mare recognises it has her own.

As a sense of smell is so important to horses, they should be encouraged to use it when settling into new pastures or yards. Lead them around their new home and let them have a good smell. This will help them to settle sooner.

Try not to keep moving horses from one stable to another and try to find a yard where they have a low turnover of horses, so that the horse has time to bond and make friends with other horses and its own environment.

Chapter 12
The circulatory system

All large animals need a system to supply all their cells with food, oxygen and other materials. The main transport system of the mammal is the circulatory system (Figure 12.1), sometimes known as the vascular system. This carries blood out from the horse's heart to all the body cells before returning it back to the heart.

The circulation of the blood has two distinct parts:

- pulmonary – carries blood from the heart to the lungs to pick up oxygen and back again
- systemic – carries oxygenated blood around the rest of the body and back again.

The circulatory system consists of a four-chambered pump, the heart, and a system of tubes, the blood vessels, which circulate the transport medium, the blood. As a general rule, the vessels, which carry blood away from the

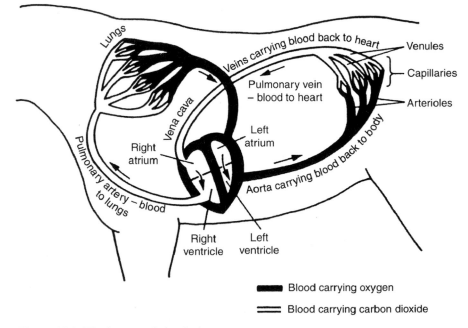

Figure 12.1. The heart and circulation.

heart, are known as arteries, whereas the vessels that carry blood back to the heart, are known as veins. In addition, there is a system of vessels that carry lymph or tissue fluids to the large veins, and these are known as lymph vessels.

The heart

This is central to the circulatory system, and is basically a large muscular pump that has the ability to contract and send blood through the network of vessels that supply the tissues of the horse's body.

The heart of a 16 hand's high horse would weigh approximately 4 kg (9 lb). As the horse gets fitter, the heart size may increase to over 5 kg. A large heart has been associated with great racehorses such as Eclipse and Pharlap.

The heart is surrounded by a sac known as the pericardium or pericardial sac. This is a completely closed sac, which contains a small amount of fluid for lubrication.

The heart is divided into four hollow chambers. The right-hand side is separate from the left-hand side, so that blood does not mix between the two. The right-hand side of the heart is responsible for moving blood that has had most of its oxygen removed as it travelled around the horse's body. Veins carry this deoxygenated blood, via the body's largest vein the vena cava, to the right side of the heart into the auricle or atrium. Once full the right auricle contracts and blood is pushed into the more muscular right ventricle. The tricuspid valve snaps shut to prevent any backflow of blood. This is the first noise of the heart sounds that can be heard using a stethoscope, the 'lub' part of the characteristic 'lub-dub'. The right ventricle then contracts, pushing blood into the pulmonary artery that takes blood to the lungs.

It is important to note that the pulmonary artery and vein are the exception to the general rule that arteries carry oxygenated blood and veins carry deoxygenated blood. The pulmonary artery carries deoxygenated blood to the lungs and the pulmonary vein carries oxygenated blood from the lungs to the heart.

Once in the lungs, the blood comes into close contact with the alveoli and the carbon dioxide it carries is exchanged for oxygen by a process known as gaseous exchange. The newly oxygenated or arterial blood then returns to the heart via the pulmonary vein to the left auricle.

The left ventricle has the thickest muscular wall of any of the four heart chambers. This is necessary because blood from the left ventricle is forced at great pressure into the aorta, which is the largest artery in the body. Blood from the left ventricle has to travel a greater distance to all parts of the horse's body and not just the lungs, hence the thicker muscular wall.

Valves at the entrance of the aorta, known as semi-lunar valves, prevent backflow and lead to the second sound of the heart beat, the 'dub' part of lub-dub.

The heartbeat therefore has four phases involving the filling and contraction of each of its four chambers, however because the auricles and ventricles empty almost simultaneously, often only two phases can be heard on an ordinary stethoscope. All four may be heard when the resting heart rate is low.

Regulation of the heartbeat

The heart is essentially a self-contained organ that can carry on working without the direct intervention of the voluntary or involuntary nervous system. This explains why isolated hearts can continue to beat for a long time if kept in the correct environment. The heartbeat is the regular contraction of the heart muscle to pump blood around the horse's body. The sequence is called the cardiac cycle and has two phases:

- systole: heart muscle contracts
- diastole: heart muscle relaxes.

The heart does have a nervous supply, but it is not responsible for starting the heartbeat. Its role is to modify the rate and force of contraction of the heart according to the needs of the horse at the time.

Blood vessels

Arteries

Blood is carried from the heart to the tissues of the body in vessels known as arteries. If an artery is cut, bright red blood will spurt from the wound in time with the heartbeat.

These arteries gradually decrease in size and form branches as they become further away from the heart. This leads to a reduction in blood pressure as blood moves into the tissues.

The larger vessels give rise to smaller ones that have smooth muscle in their walls. These are known as arterioles. Because they are able to contract, they can regulate blood flow to various organs within the horse's body. The arterioles then supply the capillaries with blood. These are very thin-walled vessels having walls of only one cell thickness. Here the blood gives up its oxygen, nutrients and hormones and collects waste products such as carbon dioxide. The capillaries then converge to form very small veins or venules and then progressively larger veins.

Veins

Veins have a similar structure to that of arteries, but the walls are much thinner and the proportion of muscular tissue is less. The larger veins contain valves to prevent the backflow of blood. Muscular contractions of the horse's body helps to keep blood moving towards the heart. This can explain why horses often develop filled legs when standing in a stable for a long time. This forced inactivity inhibits the venous return to the heart and once the horse starts walking again the swelling will often disappear. Eventually venous blood will enter the great veins or vena cava and be returned to the right auricle of the heart.

If a vein is cut, dark red blood will trickle from the wound.

The horse's normal resting heartbeat is 36–42 beats per minute. This can be measured using a stethoscope or by feeling for the pulse where an artery passes over bone, for example, under the jaw.

When the horse is exercised, the demand or oxygen increases so that it can produce the energy required for contracting muscles and motion. In order to transport this oxygen to the cells that require it, the heart has to beat faster to pump the blood to the tissues. The heart of a galloping horse can reach rates of up to 240 beats per minute. With this heart rate it only takes 5 seconds for a red blood cell to go around the entire body. Compare this to humans whose resting heart rate is about 60 beats per minute, rising to a maximum of only about 180.

Heart abnormalities in horses

Unlike humans, horses seldom die from heart disease. However, certain abnormalities of the equine heart tend to be quite common. It has been suggested that approximately 50% of all horses have a heart that makes some odd noise or beats rather unevenly, but most of these horses seem to perform quite well.

Heart abnormalities in horses tend to be placed into one of two types: arrhythmias (unevenness of beat) and murmurs (unusual noises).

Arrhythmias

Arrhythmias tend to be more likely to upset the horse's athletic performance than heart murmurs. Arrhythmias may be detected with a stethoscope, but more often using an electrocardiogram to record the electrical activity of the heart muscle cells.

Perhaps the most common arrhythmia is the dropped beat, i.e. just a 'lub' is heard instead of the normal 'lub-dub'. This is fairly common phenomenon in fit horses at rest and when these horses work the normal heart rhythm kicks into play. This is probably why most veterinary surgeons attach little significance to this condition.

Atrial fibrillation is a more serious arrhythmia. The atria or auricles empty themselves by a series of flutters that fail to stimulate the ventricles properly. These then contract infrequently. This condition will produce a sudden drop in the horse's athletic performance. It is essential that the horse is given veterinary treatment in the form of drugs and rested until the heartbeat returns to normal. This condition is also frequently seen in stressed humans. It is possible that stress may also be involved in horses, but other known causes include infections such as strangles, influenza and herpes. These infections can produce inflammation of the heart muscle itself and this is known as myocarditis.

Murmurs

Murmurs are without doubt the most common heart abnormality in horses and they are often found during routine veterinary examinations, for example, during the pre-purchase examination. Again, these murmurs can be found using a stethoscope. A horse with a murmur will be heard to have one or more additional sounds during the normally quiet phase of the cardiac cycle. The interpretation of these abnormal sounds requires considerable expertise and experience.

Some murmurs are benign in nature, in that they have no effect on the horse's performance. Others are pathological and may severely affect the horse's health as well as performance.

Heart murmurs are a result of turbulence within the normal flow of blood through the heart. A common cause seems to be a lesion on one or more of the heart valves. Some murmurs are fairly quiet, whereas others are quite loud. A grading system has been established to describe the loudness of murmurs. The scale ranges from 1 (faint murmur) to 6 (very loud).

Once detected, it is important to have a heart murmur investigated by the vet to establish its significance on the horse's performance.

Heart monitors

Many trainers and owners of performance horses measure their horse's heart rates to monitor fitness. Obviously, it is not possible to use a stethoscope while the horse is moving. Heart monitors or cardiotachometers are now available that are able to display the cardiac cycle at a given time. They have been developed so that they can record the heartbeat at fast speed for playback later. These machines are small and portable. Electrodes are placed in contact with the horse's skin and the machine is attached to the rider by a belt or is strapped to the horse's neck or saddle.

These heart monitors give a basic electrocardiograph (ECG) reading and can be very useful indeed in the training process. The readings from an ECG can be used to measure heart rate, rhythm and changes in conduction of impulses where heart problems are suspected.

Blood

The blood is the body's transport system and it consists of a fluid called plasma, in which are suspended red cells, white cells and platelets. It carries gases, nutrients, hormones and salts in solution and acts as a communication system reaching the whole body. A summary of blood's constituents is shown in Figure 12.2.

Blood consists of:

- plasma
- blood cells: red cells (erythrocytes) and white cells (leucocytes)
- platelets.

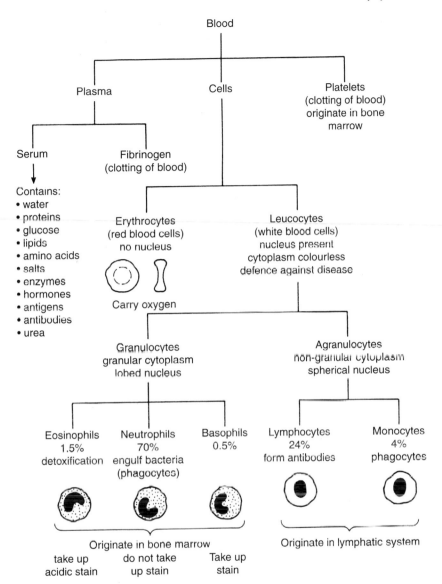

Figure 12.2. Summary of the constituents of blood.

Plasma

Plasma is composed mainly of water (about 90%), with many substances dissolved in it such as glucose, amino acids, hormones, salts, plasma proteins and antibodies. Plasma is often referred to as the 'internal environment' that bathes all the cells of the body.

Blood cells

The blood contains two types of cells:

- red blood cells (erthrocytes)
- white blood cells (leucocytes) – different types include granulocytes and agranulocytes.

Red blood cells

Red blood cells are button-shaped cells containing a red pigment, haemoglobin, that mostly carries oxygen and some carbon dioxide around the body. They do not have a nucleus and are smaller than white blood cells. Because they do not have a nucleus, they have a limited life span of about 3–4 months. Red blood cells are made in the red bone marrow.

White blood cells

White blood cells are larger than red blood cells and mostly are involved in fighting disease and infection. White blood cells are made in the bone marrow and lymph nodes. There are several types of white cell that respond to different disease challenges.

Most of the white cells contain tiny grains in their cytoplasm and these are called granulocytes.

There are three types of granulocytes:

- neutrophils: 70% of white blood cells – engulf and clean up invaders
- eosinophils: 2% of white blood cells – detoxification of foreign proteins
- basophils: quite rare – involved in inflammatory response.

Other white cells are known as agranulocytes and show few grains or granules in their cytoplasm. These include:

- monocytes: engulf and clean up invaders
- lymphocytes: produces antibodies.

Platelets

Platelets are tiny fragments of cells that are involved in the blood clotting process.

Blood tests

Many horses are routinely blood tested. Blood testing will provide answers to some questions, but not all: results will depend on which analytical tests are carried out. A list of the various tests is given in Table 12.1.

The horse's blood changes quickly in response to disease, fluid balance changes, fitness and stress.

Table 12.1. Haematology and plasma biochemistry tests

Blood test	Function	Normal range (SI units*)
Haematology		
Red blood cells (erythrocytes)	Oxygen-carrying capacity	6.5–12.3
Haemoglobin	Low = anaemia	11.2–16.2
Haematocrit (packed cell volume)	Proportion of cells to plasma Low – unfit or disease High = electrolyte imbalance or exhaustion	0.32–0.43
Mean corpuscular volume (MCV)	Size of erthryocytes. New ones are larger than older ones High = red worm damage	36–46
Mean corpuscular haemoglobin concentration (MCHC)	A guide to the oxygen-carrying capacity of blood Low = severe anaemia	29–37
Total white blood cells	Vary in response to disease Low = viral High = bacterial infection	5–10.5
% neutrophils to total white blood cells	High shows bacterial infection	60
Neutrophilis	High = bacterial infection	Normal = 6 Range 2–7
Lymphocytes	High = chronic bacterial/viral infection	Normal = 4 Range 1–6
Monocytes	Seen in some viral infections	0–0.4
Eosinophils	Seen in allergic response and parasitic infections	0–0.3
Basophils	A sign of inflammation	0–0.1
Plasma biochemistry		
Total protein albumins	Shows nutritional status and gut function. Reflects feed quality	60–80 g/l
	High = rhabdomyolysis Low – poor liver function, poor feeding or intestinal disease	27–40 g/l
Globulins (antibodies)	Increase with infection	17–34 g/l
Plasma viscosity (PV) or erythrocyte sedimentation rate (ESR)	Measure of blood condition High = unfit or viral infection or poor performance syndrome	1.4–1.7 centipoises
Plasma fibrinogen	Chronic infection, internal parasites	0–3.0 g/l
Calcium (Ca)	Vital for bone health and muscular function. Low Ca may be due to stress, laminitis of muscular problems	2.6–3.9 mmol/l
Phosphorus (P)	Bone health	0.8–1.8 mmol/l
Ca:P ratio	Phosphorus should be lower than calcium	3:1
Urea	High = kidney problems	3.5–7.3 mmol/l
Bilirubin	Bile salt	10–40 mmol/l
Enzymes – body function tests		
Aspartate aminotransferase (AST/SGOT)	High = rhabdomyolysis, liver problems	0–250 u/l
Creatine kinase (CK/CPK)	Muscle enzyme – rises with muscle breakdown, tying up	0–100 mmol/l

*Measured in standard SI units.

Early signs of problems may show up in the blood before physical symptoms appear in the horse. This gives the owner time to rest or delay work with the horse until recovery has taken place.

Each horse is unique and will have an individual blood picture. Taking regular blood tests from the same horse will therefore allow a normal profile for that horse to be ascertained. This information can be kept with the health record of that horse.

Blood tests should be taken when the horse is completely rested, preferably first thing in the morning.

Blood tests fit into one of two categories:

* haematology (study of cells within the blood plasma)
* biochemistry (soluble chemicals dissolved in the plasma).

A thorough, full haematology and biochemical profile would involve endless tests and would be prohibitive financially, so most veterinary practices and laboratories will select a series of tests in the expectation that these will produce the information required.

Haematology

Haematology provides the basis for fitness tests and this is often known as the haemogram. This includes:

* haemoglobin
* packed cell volume
* red blood cell count (erythrocytes)
* mean corpuscular haemoglobin content
* mean corpuscular volume
* white cell count (leucocytes)
* erythrocyte sedimentation rate or blood thickness.

Haemoglobin (Hb)

This simply measures the amount of haemoglobin in the sample. Haemoglobin is important for carrying vital oxygen to the tissues and, most importantly, the muscles.

Packed cell volume (PCV)

This is measured by placing a sample of blood in a centrifuge. Spinning the sample separates the blood cells to the bottom and the plasma to the top. From this a reading of the proportion of cells to plasma can be obtained. The levels tend to be higher in stressed horses or those suffering from exhaustion and/or electrolyte imbalances. Excited horses will also show higher levels, so horses must be kept calm when sampling is undertaken. Unfit horses tend to have a lower PCV result.

Red blood cell count (RBC)

Red blood cells, otherwise known as erythrocytes, are measured by electronic cell counters. Low RBC may indicate anaemia. RBC and Hb are important indicators of a horse's fitness.

Mean corpuscular haemoglobin content (MCHC)

This is a combination of RBC and Hb and is normally stable. The results are lower in horses that are stressed or anaemic.

Mean corpuscular volume (MCV)

This is a combination of RBC and PCV: it gives the average size of the red blood cells. Interestingly enough, these are smaller in horses than humans. With horses, red blood cells have a lifetime of about 140 days compared with 40 days in humans. Newly produced red blood cells are larger and more efficient than older ones.

An increase in the MCV result indicates an increased turnover in red blood cells, often seen in red worm infestation, internal/external bleeding and ulcers among other problems. This may rise in stressed horses.

White blood cells or leucocytes (WBC)

Again, this is measured by electronic cell counters. White blood cells are important for defence against disease. A normal result indicates the horse is not fighting any infections. A low result may be seen in early stages of viral challenges and high levels in bacterial infections.

Erythrocyte sedimentation rate (ESR) or blood thickness

For accuracy, this test must be carried out within a few hours of sampling. A high result may be seen in unfit horses and in horses suffering from viral infection or poor performance syndrome. This may be post-viral.

Biochemistry

There are several biochemical tests available, and those discussed below are probably the most common:

- serum proteins: albumens and globulins
- plasma electrolytes
- enzymes – aspartate aminotransferase/serum glutamic-oxaloacetic transaminase (AST/SGOT), creatine phosphokinase (CPK), gamma-glutamyl-transferase (gamma GT).

Serum proteins

Albumens and globulins are dissolved within the plasma. High readings may indicate high levels of nutrition or overfeeding whereas low readings may show poor nutrition, ulcers, reduced liver function or parasitism in the gut (worms).

Globulins tend to rise in response to disease challenges to help the horse's body fight infection.

Plasma electrolytes

These are important substances dissolved in the blood, such as calcium, phosphorus, sodium, potassium, chloride and bicarbonate. Fluid imbalances can be a response to exhaustion following racing in hot environments. Horses lose tremendous amounts of sweat when they work hard and these body salts have to be replaced usually through electrolyte preparations. Racehorses on low forage rations are more likely to suffer from electrolyte problems.

Plasma enzymes

These are vital and mainly involved in the metabolism. Increased levels in the blood normally indicate problems with these enzymes in certain tissues, for example, the muscle or liver tissue.

AST/SGOT. These enzymes are found in all tissues, but especially in muscles. Very high readings are seen in rhabdomyolysis (tying up). High readings may indicate liver problems.

CPK. This enzyme also increases dramatically with tying up and may also be seen in horses with heart problems or in respiratory distress.

Gamma GT. An enzyme found in the liver. Increased readings follow increased training, but can be too high when horses are overtrained or stressed.

Disorders of the circulatory system

These include:

- anaemia
- dehydration
- heat stroke and exhaustion.

Anaemia

Anaemia is a symptom of a disease but also a condition of the blood, so it is important to find the cause before treatment.

Causes include:

- bleeding, external or internal
- nutritional deficiency; iron, cobalt or copper deficiency
- overtraining/stress may lead to reduced red cell production
- worms.

Signs include:

- pale mucous membranes
- pale conjuctiva
- weakness

- lethargy and depression
- poor coat.

Treatment will depend on the original cause and may include nutritional tonics including folic acid, vitamin B_{12} and copper.

Dehydration

Horses sweat freely and are very susceptible to dehydration. Dehydration may also follow diarrhoea (see Chapter 17).

Dehydration may be assessed by a pinch test or a biochemical blood test.

The pinch test involves pinching a fold of skin on the horse's neck and seeing how long it takes to return to normal.

Symptoms

A fold of skin pinched up will be slow to flatten out. After exercise, the horse is slow to recover its normal pulse and respiration rate. It is dull and lethargic. Prolonged stress such as a long journey or an endurance ride in hot weather can produce an audible diaphragm spasm ('the thumps'). This is a serious condition, the horse being near collapse, and it requires urgent veterinary attention.

Causes

Causes can be a shortage of water, from the horse not drinking enough, or a loss of fluid through scouring or excessive sweating from exertion, travel in a confined space or fever.

Treatment

Ensure that the horse has access to water at all times. Check that the water is pleasant for the horse. Salt in feed may encourage it to drink more. The cause of any scouring or looseness in the droppings must be treated.

Performance horses that will be competing in hot weather and sweating heavily should be given electrolytes at the recommended rate immediately before, during and after competition. Electrolytes are sometimes given during endurance rides by syringing concentrated electrolyte solution into the horse's mouth, but this must never be done before the horse has started to drink well, or it will cause fluid to be drawn into the stomach from the tissues and dehydrate the horse even more.

When dehydration is due to lack of available water or after exercise, the horse should be allowed to drink small quantities of water (no more than half a bucket) every 10 minutes until thirst is quenched. Once the horse has started to drink, electrolytes can be offered dissolved in water to replace the body salts that have been lost. In severe cases, however, the horse may be given electrolytes intravenously so that the body is rehydrated as quickly as possible.

Heatstroke and exhaustion

Prolonged exercise undertaken in hot and humid conditions will result in heat stroke or exhaustion. This occurs when the internal body temperature reaches 43°C (109.5°F). Heart and respiratory rates fail to return to normal and irregularities in heartbeat may be detected.

These horses must stop exercise immediately and be placed in a cool box, or shade and cold hosed. If the horse will drink, small amounts of water should be offered. Severe cases will need veterinary treatment of intravenous fluids and electrolytes.

Chapter 13
The respiratory system

The main task of this system is to get oxygen into the blood. Without oxygen, all heat production and activity will cease. If the respiratory system falters, the horse will die within a few minutes. Of the horse's three major requirements, food, water and oxygen, the latter is the most crucial in the shortest time. A horse can go several days without water; it can go weeks without food; but death will occur if it is deprived of oxygen for a matter of minutes.

The functions of the respiratory system include:

- provision of oxygen to the body
- removal of carbon dioxide from the body
- temperature control (breathing out warm air, taking in cool air)
- removal of water
- communication (through the vocal cords)
- sense of smell and touch (sensory hairs on the nose)
- filter out airborne invaders.

Air passages and the lungs

Head

Oxygen is taken down into the lungs along a highly specialised route. The extremity of this route consists of the nostrils, which are large, soft, gentle and inquisitive. They change in shape according to the horse's needs. The horse draws air in only through the nostrils and not the mouth. They are easily dilated and form part of the horse's facial expression, showing when it is inquisitive or angry. Facial expressions are backed up by air blown from the nostrils and expelled as a blow or a snort. The hairs between and below the nostrils combine with the animal's sense of smell to investigate strange objects at close range. The airways in the head are shown in Figure 13.1.

The nasal cavities – one for each nostril – are divided from each other by a piece of cartilage. They are separated from the mouth by the hard palate and, higher up, by the soft palate. The cavity is partially filled with wafer-thin, curling bones, called the turbinate bones, designed to have a large surface area. This, like the rest of the cavity, is covered by mucous membrane that helps to warm incoming air so that it is not too cold on reaching the lungs. In warming

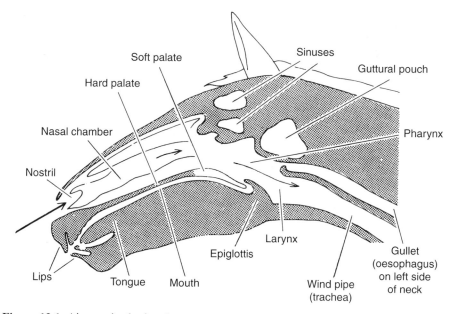

Figure 13.1. Airways in the head.

the air in this way, the body loses heat when the air is expelled. This membrane, in the higher part of the cavity, contains the olfactory nerve endings to detect smells.

In the skull at the front are air-filled cavities called sinuses, connecting with the nasal cavity. The maxillary sinus is above the molar teeth, and the others are called the frontal, the sphenopalatine and the ethmoidal sinuses. All exist in pairs, one on each side, and they give the skull strength and form, without excessive weight.

The pharynx or throat is the common passage for food and air, each coming from a different place and going down a different tube, with a crossover mechanism which shoots the food to be swallowed up and over the windpipe and into the gullet. When stomach-tubing a horse, it is necessary to pass the tube up the nostril because of the arrangement of the pharynx. Care must be taken to ensure that the tube goes down the gullet and not down the windpipe.

The Eustachian tubes come into the top of the pharynx. They allow air to pass to the middle ear, and connected to them are the guttural pouches sited just above the pharynx.

Within the neck

Air passes from the pharynx through the larynx, the organ producing the voice. It is a box of jointed cartilage and the surrounding muscles can alter its calibre. The function of the larynx is to control the air going in and out, monitoring it for foreign objects that must be rejected. It is sited in the throat between the branches of the lower jaw, where it may be readily felt. Food and water pass over its opening (the glottis) on the way down the gullet, and it has a lid (the epiglottis) which closes automatically when the horse swallows. Problems with the glottis or epiglottis may cause coughing.

These organs and the vocal cords (which are thick and elastic) produce the horse's sounds of communication or voice. The larynx is thus commonly called the 'voice-box'. The horse can squeal, nicker, whinny and groan. The muscles that retract or draw back these cartilages are controlled by a branch of the vagus nerve which, curiously, is much longer on the left than on the right side. This nerve sometimes malfunctions so as to give wind problems, which are often confined to the left side of the larynx. Despite the larynx's function as a filter, some dust is inhaled by the horse, particularly when eating dry hay or when straw is shaken up when bedding down.

The windpipe (trachea) runs from the larynx to the lungs. It runs along the lower border of the neck and can easily be felt as far down as the entrance to the chest. It is a tube reinforced with rings of cartilage with overlapping ends. The lining of the trachea produces sticky mucus to trap any foreign particles that may enter the tube. The particles are wafted up the trachea to the larynx by a carpet of microscopic hairs called cilia. The mucus is then coughed up and swallowed.

Within the chest

The windpipe divides into two bronchi at the entrance to the chest, one branch going to each lung. From this point they divide and subdivide into bronchioles, which end as alveolar sacs. These in turn are subdivided into many tiny alveoli – like grapes in a bunch – in order to give a maximum surface area (see Figure 13.2).

The surfaces of the bronchi and bronchioles are protected by mucus and cilia. The bronchioles have fine muscle fibres in their structure enabling the diameter to be changed.

The lungs are two large, elastic organs. The horse's right lung has an extra lobe, but the shape of the lungs is not important as they completely fill the cavity of the chest (except for the cavity occupied by the heart) below the backbone and are enclosed by the ribs and the diaphragm. The lungs are surrounded by a covering (the pleura), which is a smooth and slippery membrane that prevents friction.

The pulmonary artery brings blood to the lungs from the heart. This blood is described as deoxygenated as it has given up oxygen deep in the tissues of the horse so that normal body processes can take place. In return, the blood carries away a by-product of these processes, carbon dioxide. See Chapter 12 for a fuller description of the pulmonary system.

The diaphragm separates the chest from the belly. It is a strong and thin sheet of muscle attached to the inner sides of the ribs. It begins just in front of the loins, high under the backbone, sloping downwards and forwards to the breast bone. The major blood vessels and gullet go through it as they come from the chest, and like the lungs (which it touches) it is covered with pleura.

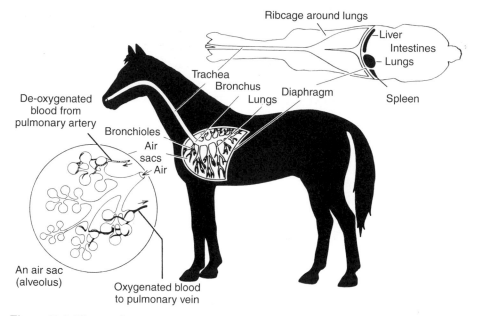

Figure 13.2. The respiratory system.

Breathing

Breathing is taking the air down into the lungs so that gaseous exchange with blood is possible. It is one aspect of respiration. The second aspect is the activity in the body tissues where the oxygen is used.

The horse draws in air through its nostrils. The pair passes through the larynx, down the windpipe and into the lungs. There, air and blood exchange the required elements and, after a slight pause, the used air is expelled. The process is repeated.

Air is dawn into the lungs by muscular expansion of the thorax or rib cage, and is expelled by elastic recoil of the rib cage. In the horse the rib cage is a single cavity whereas in many animals it is divided into two, with a separate lung in each. It is surrounded by ribs and separated from the abdomen by the diaphragm, which is dome shaped, with the top of the dome nearest the front of the horse. When the diaphragm muscles contract, the dome is pulled flatter and this increases the size of the chest cavity. This diaphragm activity is important for deeper breathing. However, if the stomach and intestines are full, the movement of the diaphragm is impeded. This is why a racehorse has little hay and only a small feed on the morning of a race day.

When the horse is relaxed and at rest, the amount of air taken into the lungs is about one-fifth of the amount taken in when the horse is at full exertion. At rest, the horse has a respiratory rate of 8–16 breaths a minute, the rate being higher for younger stock. After prolonged rapid exertion, this rate may be increased to 120 breaths a minute. Other factors that will cause an increase in the respiration rate include excitement, high altitude, high ambient temperature, high humidity and obesity. The lungs never empty totally, but take in and expel more air when the horse is exerted.

The rate of breathing is linked to the horse's gait. At gallop the stride rate equals the respiration rate. This means the muscles of breathing and movement do not work against each other. As the galloping horse lifts its legs, the head is raised, the gut moves back and it breathes in. As the horse lands, the head drops, the gut moves forward and it breathes out (see Figure 13.3).

Healthy breathing

Signs of healthy breathing are:

- quiet, relaxed breathing in regular rhythmic fashion
- nostrils relaxed and clean (although there may be some clear fluid)
- no abnormal sounds such as coughing or wheezing.

Breathing problems

Signs of breathing problems are:

- coughing or abnormal sound at rest
- increased breathing rate or laboured breathing at rest
- irregular breathing
- reduced exercise tolerance
- prolonged recovery rate after exercise.

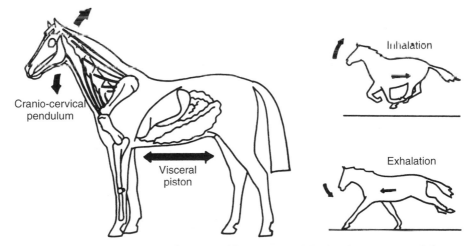

Figure 13.3. Synchronisation of stride and breathing. As the head moves up and the gut back, the horse breathes in, the head moves down as the horse lands, the gut moves forwards and the horse breathes out.

Disorders of the respiratory system

Respiratory disease

Respiratory disease falls into three main categories: infection, inflammation and allergy.

Infection

Many horses travel widely to competitions and mix with other horses making them particularly vulnerable to viral infection. A horse will recover from a simple, uncomplicated viral infection in about a week. However, the virus will have damaged the cells lining the airways making the horse much more susceptible to a secondary bacterial infection, which may take much longer to clear up and cause further damage to the lining of the airways. These infections are often described as chills or colds and the vet will refer to them as upper respiratory tract (URT) diseases.

Inflammation

A condition known as small airway disease is associated with local inflammation. This may follow infection, irritation or allergy. Inflammation leads to a swelling of the lining of the airways so that the internal diameter is reduced, making breathing less efficient.

Allergy

Blood cells attracted by the inflammation may meet fungal spores that have been inhaled by horses being fed mouldy hay. This causes the muscle of the airways to go into spasm, thus reducing the diameter even further. Dead cells and mucus from the inflammatory reaction accumulate, physically blocking the air flow. Once the mucous linings of the small airways of the lungs have been damaged they may become 'sensitised' to environmental influences, to which they develop an allergy. This is called chronic obstructive pulmonary disease (COPD). Horses can become allergic to the fungal spores found in hay, while some horses may be allergic to pollens, causing a hay-fever-type condition.

Respiratory disease is usually progressive; horses rarely develop COPD overnight. There is a build-up of stress on the respiratory system, infection, poor environment and exercise all contributing to inflammation and damage until the lung becomes hypersensitive and COPD results.

Signs of respiratory disease

Increased respiration rate, the effort made in breathing out or on expiration, becomes more noticeable, and in severe cases the horse will develop a 'heave line' – the muscles of the abdomen involved with breathing out become enlarged and the horse can be seen making an additional exhalatory effort. There may be an abnormal discharge from the nose and/or eyes; in the early stages of a viral infection this will be watery, but becomes thick and purulent, indicating a secondary bacterial infection. The early stages of a viral infection usually cause a sharp rise in body temperature [normally 38°C (100.5°F)], but this is often very short lived and is easily overlooked. Where high performance is essential, temperature should be taken routinely morning and evening. The horse may go off its feed for a few days and this usually coincides with the fever. A cough will develop – this may be an occasional cough in the stable, becoming more severe during and after exercise. All of these factors will combine to stop the horse working as efficiently: indeed, the first thing the rider or trainer notices may be the fact that the horse seems 'not himself'. Temperature-taking may indicate a problem before the horse shows any clinical signs.

Treatment of respiratory disease

There is no single cure for respiratory disease, but all of the following have an important role to play.

Rest
In the acute stage it is important to allow the horse complete rest. Fresh air is necessary but draughts, cold winds and rain should be avoided.

Antibiotics
The bacterial infection that moves into the cells damaged by the viral infection can be readily and effectively treated with antibiotics.

Getting rid of the mucus
In respiratory disease the cilia that waft away the mucus are reduced in number, and more mucus is produced which is more viscous than usual. If a cough suppressant is used the horse stops coughing and large particles of debris will be left in the airways to cause damage. In the early stages it is better to give the horse a mucolytic agent that helps move the mucus by making it more liquid. Consequently, coughing is reduced because the horse can clear the mucus far more easily.

Relieving the bronchospasm
Horses with respiratory problems may suffer bronchospasm: the small airways contain smooth muscle, which in response to irritant substances present in the airway contract causing a narrowing of the passages. This can cause quite severe distress in the horse that will have real difficulty in taking in enough air to breathe – this is equivalent to an asthma attack in humans. The veterinary surgeon can prescribe a spasmolytic drug that acts by causing the smooth muscle to relax, opening the airways and allowing more air to pass into the lungs. This can be life threatening.

Stable management
Respiratory disease must not be allowed to progress into COPD, the environment should be as dust- and fungal-spore-free as possible. In severe cases change

to a fungal-spore-free alternative such as: haylage, good silage made for horses, barn-dried hay, alfafa, grass nuts, hydroponic grass or high-fibre cubes. Otherwise hay needs to be soaked by fully submerging it in water for 20 minutes and no longer. This is an adequate period of time for the fungal spores to swell up and be swallowed instead of inhaled.

Dust-free bedding should be used; wood shavings, although often dusty, contain few spores – let the dust settle after putting in new shavings before returning the horse to its box. Bedding should be kept scrupulously clean. Bad drainage means a damp bed – paper and peat are very prone to dampness. A damp bed produces ammonia, which irritates the lungs and paralyses the hair-like cilia that waft the mucus away from the alveoli and up the bronchial tree.

Fresh air is essential. The stable should be draught-free having air vents in the roof apex that are large enough to carry away stale air. The air inlets – half door and window – should be on more than one side, so that air movement outside will always get into the stable. Air movement around the stable should be free – buildings, hedges and trees can all obstruct air flow.

The stable should be kept as clean as possible: the dust from floor to ceiling should be vacuumed or washed away – dust, cobwebs, ledges and cracks all harbour spores. The hay fed to the rest of the horses in the yard should also be soaked – spores can be blown on the wind and the position of the muckheap and hay and straw storage must all be away from the stabling.

The horse should be turned out as much as possible, especially in acute cases of COPD, regardless of the weather and time of year – you will have to invest in a sturdy New Zealand rug.

If exposure to the allergens responsible for a horse's 'asthma attack' is unavoidable, a spasmolytic drug can be given as a liquid that can be inhaled using a mask and a nebuliser. Treatment by inhalation on 3 or 4 successive days will protect a horse for up to 3 weeks and can be given in anticipation of exposure to fungal spores if, for example, being stabled away from home.

See Chapter 5 for more information on equine influenza or flu, EHV 1–4 and lungworm.

Epistaxis or nosebleed

This is also known as exercise-induced pulmonary haemorrhage (EIPH). Horses may bleed from one or both nostrils. The source of the bleeding may be the mucous membrane of the nasal passage, throat, guttural pouches or lungs. Bleeding may occur for several reasons:

- guttural pouch infection
- damage to capillaries in the lungs following prolonged or fast exercise
- inadequate recovery time following respiratory virus
- ethmoid haematoma.

There is no reliable cure for epistaxis, although some coagulant drugs, vitamin C and antibiotics may help. Rest is essential to allow lesions to heal.

Laryngeal paralysis or hemiplegia

Common terms include whistling and roaring. This condition is caused by an obstruction in the airway causing an abnormal noise.

The left recurrent laryngeal nerve, which supplies the muscle of the left side of the larynx, degenerates. The muscles then fail to open the left side of the larynx properly causing an obstruction of the airway during fast exercise.

The condition is most common in horses over 16 hands and is usually apparent by the time the horse is 6 years old.

Symptoms include abnormal noise at canter or gallop and reduced tolerance to fast exercise.

Treatment

There is no cure for this problem. There are various options for correcting the condition:

* Hobday operation: tie-back operation to pull the paralysed side of the larynx out of the airway.
* Abductor muscle prosthesis: the paralysed muscle is replaced with a prosthesis.
* No treatment: horses are able to continue work, while making a noise. This is not the case for performance horses.

Chapter 14
The skin

The skin is the body's largest organ. Skin is a protective layer shielding the horse's body from weather and infection, and helps maintain the correct temperature.

Functions of the skin include:

- protection
- heat loss and conservation
- elimination of waste products
- camouflage
- vitamin D synthesis
- sense receptor for touch, pressure, cold heat and pain.

The thickness of the skin varies with both breed and area of the body. The skin of the Thoroughbred and Arab is thinner than that of the heavier breeds. The skin on the horse's back is thicker than on the face.

Skin colour varies due to the pigment melanin. The more melanin, the darker the skin. The skin is also a good indicator of the horse's health. Movement of the skin over the ribs shows the presence of subcutaneous fat, even in a fit horse. Similarly, a pinched-up fold of skin on the horse's neck may be an indication of dehydration, if the fold is slow to disappear.

Structure

Skin

Skin (see Figure 14.1) is the tissue forming the outer covering of the horse's body. It consists of two layers: the inner, known as the dermis, and the outer, the epidermis.

The epidermis is covered with hairs to form the coat, and it is modified at the extremities of the horse's limbs to form the hooves. It is a superficial layer that is being shed constantly in the form of scurf because, like many cells within the body, its cells are continually dying and being replaced. The scurf needs to be groomed from the body so that it does not litter the surface and impede some of the skin's other functions.

Horses in the wild do not need grooming. It is not in their nature to dash around working up a sweat. In the wild, the dead cells mix with grease, mud and

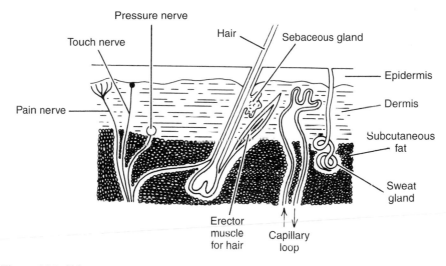

Labels on figure: Pressure nerve, Touch nerve, Hair, Sebaceous gland, Pain nerve, Epidermis, Dermis, Subcutaneous fat, Sweat gland, Erector muscle for hair, Capillary loop

Figure 14.1. Skin.

so on, and the accumulation gradually falls off. In contrast, the ridden horse is being asked for sustained activity and high performance. Regular grooming increases the power of the skin to work at high pressure as well as being an aid to cleanliness to prevent disease.

The dermis, or inner layer, of the skin is deep and sensitive. It contains blood vessels, nerve fibres, glands producing sweat and oil, and hair roots. The hairs and the tubes of the oil and sweat glands pass through the epidermis to the surface, where their openings are known as pores.

The skin is very elastic, varying in thickness according to the amount of protection required. It moves freely over the horse's flesh and should feel loose when handled. The inner layer is seated on a thin layer of subcutaneous fat.

The sweat glands lie deep in the skin, and are small, coiled tubes continuing to the surface by a thin duct through which the sweat is discharged. They are constantly working, although this will not be visible when the horse is at rest.

Hairs

Almost the whole of the horse's body is covered by hairs. They grow from the hair bulbs, set deep in the skin, and come out at an acute angle with the surface so that the coat lies flat and smooth. The skin carries several kinds of hair: permanent hair such as the long hair of the mane, tail and heel 'feathers', tactile hairs of the lips, nostrils and eyes, and the temporary hair of the coat which is shed and changed for a new growth in spring and autumn, the length of the new growth depending on the season. Hair is also shed, a little at a time, constantly throughout the year, being replaced by new growth. Each hair is lubricated by oil that exudes from a small gland at the base, and has a tiny muscle that can pull it into an upright position. The hair is part of the mechanism for stabilising body heat. Some hairs, such as the whiskers on the muzzle, are modified so as to act in a sensory capacity, rather like antennae.

The colour of the hair is due to a single pigment which, by its variation in quality and grouping, gives the colour range with which we are familiar. Ranging from grey, through chestnut to black, or almost any combination of these colours. There is no pigment in white hairs. A roan-coloured horse has a mixture of white and coloured hairs, mixed to one side of the hair. In an albino there is no pigment in either the hair or the skin: the pinkness comes from the blood inside the skin.

Protection

The colour of the skin and the coat offers protection from sunlight. The skin is not necessarily the same colour as the coat, as in the case of a grey. The albino, being devoid of pigment, is more vulnerable to exposure to sunlight and often has a lower resistance to infection. The coat also gives protection from thorns, brambles and the like. The skin is tough in its outer layer, is attached loosely and is free-moving so as to minimise the risk of its tearing. It keeps water out, and yet is able to expel excess moisture as required. This is done through the sweat glands. The subcutaneous fat under the skin acts as padding to protect the horse's body from minor bumps.

Stabilising body heat

The muscular activity of the body generates heat, which is then lost from the body by radiation and the evaporation of sweat. If the weather is hot, or there is intense muscular activity (as in galloping), the blood vessels in the skin expand to radiate more heat and to stimulate the sweat glands to greater activity. This is then noticeable as 'lathering up', particularly in Thoroughbred horses.

The skin is cooled by the action of the sweat evaporating off the skin. The hairs of the coat lie flat against the skin, so trapping the minimum amount of air and allowing the sweat to evaporate as quickly as possible. Sweat evaporates more slowly in very humid conditions and so the cooling effect is then less. Horses that have sweat dripping off them are creating sweat faster than it can evaporate; it is likely that they are not losing heat effectively as evaporation may be slow. To work a horse hard and long in hot and humid conditions creates the serious problems of overheating and dehydration, causing unacceptable distress to the horse. In extreme circumstances this can result in death.

The horse needs to conserve its body heat in cold weather and therefore the blood vessels in the skin contract. Less heat is then lost by radiation. When the horse is ill, there is often a battle between the invading germs or bacteria and the body's defences, and this leads to sweating.

The horse's coat keeps the body warm, and the oil produced by the glands under the skin's surface greases the hairs and renders the surface waterproof. In cold weather the hairs stand on end, so increasing the amount of air trapped in the coat which also grows longer, thus providing yet more protection. In hot weather the hair lies flat and is much shorter, replacing the long coat that has been shed in spring. Horses of Eastern origin, such as the Arab and the Thoroughbred, have a shorter and finer coat than British native stock.

When the horse is debilitated, the subcutaneous fat is reduced and so the horse gets cold. To cope the horse tends to make the hairs of the coat stand up or 'stare'. Want of condition, neglect or ill health will also cause the coat to look dull and feel harsh. In good health, the coat lies flat, feels quite smooth and has a good gloss.

Where a horse is clipped out, as is the hunter during the winter, the balance must be put right by the provision of rugs, blankets and food. Clothing on horses stops the hair growing as quickly by reducing the need for a warm coat.

Waste disposal

The function of eliminating waste products in solution with the sweat is particularly important for the horse under stress. Where horses sweat a lot for other reasons, it is evident that they will get rid of more salts from the body than are surplus to requirements. In such circumstances, therefore, greater care must be taken with nutrition to make good the deficit. Extreme cases of such losses of essential salts (electrolytes) may occur in 3-day eventing or long-distance riding in hot weather. On completing their activity such horses may need a solution of those salts that are required by the body.

For this aspect of the system to work efficiently, it is important that the pores in the skin be kept open. They have a tendency to become clogged with dirt and debris such as dead skin cells. The horse in work therefore requires efficient use of the body brush. This is most effective when the horse is still rather warm after exercise, as the pores are then open.

Camouflage

The horse's coat colour is a means of camouflage in its wild stage, enabling it to escape the notice of its enemies by allowing it to blend into the background. This can be seen in the wild ponies on both Exmoor and Dartmoor, where the coat colour tends to blend in with the bracken and other background foliage. The striped coat of the zebra, which is a member of the horse family, is another example of camouflage.

Synthesis of vitamin D

Vitamin D, known as the 'sunshine vitamin', occurs as two provitamins that need the ultra-violet component of sunlight acting on the skin to be converted to the vitamin. The main function of vitamin D is concerned with the body's ability to utilise calcium and phosphorus. Horses exposed rarely to the sun may run short of vitamin D. It is important to turn horses out without rugs in summer to allow vitamin D synthesis in the skin.

Disorders of the skin

These include:

- mud fever, rain scald, cracked heels
- lice
- ringworm
- sweet itch
- urticaria (nettle rash)
- warbles.

Mud fever, rain scald, cracked heels

This common problem affects horses living or being turned out in muddy conditions.

Causes. The constant wetting of the skin and irritation from mud allows infection to set in by the bacterium *Dermotophilus congolensis*.

The back of the pastern and heels are affected most and white legs seem more susceptible. The belly back and quarters may also be affected. (If the back and quarters are affected it is termed rain scald – see Figure 14.2.) Mild cases show a few, small scabby areas of skin. Without prompt attention they may develop

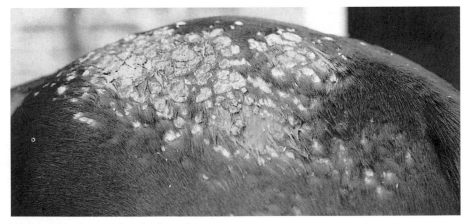

Figure 14.2. A example of rain scald.

into the more severe form with large areas of skin becoming inflamed. Serum may ooze, which mats the hair. The skin is sore and there may be swelling.

Tufts of hair can be pulled off with scabs attached to the bottom.

Occasionally, an inflamed area of hard skin will crack and cause lameness, this is known as cracked heels. Treatment may require antibiotic therapy and the cleaning and drying as below.

Treatment. Affected horses should be housed, and excess feather removed, the area should be cleaned and dried. Dilute iodine may be used followed by antibiotic topical cream. Once healed, a barrier cream may be used to protect the skin when the horse is turned out. To prevent rain scald, a New Zealand, or waterproof, rug may be used.

Lice

Symptoms. Skin irritation in the mane, neck and side of the chest, especially in spring and early summer. Scratching is a sign of lice infestation (see Figure 14.3).

Causes. Lice.

Treatment. Dust with louse powder. Check general condition and improve diet if necessary. Clean coat thoroughly.

Ringworm

Symptoms. Young horses are particularly at risk, but ringworm can affect horses of all ages. Early signs are circular tufted areas of hair, about 1–2 cm in diameter, the hair falling out to reveal scaly skin which may become infected, accompanied by the formation of pus.

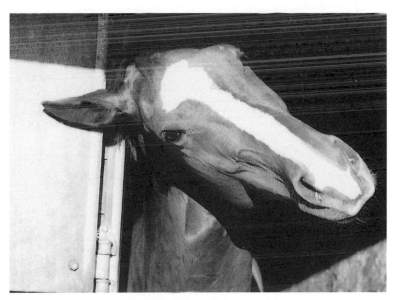

Figure 14.3. Scratching is a sign of lice infestation.

Cause. Fungal infection. Ringworm fungi are able to survive for at least a year in stables, in horse transport and on wooden fences from which horses can pick up infected hairs by rubbing themselves. Horses can also be infected by other animals, grooming kit, tack or clothing.

Treatment. The horse should be isolated, the affected area clipped with scissors to remove the hair and then treated with fungicidal dressing. An antifungal drug may also be given in the feed. Contaminated woodwork should be pressure-hosed and the horse's tack and clothing disinfected. It is advisable to take hygiene precautions such as wearing rubber gloves as ringworm may occasionally be contracted by the horse's handlers.

Sweet itch

Symptoms. The mane, back, quarters and tail look inflamed and rubbed. Sores (see Figure 14.4).

Cause. Allergic dermatitis. Midge bites cause an allergic reaction in some horses and ponies. It is found particularly in ponies, generally in spring and summer, on animals at grass. It is thought to have a genetic component.

Treatment. Stable at dawn and dusk. Keep the affected area clean. Apply the parasiticide benzyl benzote every other day. At first occurrence, get the vet to check for mange.

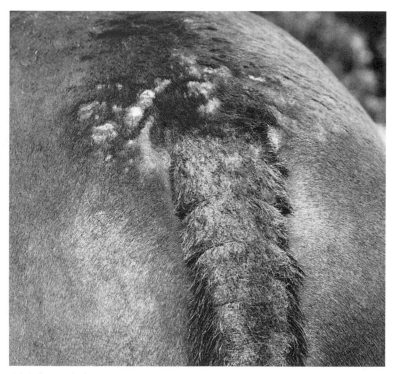

Figure 14.4. Sweet itch.

Urticaria (nettle rash)

Symptoms. Raised areas or swellings on the skin, caused by accumulation of fluid under the skin.

Cause. There are several possible causes. It may be an allergic reaction to plants, bites or stings, but it sometimes indicates an allergy to a specific protein, possibly in the diet.

Treatment. Use calamine lotion or 2 tablespoons of bicarbonate of soda in half a litre of water, applied externally. Antihistamines may be helpful. Try an exclusion diet to find the source of the allergy.

Warbles

Symptoms. Firm nodules or swellings on the back. After a fortnight or so the swellings are bigger and may have a hole in the top.

Cause. Warble-fly larvae. The fly lays its eggs on the coat, and the larvae eventually make their way to the skin, usually in spring and early summer.

Treatment. It can be dangerous to try and squeeze out the larvae. If they are squashed under the skin, for example by the saddle, a massive allergic reaction can occur. The condition is therefore best left alone. Poultices should not be used except when a grub has been squashed and an acute reaction has occurred.

Girth galls/saddle sores

These refer to sore areas developing under the girth or saddle. These are rubbing or pinching injuries that may leave a permanent scar and white hair.
Causes include:

- dirty girth with mud and sweat
- loose girth rubbing the skin
- tight girth rubbing the skin
- sensitive skin
- incorrectly fitted saddle
- overtight rollers or surcingles.

Signs include patches of rubbed skin or hair, tender, swollen areas, patches of new white hair.

Treatment

The damaged areas must be protected from further trauma or injury. The horse should be rested. If the skin is broken it must be cleaned and dried, and antiseptic ointment applied. The saddle and girth should be checked and cleaned thoroughly, if they do not fit they must be replaced.

The newly healed skin may be hardened by dabbing with surgical spirit.

Chapter 15
The digestive system

There is much confusion regarding the feeding behaviour of horses. Many domestic horses are not allowed to feed naturally, being stabled for most of the time. Some knowledge of the horse's unique digestive system is essential for the understanding of feeding horses.

The horse is a non-ruminant herbivore or hindgut fermenter. Its natural feeding pattern involves endless and varied grazing, eating small amounts often. Horses will spend up to 60% of the day grazing if allowed to do so. This is known as 'trickle' feeding and the horse's digestive tract is ideally suited to this feeding pattern.

The natural diet of horses consists of grasses and vegetation containing large amounts of substances called cellulose or hemicellulose, more commonly known as fibre. The horse is unable to digest this cellulose and requires the assistance of billions of microorganisms in its hindgut to perform this task.

The digestive tract

The function of the digestive system of the horse is to take in food, break it down and remove nutrients from it.

Nutrients are needed for:

- energy
- growth and repair of tissues
- functioning of the horse's body.

It takes approximately 65–75 hours for food to pass through the entire length of the gut. The digestive system is about 30 m (100 ft) long and is completely unique to the horse. The digestive system is shown in Figure 15.1.

The horse's digestive system tends to be referred to in two functional parts: the foregut and the hindgut (see Table 15.1).

The foregut consists of the mouth, oesophagus, stomach and small intestine. This is the area where mostly enzymic digestion occurs (i.e. enzymes are secreted into the gut to breakdown food).

The hindgut consists of the large intestine, which in turn is split into the caecum, large colon, small colon and rectum. The hindgut is the area of fermentation, where microorganisms breakdown cellulose and hemicellulose (fibre).

The gut's 30-m (100-ft) length is looped and coiled to fit into the abdominal space and there are several changes in diameter and direction. For this reason the horse's gut is prone to blockages.

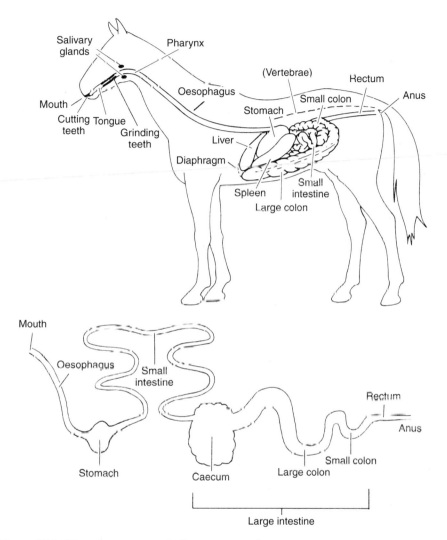

Figure 15.1. Digestive system and alimentary canal.

Table 15.1. The horse's digestive system

Foregut – mainly enzymic digestion	Hindgut – fermentation area
Mouth	Caecum
Phraynx	Large colon
Oesophagus	Small colon
Stomach	Rectum
Small intestine	Anus

Mouth

The horse grazes by carefully selecting food with its highly mobile lips and then cropping it with the incisor teeth. The food is then passed, via the tongue, to the back of the mouth where the molars start to grind down the food material by chewing. The horse's teeth differ from human ones in that they grow throughout the life of the horse. This is necessary because of the constant grinding action that wears down the molars (see Chapter 5).

Horses produce about 10–12 litres (3 gallons) of saliva per day. Although it has little, if any, digestive activity, saliva wets and lubricates the food as it is swallowed via the pharynx and passed into the oesophagus on its way to the stomach. The pharynx helps to guide food into the oesophagus during swallowing.

Food or water cannot return to the mouth from the oesophagus because the soft palate blocks its return. The epiglottis (a muscular flap) also closes over the top of the trachea to prevent food going into the lungs.

The horse has three salivary glands: the parotid, sublingual and submaxillary salivary glands.

Saliva also contains bicarbonate, which is alkaline and helps to neutralise or buffer the acid produced by the horse's stomach.

The bolus of food after it has been swallowed, moves along the digestive tract by waves of muscular contractions known as peristalsis. These waves are usually irreversible. Occasionally, food becomes lodged in the oesophagus and this is known as choke.

Stomach

A muscle known as the cardiac sphincter regulates the opening of the oesophagus into the stomach. Once food has passed into the stomach it cannot be regurgitated back, so the horse is unable to vomit, unlike humans.

The presence of food in the nostrils may indicate a ruptured stomach an extremely serious condition.

The stomach of the horse is small compared to that of other animals. It comprises about 8–10% of the total digestive tract and holds about 7–9 litres (2 gallons). The empty stomach is roughly the same size as a rugby ball.

Feeding too large concentrate feeds to a horse can lead to severe problems such as:

- laboured breathing and fatigue
- laminitis
- colic
- ruptured stomach.

The small stomach simply does not have the capacity to, nor is it designed to handle a large feed. If too much feed is given at one time, then it will be pushed out of the stomach too quickly, before it has time to mix thoroughly with the gastric secretions, which help to begin digestion.

Feeds begin to break down due to enzymic and microbial digestion in the stomach. The stomach does have a small microbial population enabling a small amount of digestion to take place. Acid secretions help to kill any bacteria that may have been eaten with the food.

Food material is only in the stomach for a short time and this limits the amount of digestion that can take place. It is in the less acidic regions of the stomach that some bacterial breakdown of food (or fermentation) occurs resulting in a small amount of lactic acid. The food material produced by the stomach is then poured into the first part of the small intestine.

Small intestine

The length of the small intestine in the horse is approximately 20–27 m (65–88 ft) with a capacity of 55–70 litres (12–16 gallons). It runs between the stomach and the caecum.

The small intestine is split into three different sections:

- duodenum
- jejunum
- ileum.

The duodenum is about 1 m (3 ft) long. It forms an S-shaped bend, which contains the pancreas. The jejunum is 20 m (65 ft) long and the ileum is 1–1.5 m (3–5 ft) long.

The small intestine can move quite freely within the abdominal cavity except at its attachment to the stomach and the caecum. It lies in several coils with the small colon. This area of the gut is the major site of enzymic break down of food, such as starch, protein, fat, vitamins and minerals, and their absorption.

The fibre part of the diet is digested further along the digestive tract, mainly in the hindgut.

The enzymes of the small intestine require alkaline conditions. This alkalinity is produced mainly by the pancreatic juice from the pancreas and bile from the liver. The horse does not have a gall bladder in which to store bile, instead bile trickles continuously into the duodenum from the liver via the bile duct.

Pancreas

The pancreas is a gland that lies alongside the duodenum and empties into it by means of one or more pancreatic ducts. The pancreas produces digestive enzymes to break down food and sodium bicarbonate to neutralise acid entering the small intestine from the stomach.

The pancreas also produces the hormone insulin, which passes into the blood stream.

The rate of passage of food through the small intestine is rapid, relatively speaking, and food will reach the caecum in just over an hour. Substantial digestion of non-fibrous, soluble foods will occur in this short period through the action of digestive enzymes.

Large intestine

This is made up of the caecum, the large colon, the small colon and the rectum. The large intestine is approximately 8 m (25 ft) long. Although the foregut of the horse is similar to other simple stomached animals, the hindgut is remarkably different. It is in the horse's hindgut that the complex insoluble carbohydrates (cellulose and hemicellulose) are broken down. Cellulose and hemicellulose are substances that make up all plant cell walls and are more commonly referred to as plant fibre. The horse does not have enzymes such as cellulase that could break down these complex substances itself.

Some microorganisms, however, are able to breakdown cellulose and hemicellulose by a process of fermentation. The horse has a greatly enlarged large intestine that accommodates a vast number of microorganisms, and these are able to release the 'locked' energy providing nutrients to the horse. In return, the microorganisms are provided with a safe environment in which to live.

More than half the dry weight of faeces produced by the horse is bacteria. The amount of microorganisms in the digestive tract of the horse is huge; they number more than ten times all the tissue cells in the horse's body.

Caecum

This is a large blind-ended, comma-shaped sac situated at the end of the small intestine. The capacity of the caecum is approximately 25–35 litres (6–8 gallons).

The caecum acts as a large fermentation vat where fibrous parts of the food are mixed with the microorganisms.

Large colon

This is approximately 3–4 m long (10–13 ft) and has a capacity of 90–110 litres (20–24 gallons).

The large intestine is only held in place by its bulk. At certain points, the large intestine changes in direction and narrows at the same time. These points are known as flexures and not surprisingly they are vulnerable to blockages.

The digesta reaches the caecum approximately 3 hours after a meal and remains in the large intestine for 36–48 hours.

Small colon

This is 3–4 m long (10–13 ft) but is narrower than the large colon. The small colon lies intermingled with the jejunum and as it is fairly free to move it can lead to abdominal crises such as a twisted gut.

Rectum

This is a relatively short, straight tube connecting the small colon to the anus. It acts as a storage area for faeces before being evacuated as dung.

Fermentation

The digestion of fibre is reliant entirely on microorganisms that ferment insoluble carbohydrate, such as cellulose, to energy-producing substances known as volatile fatty acids (VFAs). The principal VFAs produced are acetic, propionic and butyric acids. These are absorbed into the bloodstream and converted into energy. This allows the horse to thrive on its natural forage diet.

Ailments related to feeding or the digestive tract

Equine nutrition in not a precise subject and the condition of the horse will rely to a great extent on other factors, including the management programme and the owner's ability to assess when the horse is not 100% and take the appropriate steps to resolve the problem.

Poor feeding practice can have a drastic effect on the horse and problems such as colic may even result in death.

Poor nutritional management will eventually result in reduced performance of the horse, resistance to disease will be impaired and the horse will simply not be able to cope with the work being asked of it.

Other factors also affect the way in which the horses uses its feed. For example, a heavy worm burden will reduce the horse's ability to digest and absorb vital nutrients effectively (see Chapter 5).

Colic

Colic is common. This is particularly the case in performance horses, mainly due to the increased stresses imposed on them.

Colic is a general term for abdominal pain and it should always be treated as an emergency.

Managing and feeding the horse in a consistent and natural manner will help to reduce the incidence of colic. For example, any changes made to the diet should be made over a period of 10–14 days so as to prevent upset to the horse's digestive system. The stabled horse, if at all possible, should be turned out to pasture for a few hours a day to prevent the horse becoming upset at being confined. This helps to keep even fit horses calm and even-tempered.

Predisposing factors for colic

- Sudden access to large quantities of rich feed, e.g. grass clippings, cereals, fallen apples.
- Change in routine, new stable, new surroundings.
- Irregular work, change in feed time.
- Exhaustion.
- Feeding/watering too soon after fast work.
- Mouldy feed.
- Sudden change of diet.
- Greedy feeders.

Signs of colic

- Kicking at the belly.
- Loss of appetite.
- Lethargy.
- Looking at the flanks.
- Pawing the ground.
- Patchy sweating.
- Getting up and lying down repeatedly.
- Rolling.
- Increased respiratory rate.
- Increased heart rate.

If colic is suspected, generally the vet should be called, feed and hay should be removed and the horse should be left alone but observed at regular intervals. Most cases of colic will recover in a couple of hours but some require urgent attention.

There are several types of colic:

- spasmodic
- impactive
- gas, tympanitic or flatulent
- sand
- twisted gut/internal catastrophe.

Spasmodic

Caused by spasm of the muscular intestinal wall. Horses with spasmodic colic may be moderately distressed, constantly get up and lies down, and look at their flanks. They may roll and sometimes get themselves cast. The pulse and respiratory rates and the horse's temperature may increase. If this persists the vet will administer a relaxant drug that usually relieves the problem quickly.

Impactive

As the name suggests this is caused by food getting impacted within the horse's intestine. The horse's gut is coiled and looped within the abdomen and there are several changes in diameter and direction. At these points blockages may occur. Affected horses rarely show extreme signs of pain, but look uncomfortable and roll more than usual. The vet will assess where the blockage is and administer liquid paraffin via stomach tube to lubricate and move the blockage.

Gas, tympanitic or flatulent

This type of colic is caused by a build up of gas within the gut and is very painful. The horse will often react violently, rolling and sweating profusely. Veterinary attention is essential when the problem will be assessed and then treated.

Sand

Some horses when out at pasture with a sandy soil base may take in large quantities of sand while grazing. This may lead to an impaction and therefore colic. The treatment is the same as for impactive colic.

Twisted gut/internal catastrophe

This is the most serious and dramatic form of colic. The intestine can become twisted or telescoped within itself resulting in an obstruction of the blood supply. The horse will be in extreme pain and veterinary attention is extremely urgent. Abdominal surgery is necessary if the horse has any chance of survival, but this is often a fatal form of colic.

Laminitis (founder)

Laminitis is a severe disease of the horse's foot.

The term laminitis refers to inflammation of the sensitive laminae of the horse's foot. These laminae are situated between the pedal bone and the hoof wall.

Laminitis is, in fact, the end result of a chain of events that may be started by a number of different trigger factors.

Trigger factors

- Carbohydrate overload – overeating grain or concentrates.
- Grazing lush, spring pasture.
- Excessive fructans intake from pasture.
- Drug induced – corticosteroid treatment may develop laminitis.
- Road work – excessive concussion to the feet.
- Toxaemia – retained placenta in the mare following birth, severe diarrhoea or colic.
- Pituitary tumours (Cushing's syndrome) – occurs sometimes in old horses.

One of the above trigger factors leads to a chain of events, eventually resulting in an increase in blood pressure. The blood supply to the hoof shunts through the coronary band area, bypassing the hoof itself. This reduces or stops the blood supply to sensitive laminae resulting in inflammation and severe pain.

Unless the cause is removed to prevent further damage, the pedal bone may separate from the laminae and this combined with the pull of the deep digital flexor tendon will cause the pedal bone to rotate and the sole to drop. X-ray analysis will be required to determine the extent of rotation of the pedal bone.

Horses with laminitis show a characteristic laminitic stance, leaning backwards in an attempt to transfer weight away from the painful toe part of the hoof and rest on the heels. They have a bounding digital pulse and their temperature and respiratory rate may increase.

Laminitis is characterised as acute or chronic:

- acute: extreme pain and therefore acute lameness
- chronic: follows initial acute episode, intermittent lameness, diverging growth pattern around hoof wall (laminitic rings).

Treatment

Veterinary attention is required urgently for acute laminitic cases. The horse should be stabled on a deep shavings bed to support the hooves. The horse should *not* be moved as the old treatment of walking the horse will result in further damage.

The concentrate ration should be withdrawn and a diet provided of hay plus a good vitamin/mineral supplement. The horse may need pain relief and it is important to keep the horse comfortable. Prevention is important and good management plays a vital role.

- Feed a high quality fibre, low starch, low energy diet, try to avoid feeding cereal grains even within mixes. If energy is required use oil as an energy source.
- Limit time out at grass to no more than 4 hours per day on short pasture.
- Aim to slowly reduce the bodyweight if the horse or pony is very overweight. Do not put on a drastic diet.
- Add a performance-level broad spectrum vitamin and mineral supplement to support repair or hoof tissue. Preprobiotics are also useful.

Diarrhoea

This is often caused by infectious disease, but may also be caused by many other factors including poor nutrition, worms or worm damage. Diarrhoea may be mild and self-limiting or severe.

Diarrhoea results from disturbed fluid transport across the gut lining. Fluid, which would normally have been resorbed into the horse's body, passes out with the faeces, making it loose and very wet. A small pony may absorb about 30 litres (6 gallons) per day from the bowel.

Depending on the amount, this fluid loss may be catastrophic, particularly in foals. These foals dehydrate quickly and may die within a few hours of acute onset.

Also, excessive secretions of fluid into the gut will lead to wet droppings or diarrhoea. Diarrhoea is considered to be a sign of a problem with the working of the colon. Mild diarrhoea may even be due to an imbalance of the hindgut microorganisms resulting from a change of diet.

The underlying cause needs to be found if the correct treatment is to be given. Causes include:

- sudden change in diet, access to rich grass
- worms/worm damage
- *Salmonella*
- *Clostridium*
- antibiotic treatment
- tumours
- poisoning
- excitment, nervousness
- toxins.

Treatment

Remove the cause, give fluid and electrolytes where necessary, restore the natural gut microorganism population with preprobiotics or probiotics. Make sure plenty of clean fresh water is always available.

Grass sickness

This results in a breakdown of the nerves leading to paralysis of the digestive tract. It is most common in horses aged 3–7 years and affects horses at grass. Horses turned out after winter stabling seem to have a slightly higher risk. Fields where grass sickness has occurred previously are a high risk for reoccurrence.

The cause is still unknown and there is no cure. Horses may develop acute, subacute or chronic forms but the outcomes are the same. The prognosis is extremely poor.

Choke

Choke occurs when food material becomes lodged in the oesophagus. Signs include:

- coughing
- holding the head and neck low and extended
- difficulty in swallowing

- green or brown fluid tricking from the nostrils
- saliva drooling from the mouth.

Causes include bolting of food, sharp teeth or a sore mouth. Cubes and odd-shaped pieces of carrot or apple may become lodged. Inadequately soaked beet pulp if bolted down, may be a problem.

Horses suffering from choke should be moved to a stable, not given water or food and kept under observation. If not resolved within 5–10 minutes the vet should be called. The vet will be able to administer drugs to relax the oesophagus.

Horses that choke should be given very wet feed and encouraged to chew the feed by adding short cut forage to the concentrate feed. If cubes caused the problem, then these should either be soaked prior to feeding or a coarse mix fed instead.

Chapter 16
The theory of feeding

The horse is an athletic animal. It evolved to have the ability to evade predators and can reach top speeds of up to 60 km/hour (40 mph).

Domestication has resulted in many horses that have been bred for performance, such as the Thoroughbred; however, their digestive tracts have not changed at all. Horses are dependent on humans to meet their nutritional needs and it is important to supply required nutrients while maintaining as natural a diet as possible.

The population of horses shows huge variation among large numbers of breeds and cross-breeds, and this results in some difficulties when discussing balanced rations for horses. Research carried out on nutrient requirements does not tend take into account the individual horse's temperament and breeding.

A balanced ration provides the horse with carbohydrates, protein, fat, minerals, vitamins and water in sufficient quantities to maintain life and allow it to do work, reproduce or grow depending on the particular demands at the time.

The nutrient demands of the horse will depend on such factors as:

- bodyweight
- condition
- work level
- appetite
- age
- health
- reproductive status
- environment
- management.

Bodyweight

Larger horses require more food than smaller ones; this refers to bodyweight and not height. The first step in determining a horse's nutrient requirements and then producing a ration is therefore to determine the horse's bodyweight.

There are several methods of determining bodyweight:

- weighbridge
- tape measure and calculator
- weigh-tape
- table of weights.

The weighbridge is the most accurate, but few horse owners have access to this piece of equipment. Many training yards and studs have a weighbridge as it is vital to their daily management and training routines.

An equation has been produced that gives the bodyweight based on the horse's heart girth and length from point of shoulder to the point of buttock:

$$\text{Bodyweight (kg)} = \frac{\text{heart girth (cm)}^2 \times \text{length (cm)}}{8717}$$

or

$$\text{Bodyweight (lb)} = \frac{\text{heart girth (in)}^2 \times \text{length (in)}}{241}$$

Weigh-tapes are also available which use the horse's heart girth measurement to give an approximate bodyweight. These are quite useful in measuring weight loss and/or gain if used consistently.

Ration analysis

To make a successful ration two factors must be taken into account: first, the nutrient requirements of the horse and, second, the nutrient values of the feeds being given to the horse.

The nutrient values of feeds can be measured in a laboratory using many different analytical procedures. The dry matter, for example, involves all the water being removed from the food material by drying it in an oven and then repeated weighing until the weight remains constant.

Grass contains a large proportion of water and therefore has a low dry matter value when compared with cereals such as oats or barley, which contain little moisture and have a higher dry matter value.

Horses therefore have to eat much greater quantities of grass as it contains so much water. Haylage also contains more water then hay and this must be taken into account by when swapping from hay to haylage.

Further tests can then be performed on the dried food material to determine the levels of nutrients such as protein, energy, fibre and oil content.

Carbohydrates

Carbohydrates provide the energy needed for all cell processes and basic functions such as breathing and the beating of the heart. They also provide energy for muscle contraction.

Energy from a feed is derived from various sources including sugar, starch and fibre. Once the energy content of feedstuffs (determined by chemical analysis) is known then this information can be used to calculate rations for horses.

Table 16.1. Energy values of some common horse feeds

Feed	Digestible energy (MJ/kg dry matter)
Oats	11–12
Barley	13
Maize	14
Extracted soyabean meal	13
Wheatbran	11

Carbohydrates may be roughly divided into two groups:

- Soluble carbohydrates (non-structural): starch, sugars (grass, cereals).
- Insoluble carbohydrates (structural): cellulose, hemicellulose (fibre).

Grains such as oats, barley and maize contain large amounts of starch, whereas hay contains more fibre, which is still an excellent slow-release energy source for horses. See Table 16.1.

The energy content is stated as the number of kilojoules present – joules are simply metric calories. Horse feed energy values are normally given as megajoules (1 megajoule = 1,000,000 joules) of digestible energy per kilogram. Digestible energy refers to the amount of energy in the feed, which is actually digested for use by the horse. Some will be wasted.

Fat

Horses diets are normally low in fat, however fat contains two and a quarter times more energy than carbohydrate, and so many hard-working horses are given high fat rations. Fat has been used for some time to supplement diets of endurance horses with much success.

Just as excess glucose can be converted to fat, then fat can be converted to glucose (the main energy source for all living cells). Fats contain fatty acids, some of which are essential to the horse's health.

The addition of 0.3 litres (1 cup) of oil to each of three feeds supplies the equivalent amount of energy as 1 kg (2 lb) of oats. The oil should be a polyunsaturated one of vegetable origin such as soya, corn or vegetable.

Protein

Protein is an important structural component of all animal tissues. The need for protein is greatest in the young horse, as it is still growing. When maturity is reached, the protein requirement is reduced and only enough is needed to replace worn body tissues and support the slow growth of tissues such as skin, hoof and hair. It is highly unlikely that a mature horse will be deficient in protein, particularly if it has access to good grazing.

The horse's dietary requirement for protein is not greatly increased by work; in fact, feeding excess protein to working horses can be detrimental.

Proteins vary widely in composition, but their basic structure is made up of simple units called amino acids, more than 20 of these amino acids occur naturally. The horse can make some amino acids within its body and these are therefore known as 'non-essential' in that they are not required in the diet. Others which cannot be made in the body, and need to be supplied in the diet, are known as 'essential' amino acids. The most important essential amino acids are lysine, methionine and tryptophan. Lysine is most likely to be deficient in the horse's diet, particularly when a cereal or 'straight' ration is being fed and the horse has limited grazing.

Some proteins contain more of the essential amino acids and these are referred to as higher 'quality' proteins.

Unlike carbohydrates, excess proteins cannot be stored in the horse's body for future use. Any excess has to be broken down and some of it is excreted through the urine and the rest used as an energy source, but it is a highly wasteful and inefficient one. Contrary to popular belief, protein is not a major energy source, except during starvation.

Horses in hard work need more carbohydrate and or fat to provide the energy required, not protein.

Vitamins

Vitamins are a group of chemical compounds that are vital for life. They are required in minute quantities for the normal healthy functioning of the horse. Nevertheless, a deficiency in the diet will eventually result in clinical disease. There are approximately 15 vitamins known to be essential to the horse. Vitamin requirements depend on several factors such as pregnancy, growth, age and level of work.

Vitamins are divided into one of two groups: fat-soluble vitamins (A, D, E and K) and water-soluble vitamins (C and B-complex). See Table 16.2.

Table 16.2. Vitamins required in the horse's diet

Water-soluble vitamins	Fat-soluble vitamins
C	A
B_1 (thiamine)	D
B_2 (riboflavin)	E
B_3 (niacin)	K
B_5 (pantothenic acid)	
B_6 (pyridoxine)	
B_{12} (cyanocobalamin)	
B_{15} (pangamic acid)	
Folic acid	
Choline	
Inositol	
Biotin (vitamin H)	

The fat-soluble vitamins can be stored in the body, particularly the liver. Most of these can be found in abundance in fresh green herbage, therefore a horse can take in plenty over the summer months and store them for later use over the winter months when grass is in short supply. If too many fat-soluble vitamins are fed then toxicity may result, particularly from overenthusiastic supplementation of these vitamins. Most of the water-soluble vitamins can be made by the microorganisms in the horse's gut. Excess water-soluble vitamins in the horse's body are broken down and excreted, and for that reason toxicity symptoms are unlikely to occur.

Minerals

Feral horses are able to meet their mineral needs by selectively grazing and roaming over huge areas of land with different soil types. The domesticated horse is confined at pasture or stabled and therefore relies on good feeding programmes and pasture management.

Minerals are inorganic substances found throughout the horse's body and are essential for health and development. At least 21 minerals are known to be essential in the horse's diet. Some minerals are required in larger amounts and are known as macro-minerals, or major minerals, whereas those required in concentrations below 50 mg/kg are known as trace elements or trace minerals.

Most body processes require minerals to function properly and there are many interactions between different minerals. A deficiency or abundance of one can severely affect another. The need for a strong skeleton, muscles, tissue repair and efficient metabolism in the working horse results in a higher requirement for minerals in their diets.

Factors affecting the amount of minerals available in grains and forage include soil deficiencies, mineral interactions and poor availability. For example, high levels of molybdenum may result in reduced copper availability. See Table 16.3 for a list of essential minerals.

Table 16.3. Minerals (the letters in brackets are the chemical symbols)

Major minerals	Trace minerals
Calcium (Ca)	Copper (Cu)
Phosphorus (P)	Zinc (Zn)
Magnesium (Mg)	Manganese (Mn)
Potassium (K)	Iron (Fe)
Sodium (Na)	Iodine (I)
Chloride (Cl)	Selenium (Se)
	Cobalt (Co)
	Molybdenum (Mo)

Water

Approximately 70% of the horse's bodyweight is water. Water is required for many different life functions such as:

- temperature regulation
- medium in which chemical reactions can take place
- solvent in which substances may be dissolved and transported
- gives cells their shape
- excretion in the form of urine
- milk.

Horses must have a clean supply of fresh water at all times. All horses should have free access to water except after hard exercise. These horses should be cooled down for 10–15 minutes before being given access to water. Alternatively, allow only a couple of litres initially and repeat after 10 and 20 minutes.

Nutrient requirement for horses

The horse's nutrient requirements are given in Table 16.4.

Rationing

When deciding on the feed for a horse it is wise to bear in mind the theory of rationing. Horses are fed for maintenance, i.e. to maintain them in their present state. Their food provides energy for the muscles of the internal organs and for

Table 16.4. Nutrient requirements based on the National Research Council Nutrient Requirements of Horses 1989

	Weight (kg)	Crude protein (g)	Lysine (g)	Ca (g)	P (g)	Mg (g)	K (g)	Vitamin A (IU, 000s)
Mature horses								
Maintenance	500	656	23	20	14	7	25	15
Stallions	500	820	29	25	18	9.4	31	22
Pregnant mares								
9 months	500	801	28	35	26	9	29	30
10 months		815	29	35	26	9	30	3
11 months		866	30	37	28	9	31	3
Lactating mares								
Foaling to 3 months	500	1427	50	56	36	11	46	30
3 months to weaning	500	1048	37	36	22	9	33	30
Working horses								
Light work	500	820	29	25	18	9	31	22
Moderate work	500	984	34	30	21	11	37	22
Intense work	500	1312	46	40	29	15	50	22

grazing, maintains body temperature and continuously replaces cells to keep the body in good order. Horses are also fed for production. This can be broken into different categories:

- Growth from the day the horse is born until it stops growing at 4–7 years old.
- Lactation of the brood mare from the day her foal is born until the day it is weaned.
- Growth of the embryo into a foal within its mother (most of this growth occurs in the final third of the pregnancy).
- Body repair, regrowth after major injury or disease.
- Fattening.
- Work (this can be broken down into light work, medium work, heavy work or fast work).
- Build up muscle for performance.

To feed for maintenance, the main criterion is the size of the animal: bigger animals need more food. In practice, maintenance for the horse in the field is produced by grass supplemented with hay or straw and possibly some hard feed in winter. Maintenance for the stabled horse comes from hay or other forms of conserved grass. If the horse requires a large quantity of food for production, the hay must be of high quality. There is a limit to the gut capacity of a horse, and if a performance horse is filled up with large quantities of low-quality maintenance food, it will have neither room for adequate production rations nor energy.

To feed for production, the main criterion is the amount of production required. Thus, with the pregnant mare, the extra feed may be increased gradually through the last third of the pregnancy. With the competition horse, the feed is increased as the horse becomes fitter and is able to work harder. Production rations are mostly based on cereals or high digestible fibre and oil. Good grass or very high-quality hay will produce a little above maintenance and therefore contribute to energy needs.

The horse can eat, each day, hay and concentrates weighing about 2.5% of its body weight (2% for ponies and up to 3% for young stock).

Ratio of forage to concentrates

The relationship of forage to concentrates in the horse's diet has a clear bearing on the energy in the diet. More concentrates means more energy. Therefore the horse's diet is related to its work. A horse that is not working should be able to thrive on hay alone. A working horse, burning up energy, will need to have concentrates added to the ration.

This means that a 500 kg (1100 lb) horse in medium work has an appetite of 12.5 kg (27.5 lb) and is fed 40% concentrates and 60% forage, resulting in a ration of 5 kg (11 lb) of concentrates and 7.5 kg (16.5 lb) hay.

It is best to feed a horse slightly below appetite so that it is always eager for the next concentrate feed and has always finished the hay net when it comes to be filled again. Beware of the *ad libitium* feeding system; often the hay rack is

Table 16.5. Ratio of forage to concentrates

Work level	Hay/haylage (%)	Concentration (%)
Resting	100	0
Light	75	25
Medium	60	40
Hard	50	50
Fast	50	50

constantly topped up so that the hay at the bottom becomes mouldy, and the horse becomes over-fussy and wasteful. If you feed a weighed ration of hay and concentrates, within the horse's appetite, it should always eat up. If the horse does not eat all its hay and concentrates it may indicate that the quality of the feed is not up to scratch or that the horse is off-colour (also see Table 16.5).

In order to design a practical ration that supplies the energy and protein requirements of an individual horse, and fits within its appetite, we can follow the eight steps involved in the rules of rationing. For our example we use a 16 hands high, middleweight novice event horse.

The rules of rationing

Step 1: estimation of bodyweight

Several methods are available:

- table of weights
- calculation
- weight-tape (see Figure 16.1)
- weighbridge.

Our 16 hands high, novice event horse will weigh 500 kg. See Table 16.6.

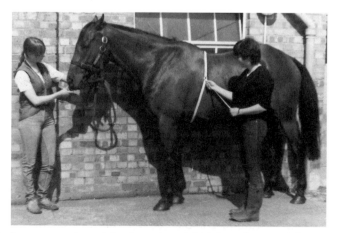

Figure 16.1. An easy way to watch a horse's weight is by using a weight-tape.

Table 16.6. Approximate bodyweights

Height (hands)	Bodyweight (kg)	Bodyweight (lb)
11	120–260	264–572
12	230–290	506–638
13	290–350	638–770
14	350–420	770–924
15	420–520	924–1144
16	500–600	1100–1320
17	600–725	1320–1595

Note. The values in this table are averages and only approximate.

Step 2: the horse's appetite

An adult working horse's appetite is about 2.5% of bodyweight. Foals and lactating broodmares may compensate for high nutrient requirements by eating more than this.

$$\text{Appetite (kg)} = \frac{\text{bodyweight}}{100} \times 2.5$$

Appetite of 500 kg horse $= \dfrac{500}{100} \times 2.5 = 12.5\ kg\ (27.5\ lb)$

A 500 kg horse can eat up to 12.5 kg of dry matter per day. Remember that different feeds have different amounts of dry matter in them, so a horse will eat much more than 12.5 kg of grass a day because of its high moisture content.

Step 3: calculating the energy for maintenance

The horse requires a minimum amount of energy a day just to stay alive, this is related to the bodyweight of the horse – bigger horses need more feed than smaller ones.

$$\text{Energy required for maintenance} = 18 + \frac{\text{bodyweight}}{10}$$

Energy required for a 500 kg horse to maintain its bodyweight.

$$(MJ\ DE/day) = 18 + \frac{500}{10} = 18 + 50 = MJ\ DE/day$$

A 500 kg horse will require 68 MJ of digestible energy (DE) per day to stay alive and to keep its bodyweight constant. (The above formula and this system of ration calculation were devised by Jeremy Houghton Brown, based on comparison of feed trials around the world.)

Table 16.7. Work scoring

Type of work	Work score (MJ DE)
1 hour walking	+1
1 hour walking including some trotting	+2
1 hour including trotting and cantering	+3
Schooling, dressage and/or jumping	+4
Novice 1-day eventing or hunting 1 day/week	+5
Intermediate 1-day eventing, hunting 3 days a fortnight, Novice 3-day event	+6
Advanced 1-day eventing, Intermediate 3-day events, hunting 2 days a week	+7
Racing	+8

Step 4: calculating the energy for work

The amount of energy the horse needs to carry out the work we demand of it depends on the intensity and duration of the work and the horse's bodyweight. The variation in the trainer or rider's perception of how much work the horse does has been minimised by giving the work a 'work score' of from 1 to 8. Examples of types of work are outlined in Table 16.7, but these are not rigid and you should adjust to fit your horse's individual workload.

For each 50 kg of bodyweight, add the work score to calculate the horse's energy requirement for work.

A 500 kg novice 1-day event horse will have a work score of 5. The extra energy needed to carry out that work will be:

$$work\ score \times \frac{bodyweight}{50} = 5 \times \frac{500}{50} = MJ\ DE/day$$

The energy requirement for work is then added to the maintenance requirement to give the total daily energy requirement per day.

Maintenance requirement for a 500 kg horse   = *68 MJ DE/day*

Work requirement for a 500 kg novice eventer = *50 MJ DE/day*

Total energy requirement   = *118 MJ DE/day*

Step 5: the forage-to-concentrate ratio

The horses work level will determine the amount of energy to come from the forage part of the ration and the amount to come from the concentration part. Using Table 16.8 that shows forage-to-concentrate ratios, we can calculate how the energy is going to be partitioned.

Of the total energy requirement (118 MJ DE/day) for our eventer in medium work (work score 5), 60% will come from hay and 40% will come from concentrates.

Table 16.8. Forage-to-concentrate energy partition

Work	Energy from hay (%)	Energy from concentrates (%)
Maintenance – resting	100	0
1–2 light	75	25
3–5 medium	60	40
6–7 hard	50	50
>8 fast	50	50

$$Energy\ from\ hay = \frac{118 \times 60}{100} = 71\ MJ\ DE/day$$

$$Energy\ from\ concentrates = \frac{118 \times 40}{100} = 47\ MJ\ DE/day$$

71 MJ DE per day are to be supplied by hay and 47 MJ DE per day by concentrates.

Step 6: making the ration

The next step is to convert these figures into a sensible ration, using the table of nutrient values shown in Table 16.9. The energy value of food will be matched with the energy requirements of the feeds.

Table 16.9. Typical nutrient values of common feeds

	Crude protein (%)	Digestible energy (MJ DE/kg)
Hay		
Average	4.5–8	7–8
Good	9–10	8
Poor	3.5–6	6–7
Haylage	9–12	9–11
Concentrates		
Oats	10	11–12
Barley	9.5	13
Maize	8.5	14
Extruded soyabean meal	44	13
Peas	23	14
Wheatbran	15	11
Sugar beet pulp	9.5	10.5
Vegetable oil	0	35
Cubes		
Horse and pony	10	9
Performance	13	13
Stud	15	11

The 500 kg event horse is to receive 71 MJ DE per day from average quality hay containing 8 MJ DE per kg.

$$Weight\ of\ hay\ to\ be\ fed/day = \frac{71}{8} = 9\,kg\,(20\,lb)$$

The horse is to receive the remaining 47 MJ DE as concentrates. This can be done by feeding a performance horse cube with an energy content of 13 MJ DE/kg.

$$Weight\ of\ cubes\ to\ be\ fed/day = \frac{47}{13} = 3.5\,kg\,(8\,lb)$$

This simple ration is perfectly adequate but could be enhanced with fresh apples or vegetables, etc. For those who like to make their own mix, the ration could be as shown in Table 16.10.

Along with his 9 kg (20 lb) of hay our event horse is going either to be fed 3.5 kg (8 lb) of performance cubes or 2 kg oats, 1 kg cubes, 0.5 kg bran and 0.5 kg beet pulp with a vitamin and mineral supplement.

The first ration falls within this horse's appetite of 12.5 kg. However, the second ration over-faces by 0.5 kg, because lower energy feeds are being used. In most cases this small amount may not be of consequence, but a fussy feeder may let you know that the rations are rather too much for it.

Step 7: checking the protein level

Energy is the most important aspect of a performance horse's diet, and if good quality feed is being used the protein requirements are likely to be satisfied. However, growing youngstock and broodmares will have a high protein requirement and it is important to check the protein level in any ration that you have formulated. See Table 16.11.

A horse in medium work requires 7.5–8.5% crude protein. The protein content of the ration can be worked out using the table of nutrient values shown in Table 16.12.

$$The\ percentage\ protein\ in\ the\ ration\ is\ therefore\ \frac{99.5}{12.5} = 8\%$$

Table 16.10. The final ration

Feed	Quantity	Megajoules provided
Oats	2 kg (4.4 lb)	24
Sugar beet pulp	0.5 kg (1 lb) dry weight	5
Bran	0.5 kg (1 lb)	5.5
Performance cubes	1 kg (2.2 lb)	13
Total		47.5

Table 16.11. Protein requirements of horses

Type of activity	Crude protein in ration (%)
Light work	7.5–8.5
Medium work	7.5–8.5
Hard work	9.5–10
Fast work	9.5–10
Pregnant mare – first 8 months	7.5–8.5
Pregnant mare – last 3 months	10
Lactating mare – first 3 months	12.5
Lactating mare – last 3 months	11
Stallion	9.5–10
Weanling	16
Yearling	13.5
2-year old	10

Table 16.12. Protein in ration A

Feed	Quantity (kg)	Protein content (%)	Protein in ration (g)
Hay	9	6	54
Performance cubes	3.5	13	45.5
	12.5		99.5

If the oat-based ration is used the calculation would look like that in Table 16.13.

The percentage protein in the ration is therefore $\dfrac{98.25}{13} = 7.6\%$

This is adequate for a horse in medium work.

If the hay had been low in protein, say at 4.5%, then these rations would be too low in protein and would need revising by using a high protein feed like soya or a performance cube.

Table 16.13. Protein in ration B

Feed	Quantity (kg)	Protein content (%)	Protein in ration (g)
Hay	9	6.0	54
Oats	2	10	20
Cubes	1	13	13
Bran	0.5	15.5	7.75
Beet pulp	0.5	7	3.5
	13		98.25

Step 8: check and adjust the ration

All horses are individuals and must be treated as such. Once a ration has been calculated and is being fed, the horse must be monitored to ensure that the ration is suitable.

- A supply of fresh clean water must be available to the horse at all times.
- The foods must be of good quality and acceptable to the horse – is the horse enjoying its food?
- Not only must the foods satisfy the horse's nutritional requirements, the horse must also be psychologically satisfied; it must not be bored and suffer a craving for roughage.
- The horse's condition must be checked by eye, tape or weigh-bridge. The horse may be gaining or losing weight. Is this what is wanted? If not, alter the ration accordingly. Horses have an optimum performance weight and should be kept as close as possible to this weight.
- The horse's temperament and behaviour may affect the ration fed. Part-bred horses may need fewer concentrates and more bulk as they are better doers and (usually) more placid. Routine and a quiet yard may save feed as horses are not fretting in their boxes.
- The horse's environment must be monitored. In a cold spell, more food and an extra blanket may be needed. A clipped horse may need more food to maintain its condition if it is not adequately rugged up. In hot weather horses may go off their concentrate ration because their maintenance requirement has fallen; do not worry unless they start to lose condition.
- Horses must be regularly wormed and have their teeth checked for sharp edges.
- Some horses are poor doers, perhaps due to a gut damaged by worms early in life, and will always need extra attention to their feeding.

Chapter 17
Practical feeding and watering

Rules of feeding

Several rules have been developed to ensure good feeding practice:

- ensure clean fresh water is always available
- feed little and often
- make any changes gradually
- feed only good-quality dust-free feed
- feed plenty of plant fibre/forage
- keep feed utensils clean
- maintain regular feeding times
- feed according to work done, condition and temperament.

Traditional diets for horses included hay, oats and bran. Now, feed companies produce a vast array of different 'feeds' for horses, with most categories of horses being catered for. As discussed in Chapter 16, the quantity of concentrates to be given depends on many factors, such as the horse's workload, health, size, whether the horse is growing or reproducing and so on.

The choice of feeds available is almost endless and so the following factors should be taken into account when deciding on a ration:

- cost – varies widely
- individual nutrient requirements of the horse – workload, health, etc.
- nutrient content of feed – is it 'balanced', any extras required?
- availability – must be readily available so sudden changes to diet are avoided
- quality.

Feeds for horse fall into two main categories:

- forage: grass, hay, haylage, alfalfa, hydroponic grass
- concentrates: straight, compound feeds.

Beet pulp falls in between the two as it contains readily digestible fibre.

Forage

Forage is the leaves, stems and stalks of plants. In the case of horses this refers mainly to grass both unharvested in the form of pasture and harvested in the form of dried grass, grass cubes, hay, haylage, silage and commercially produced chaffs. Forage is vital for horses as a source of fibre which is essential for normal gut function, it stimulates muscle tone and activity of the gut wall. The horse cannot function efficiently without fibre in the diet and this should not be considered as a 'filler' but as an essential part of the ration. The amount of nutrients available will depend on the quality of the forage and time of harvesting.

Good pasture should be used when available, particularly in the summer months. All horses benefit from time spent grazing naturally.

In the winter months access to pasture usually allows the horse to exercise, but the nutritional value of the grass at this time of year is poor. Harvested forage such as hay or haylage can be fed.

Forage is the most natural feed for horses and should always be considered a priority. The concentrate part of the ration should balance the forage.

Feeding inadequate amounts of forage can result in colic, diarrhoea, laminitis, wood chewing, tail chewing and copraphagia (dung eating).

Grass

Horses have evolved to eat grass. It is an entirely natural feed for horses. Good pasture contains all of the nutrients required in a balanced form for horses, including carbohydrates (starch and sugar), protein and vitamins. Mineral levels do vary according to the geographical area and may be a problem for growing youngstock. A disadvantage of grass is that its nutrient value changes over the growing season. Spring grass in nutrient rich and tends to be low in fibre, as the season progresses, the grass matures and contains more fibre and less nutrients. For example, the protein level can be as high as 25% dry matter (DM) in spring grass and as low as 5% DM in older grass (autumn). Different species of grass also provide varying levels of nutrients to horses.

Hay

Hay is dried grass. It may be described as seed hay or meadow hay.

Meadow hay is made from permanent, established pasture which usually contains many species of grasses and often some herbs and other wild plants. Meadow hay is often softer and potentially contains less protein, but this is not always the case.

Seed hay is made from ryegrass-based leys, which have been grown specifically to take a hay crop from. Seed hay is generally coarser than meadow hay and often contains higher levels of protein.

The quality and nutrient content of hay depends on several factors including:

- grass species
- stage of cutting – maturity of grass
- weather conditions
- storage
- fertilisation (if any).

The quality of hay depends on how it is made. The time of cutting, which is related to favourable weather conditions, is much more important than the types of grass present, with the exception of barn-dried hay, where the weather conditions are irrelevant as hay is cut and then taken to barns for drying artificially. The drying process should aim to reduce loss of leaf to a minimum as this is where most of the nutrients can be found.

Care should be taken to ensure that poisonous plants are not cut and baled along with the grass. For example, dried ragwort is very palatable to horses but can result in death.

Storage

The moisture content of hay must be reduced to 5–15%. If the hay is baled at higher moisture contents then it may heat up. If this is excessive, spontaneous combustion may result with the hay setting alight: an extremely dangerous situation. Heat and moisture will result in the production of moulds and fungi, and mouldy hay should not be fed to horses under any circumstances. Fungal spores found in hay are a common cause of horse respiratory problems.

Hay should be stacked and stored very carefully to allow some space between bales and so allow air to circulate.

Legume hays include clover and sainfoin and more commonly alfalfa (lucerne). These are more nutrient rich than grass hays, but are not widely available in the UK. Dried alfalfa is used more commonly for chaffs.

Silage

Silage as such is not often fed to horses due to practical problems associated with it. It is made in silos, clamps or big bales.

Ensiling a crop involves 'pickling' it in its own juice. It is cut earlier in the growing season than hay and left to wilt to 25–40% dry matter. It is then placed in a silo, clamp or big bales which are air-tight and the grass undergoes a fermentation process. Big bale silage is sometimes used for large yards of horses. Once opened it needs to be used within 3 days. If well made it is virtually dust and fungal-spore free. If, when opened, the silage smells of ammonia or there are white spots on it then it should not be used. It must not be too wet.

Care must be taken with silage as its feeding has resulted in several deaths of horses in the UK. These deaths were associated with the presence of bacteria and toxins, particularly those responsible for botulism.

Haylage

This fits between hay and silage. Haylage is cut at a later growing stage than silage, but earlier or at the same time as hay. The grass is allowed to dry in the field to about 50–65% dry matter, it is then collected, compressed and packed in small, tough plastic sacks which are then heat sealed. They may also be bagged in big bales, with black or green plastic wrapping. The vitamins in haylage are also preserved, unlike hay.

Many farmers now make haylage specifically for horses and horse owners should ask the farmer for a basic nutrient analysis before purchase.

Haylage is sometimes expensive, but for horses with respiratory allergies it is essential as it is 'dust' free. Although it is richer in nutrients than hay, it also contains more water and therefore a greater weight may need to be fed to ensure the dry matter intake (actual nutrients not water).

Alfalfa

This is a legume and is rich in protein, fibre and calcium. It can be fed as hay or short chaff. It contains low levels of soluble carbohydrates (unlike spring grass) and is therefore often used for laminitic cases. It can provide a useful addition to the horses diet.

Concentrates

These tend to be split into two groups:

- straights or cereal grains
- compound feeds – manufactured.

Straights

Straights refer to cereal grains such as oats, barley, maize and wheat. The most common straights fed to horses are oats and barley. Straights are carbohydrate sources containing high levels of starch. However, the mineral balance is poor, containing low levels of calcium and high levels of phosphorus (opposite to the horse's requirements). The protein level may appear to be good, but the quality of the protein is poor, being low in lysine and other essential amino acids (see Table 17.1).

The horse is not designed to eat cereals grains, and so great care should be taken when feeding them. No more than 2.5 kg of grain should be fed at one feed, due to the horse's small stomach.

Table 17.1. Nutrient values of commonly fed concentrate feeds

	Crude protein (%)	Oil (%)	MAD* fibre (%)	Ca (g/kg)	P (g/kg)	Lysine (g/kg)	Digestible energy (MJ/kg)
Oats	10	4.5	16	0.1	0.35	3	11–12
Naked oats	13.5	9.7	3.2	0.2	0.4	5	16
Barley	9.5	1.6	7	0.05	3.3	3.1	13
Maize	8.5	3.8	3	0.2	3	2.6	14
Extracted soya bean	44	1.0	10	0.4	0.7	26	13
Wheat bran	15	4	10	0.15	1.15	0.5	11
Sugar beet	9.5	0.5	20	0.7	0.1	2.8	10.5
Vegetable oil	0	100	0	0	0	0	35
Horse and pony	9–11	2.5	16	0.7	0.35	0.4	10
Performance mix/cubes	12	3.5	5	0.9	0.45	0.75	13.5
Stud diet	15	3	8.5	1.2	0.65	0.75	13.5
Racing diet	13	8.5	8	0.9	0.5	0.6	14
Oat balancer	18	5	5	1.6	0.8	0.8	14

Forage	Dry matter (%)	Crude protein (%)	Crude fibre (%)	Ca (g/kg)	P (g/kg)	Digestible energy (MJ/kg)
Hay good	86	9–10	30	3	1.7	7–8
Hay poor	86	3.5–6	40	2.5	1.7	6–7
Silage big bale	35	10	30	5.3	2.6	9–10
Haylage	55	9–12	30			9–11
Straw	88	3	40	2	0.4	6

*MAD: modified acid detergent fibre.

Feed manufacturers use straights when manufacturing horse feed, but they balance the deficiencies by adding vitamin/mineral premixes and high-quality protein sources. Straights are generally cheaper to buy than compound feeds, but their deficiencies have to be corrected and this can prove more expensive in the long term. Advice from a nutritionist may be helpful.

Straights may undergo various types of processing aimed at increasing the digestibility of starch:

- Extrusion involves cooking at great pressure, similar to popcorn. Extrusion breaks up the starch molecules and therefore the resulting feed is more digestible.
- Micronisation involves flaking and toasting in machinery similar to microwaves. The cooking process again makes the starch more digestible.
- Rolling involves crushing the grain, they are not cooked and, once open to air, the grain will start to deteriorate and it will lose its feed value after approximately 2 weeks.
- Steam cooking and flaking involves passing the grain through heated rollers that cook and split it. Again, the starch is made more available therefore increasing the digestibility.

Oats

The traditional concentrate feed for horses. They are relatively high in fibre and have a lower energy content than barley, wheat and maize. Oats are mostly fed whole, rolled or crimped, but horses must be over 1 year old and have good teeth if whole oats are to be fed.

The fibre is due to the outer husk, which has been removed in naked oats. Naked oats are therefore higher in energy and also less 'safe' to feed to horses. Many performance horses are now fed naked oats.

Barley

Barley is higher in energy than oats and lower in fibre. It is often processed to make the starch more available, by steaming, micronisation or extrusion. Extruded barley looks nothing like the original grain, for example, barley rings.

Barley tends to be used for conditioning and it is less 'safe' than oats. Some horses have an allergic reaction to barley resulting in lumpy swellings on the skin or filled legs. The barley element should then be removed from the ration.

Maize

This is high energy, low fibre and is most often fed steamed or micronised. It is more expensive and is often used to condition horses, particularly those for showing. Maize is known as corn in the USA.

Wheat

Commonly, wheat is not used as a straight due to its high cost. It contains gluten that can form a gluey mass in the gut. Wheat is very high in starch and is usually fed as a by-product such as wheat bran. Bran is the outer husk of wheat, although relatively high in protein, the quality is poor and being high in phosphorus and low in calcium can lead to bone problems. Nutritionally, it is a poor feed for horses, having had the goodness of wheat flour removed from it. Bran mashes are not necessary and this traditional practice has no place on a modern yard. The horse should not be subjected to sudden changes in diet as the gut microorganisms are affected adversely.

Sugar beet pulp

Sugar beet is technically in between a forage and a concentrate. Sugar beet looks similar to a turnip. The beet is taken to the factory where most of the sugar is removed, all that is left is fibre and pulp. At this stage it is white in colour. Molasses are then added before it is dried and shredded or pelleted.

Sugar beet is similar in energy to oats, but the energy comes from digestible fibre and not from starch (as in the cereal grains). Sugar beet may be molassed or unmolassed. Beets should be soaked in water for 24 hours before feeding. Its benefits are often underestimated. It is rich in calcium.

Compound feeds

Compound feeds, in the form of cubes or coarse mixes, have been fed to horses for many years now. Roughly, they can be divided into the following three groups:

- complete cubes or coarse mixes
- concentrate cubes or coarse mixes
- balancers – cubes or coarse mixes, or protein concentrates.

Complete cubes or coarse mixes

These are fed alone without forage and are designed to replace all the hay and concentrates in the ration. High fibre and low energy, they tend to be used for overweight ponies or when hay is scarce. Care must be taken with complete cubes, as the fibre length is too short for horses. Horses need a minimum length of fibre for efficient gut function. Some horses on high fibre cubes have started to chew wood in their search for fibre. Such cubes should be fed with a good-quality chaff.

Concentrate cubes or coarse mixes

These provide a balanced diet for all types of horses and are designed to be fed with forage and water. Different formulations are made for horses with different needs. High-protein feeds for growing stock, high-energy feeds for working horses and low-energy feeds for resting or those in light work. The deficiencies of the straights are balanced and the guesswork is removed!

Balancers – cubes or coarse mixes

These are higher in protein and designed to balance a straight such as oats. One of the most common is the 50:50 oats-to-oat balancer mix. Half the concentrate ration is oats and the other half oat balancer. The oat balancer corrects the deficiencies in the oats and the combination results in a balanced ration when fed with forage.

Coarse mixes and pellets or cubes

Coarse mixes are very popular as most of the ingredients can be seen. These usually include micronised cereals, peas and beans, and a small vitamin/mineral pellet. Molasses or syrup are then used to reduce dust levels and increase uniformity and palatability.

One of the disadvantages of coarse mixes is that some horses can leave certain ingredients and this is usually the vitamin/mineral pellet. This will result in an unbalanced ration.

Cubes or pellets are made by first grinding down the ingredients then binding them together and pushing the ground material under pressure through a dye to form the pellet. They are cheaper to make than coarse mixes and tend to be more consistent. They should be fed with a handful of chaff to ensure the horse chews then thoroughly.

All compound feeds must, by law, declare certain ingredients, and these are a very useful reference. The following information must be given:

- percentage by weight of crude oil
- percentage by weight of crude protein
- percentage by weight of crude fibre
- percentage by weight of total ash
- amounts of added vitamins A, D E [shown as international units (IU) per kg]
- total selenium content if synthetic Se has been added (in mg/kg)
- whether an antioxidant has been added.

Sell-by dates are also printed on the label and this allows the freshness of the feed to be assessed before purchase.

Quality compound feeds are expensive due to the high costs of good raw materials, nutritionists, higher quality protein, higher specification premixes and analytical equipment, not to mention the plant machinery and quality control.

Supplements and additives

There is a vast array of supplements available for horses. Supplements are substances added to the horses diet in order to balance it or correct a perceived deficiency. Feral horses have been able to balance their own diets to a large extent by seeking out herbs and plants and even specific soil areas to correct deficiencies.

Common supplements include:

- vitamin supplements, e.g. biotin
- mineral supplements, e.g. limestone flour (calcium), selenium, copper supplements
- broad-spectrum vitamin/mineral supplements, containing a range of micro-nutrients
- body salts (electrolytes) – sodium chloride, potassium, magnesium, calcium.

An additive is a substance that is added to an already balanced ration. Common additives include:

- enzymes: biological catalysts aimed to improved digestion by various means
- herbs: a natural alternative to supplements, but nutrient specifications under debate
- cod liver oil: source of vitamins A, D and E but may make feed unpalatable
- probiotics: 'live' bacteria to help recolonise the horse's gut after stress or antibiotics
- yeasts: improves the number of fibre-digesting bacteria in the hind gut.

Most horses, if fed a balanced diet, do not need a supplement. If horses are being fed poor-quality forage (i.e. low in nutrients) as the main ration, then a supplement may be necessary. Also, if a compound feed is not being fed at the manufacturer's recommended level, then a supplement may be required.

For example, an overweight horse is fed 1 kg of horse and pony cubes per day. The recommended amount may be 3 kg per day to supply all the minerals and vitamins to the horse. Therefore 1 kg will only supply one-third of that horse's requirements (excluding the forage element) and a broad-spectrum supplement containing a wide selection of vitamins and minerals may be required.

A B vitamin supplement is often used for horses who have been ill, who are in very poor condition, recovering from surgery or who have been 'over-trained'. This is given as a tonic and is very useful. This will also help to stimulate the appetite.

Body salts (electrolytes) are essential for performance horses and are often neglected. They should be given whenever the horse has been sweating after work, but fresh water must be given alongside. Salt should be freely available as a salt lick.

Guidelines for feeding supplements

- Never mix or overdose supplements without professional nutritional advice.
- A supplement should not be necessary if the compound feed is being fed at the recommended rate.
- Split the supplement between all the feeds.
- Do not add boiling water to a supplements as this will destroy the vitamins.
- Mix the supplement thoroughly into the feed.

Herbs are quite fashionable at the moment and there is a large selection available. Some of them contain quite potent chemicals and care should be taken when feeding to pregnant mares and youngstock. Always follow the recommendations given on the label.

Common herbs include:

- dandelion: laxative, tonic
- garlic: antibacterial, fly repellent, expectorant (thins mucus in respiratory tract)
- fennel: diuretic, antispasmodic, expectorant
- peppermint: tonic, antispasmodic
- valerian: calming
- thyme: antiseptic, diuretic
- rosehip: laxative, astringent
- camomile: calming, analgesic
- comfrey: eases inflammation.

Monitoring condition (see Figure 17.1)

Once a ration has been decided on for a horse and written on the feed board it is essential to monitor that horse's reaction. Does the horse eat up?

Condition score	Back	Pelvis	Comment
0			*Starvation*: Croup and hip bones sharp and prominent. Cut-up behind. Rib cage prominent.
1			*Thin*: Bones still prominent but a little more muscle definition.
2			*Approaching normal*: Hip bones and vertebrae of back defined but not prominent. *Hunters & eventers*.
3			*Getting fat*: Bones becoming more difficult to feel. *Show horses*.
4			*Obese*: Large masses of fat carried on neck quarters and back. Can only feel ribs on pressure.

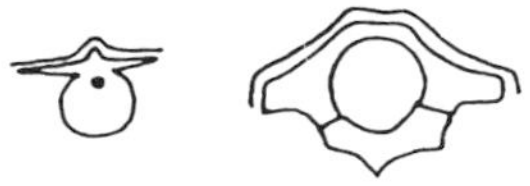

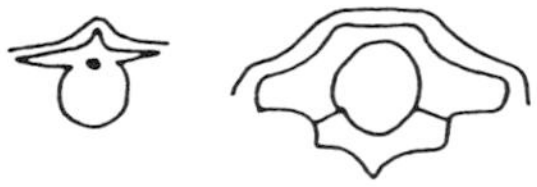

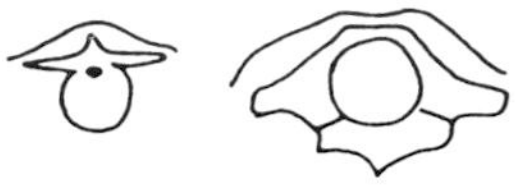

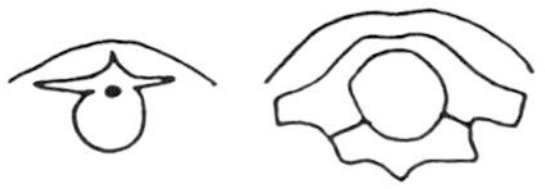

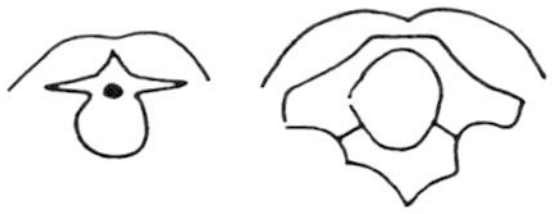

Figure 17.1. Monitoring condition.

Are temperament and performance affected? Is it gaining, losing or maintaining condition? A diet too high in starch may make the horse 'fizzy' and it will grow fatter, while too little energy will result in loss of condition and possibly a lethargic temperament. Some horses are naturally energetic no matter how little they are fed and it must be remembered that training, fitness and discipline will affect temperament. Remember as well that a horse must be regularly wormed and have its teeth checked twice a year and rasped if necessary.

Nutritional requirements of elderly horses

Elderly horses need frequent attention to their teeth, as the loss of a tooth or the formation of sharp edges and hooks can cause considerable discomfort, leading to a loss of condition. Consequently, old horses may need food that is easy to chew; stemmy hay and whole oats would not be suitable as the horse's teeth would not be able to process the food sufficiently to allow adequate digestion.

Nutrition of the sick horse

Providing the horse with a balanced ration plays an important part in the horse's ability to fight illness, and correct nutrition provides one of the body's defence mechanisms. Proper feeding of the sick horse should always be considered as an integral part of the nursing and therapeutic regime.

The task of feeding a sick horse can be difficult and tiresome; the horse's appetite is likely to be depressed, swallowing may be difficult and the function of the gut may be disturbed. Any upset in gut function may lead to dehydration and a disturbance of the electrolyte balance (the ratio of salts in the body), all of which may occur just when the horse's metabolic requirements may be substantially greater. This means that there is often marked weight loss during illness, with a resultant decrease in the horse's defence capacity and prolonged illness and convalescence.

The sick horse's diet must have several special characteristics:

- palatability
- good-quality protein
- fibre
- minerals and vitamins.

Palatability

The sick horse must be provided with the most palatable feed possible to encourage eating. Barn dried hay or haylage is ideal if the horse has previously been fed poor-quality hay. Molasses, mashes and succulents can all be fed providing that the food is fresh. If swallowing is difficult, the feeds should be soft and any carrots cut into very small pieces. If chewing is a problem the horse may need a liquid diet.

Feeding little and often is vital for the sick horse with up to eight feeds a day, including first thing in the morning and last thing at night. Any rejected food should be removed immediately. Soaking or damping the hay may help and will also mean that the horse is taking in water. Plenty of fresh, clean water must always be available, and it should be changed frequently. If the horse is using an automatic drinking system, close it off and give the water by bucket so that you can monitor the amount the horse drinks.

Good-quality protein

The protein content of the sick horse's diet is more important than the amount of energy the food is providing, because the horse is not active but protein is needed for the repair of body tissue. Good-quality grass nuts, stud cubes and soyabean meal are all high in good-quality protein. Care must be taken not to overfeed the horse as recovery proceeds. Beware of feeding high starch feeds to horses at box rest.

Fibre

Fibre is important in maintaining normal gut function, but as the fibre content of the diet increases so its digestibility falls and a compromise has to be reached. Molassed sugar beet pulp is a useful and palatable source of fibre.

Minerals and vitamins

The sick horse may become severely dehydrated and it is important to supply a suitable source of electrolytes to help restore the fluid balance of the body. A supplement of minerals, vitamins and/or amino acids may be recommended by the vet, depending on the horse's blood profile: an anaemic horse would require iron, folic acid and vitamin B_{12} as well as his normal broad-spectrum supplement. As always, calcium and salt are important. A performance level vitamin and mineral supplement is ideal.

Watering horses

Water makes up 65–75% of an adult horse's bodyweight and 75–80% of a foal's. Water is vital for life; it acts as a fluid medium for digestion and for the movement of food through the gut. It is necessary for growth and milk production, and is necessary to make good the losses through the lungs, skin, faeces and urine. Restricted water intake will depress the horse's appetite and reduce feed intake, resulting in loss of condition. Under most circumstances the horse should have free access to fresh, clean water at all times. After hard, fast work during which the horse has been denied water, care should be taken to cool the horse before allowing substantial amounts of water. Excessive consumption of cold water by hot horses can cause colic or laminitis.

The 'rules of watering'

- A constant supply of fresh, clean water should always be available.
- If this is not possible, water at least three times a day in winter and six times a day in summer.
- Water a hot or tired horse with water which has had the chill taken off it.
- If a bucket of water is left constantly with the horse, swill out the bucket and change the water at least twice a day, topping it up as necessary throughout the day. Standing water becomes unpalatable.
- Horses that have been deprived of water should be given small quantities frequently until their thirst is quenched. They must not be allowed to gorge themselves on water.
- During continuous work, water the horses as often as possible, at least every 2 hours. Hunters should be allowed to drink on the way home.

- If horses have a constant supply of fresh, clean water there should be no need to deprive the horse of water before racing or fast work. However, the horse's water can be removed from the stable 2 hours before the race or competition, if thought necessary.

The horse at grass

Access to rivers and streams can be a good way of watering horses at grass provided the river contains running water with a gravel bottom and a good approach. Shallow water and a sandy bottom many result in small quantities of sand being ingested, collecting in the stomach and eventually causing sand colic.

Ponds tend to be stagnant and are rarely suitable; usually it is best to fence them off and provide alternative watering arrangements.

Filled from a piped water supply, field troughs provide the best method of watering horses at grass. Troughs should be 1–2 m (3–6 ft) in length and about 0.5 m (18 in) deep. There must be an outlet at the bottom so that they can be emptied and scrubbed regularly. The trough should be on well-drained land, clear of trees so that the ground around the trough does not get poached and the trough does not fill up with leaves. During freezing weather troughs should be checked twice a day and the ice broken if necessary. They must be free from sharp edges or projections, such as a tap, which might injure a horse.

If the trough is tap-filled, the tap should be at ground level and the pipe from the tap to the trough fitted close to the side and edge of the trough. The best method is to have a self filling ballcock arrangement in an enclosed compartment at one end of the trough. Ideally, the trough should be sited along a fence or recessed into it (Figure 17.2), rather than at right angles to it or in front of it. If not in the fence line the trough should be at least three to four horse's lengths into the field so that there is free access all round and horses cannot be trapped behind it.

The stabled horse

Stable horses are usually offered water in buckets or automatic drinkers, both of which have advantages and disadvantages.

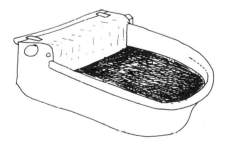

Figure 17.2. Automatic drinker.

Buckets

Buckets can be placed on the floor, in the manger, hung in brackets or suspended from a hook or ring at breast height. They should be placed in a corner away from the manger, hayrack and door, but should still be visible from the door for checking. Providing water in buckets is time-consuming, heavy work and wasteful on water; they must be emptied, swilled out and refilled at least twice a day, and topped up three or four times a day. Horses frequently knock buckets over and may damage themselves by getting a leg caught between the bucket and the metal handle. However, they have three advantages: you can monitor how much the horse is drinking – a change in a horse's drinking habits may be the first sign of illness; buckets are a very simple method of providing water which cannot go wrong; they are cheap – though the cheapest buckets will not last long.

Automatic drinkers

Although expensive to install, automatic drinkers (Figure 17.2) are an asset in a large yard, saving time and effort. They should be fairly deep so that the horse can take a full drink, they should be cleaned out regularly, sited away from the manger and hayrack, and well-insulated to stop the pipes freezing in winter. Some horses are reluctant to drink from the small noisy automatic drinkers and water intake cannot be monitored easily. Each drinker should have its own tap so that if it malfunctions, or one needs to monitor the horse's water intake using buckets, it can be switched off.

Part 4
Work in the stable yard

Chapter 18
Handling horses

Basic handling of horses

Potentially, horses are dangerous animals with a natural and inherent desire to flee from perceived danger. Handlers must be aware of this so that the horse does not become unmanageable. Also, some horses may be persistently difficult to handle and they require understanding and careful management to instil confidence.

Young foals are playful, but if not taught good manners through rewarding good behaviour, they may develop into adult horses that are dangerous. A colt foal rearing and playing with the handler will soon turn into a 3-year old with a problem. The time to instil good manners is at the foal stage.

Horses should not be taken for granted and the handler should be aware that even the most placid horse may become frightened and kick out or bolt.

Horses respond to a kind voice and when working in the stable it is important to talk to the horse in a calm manner. Tone of voice may be used as a subtle training aid, as horses have an acute sense of hearing.

Handlers should, with experience, develop a perception of potentially hazardous situations and be prepared. Talking quietly without fear to horses will calm them down.

Approaching the horse in the stable

Horses should be responsive to the handler's voice. When approaching horses the voice should be used to make them aware of your presence. This will prevent them being surprised and spooking. The horse should be taught to stand back from the door as the handler enters and certainly should not barge out through a partially open door, as this may be extremely dangerous. If the horse is standing with its head in the corner, then call the horse to you or encourage with some food.

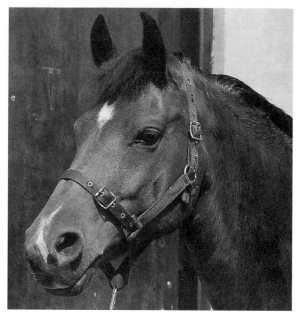

Figure 18.1. A correctly fitted headcollar.

Putting on a headcollar or halter

Control of the horse in the stable and when leading outside to the field is important. A headcollar or halter is an essential part of equipment and should be put on as follows:

- unfasten headcollar and uncoil the rope
- slip both safely over one arm
- stand at the side of the head on the near side of the horse
- place the rope gently over the horses neck, just below the poll
- hold the cheekpieces of the headcollar in both hands
- slip the noseband over the horses nose
- lift the head piece and gently flip over the poll with the right hand
- catch the end with the left hand and fasten
- tuck excess length of headpiece through the headcollar ring out of the way
- clip on the rope under the jaw with the open side facing away from it.

Figure 18.1 shows a correctly fitted headcollar.

Securing the horse

It is safe practice to tie the horse up when the handler is working in the stable. The horse should be tied with a quick-release knot to a string loop on the

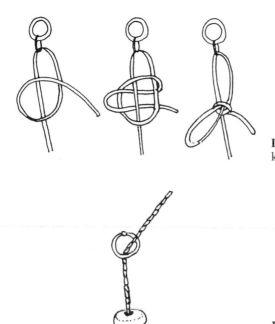

Figure 18.2. Trying a quick-release knot.

Figure 18.3. A sliding log and rope arrangement for securing a horse.

tie-up ring (Figure 18.2). The string loop is designed to break if the horse panics and pulls back. Baling twine is practically unbreakable and should not be used. Horses should never be tied to objects that may move, for example, the stable door or a gate. Mares with foals and untrained young horses should not be tied up.

Horses kept in stalls are tied to a rope that passes through a ring and is then fastened to a sliding log by means of a knot at the end of the rope. As the horse moves in the stall the heavy log takes up the slack of the rope so that there is no danger of the horse putting a leg over a loose rope (Figure 18.3). Horses may also be cross-tied using two ropes, one from each side of the headcollar, passing to tie-up rings on two posts or two sides of a stall. As this technique limits the range of movement, this is a useful way of keeping the horse still and secure while handling the horse.

The handler must speak when approaching a horse that is tied up to ensure that the horse knows that the handler is there. Do not walk straight up to the horse's bottom and pat it; let the horse see you and give reassurance before touching.

Leading a horse in hand off-road

Before taking any horse out of the stable, the handler must be sure that he or she is in control; a quiet, reliable horse can be led in a correctly fitting, sound headcollar with a leap rope (Figure 18.4). The handler should be wearing suitable shoes and gloves – nothing hurts like a rope burn – and should never wrap the lead rope around the hand. An overhand knot should be tied in the end of the lead rope. Even so, a naughty horse can quickly learn to pull a short lead out of the handler's hands and if there is any doubt about how the horse is going to behave, for example, a young horse or a horse that has been in the stable for a while, the handler should wear a hard hat and lead the horse in a bridle or head-collar with a lunge line attached.

Care must be taken when leading the horse through openings such as stable doors or gateways; do not hurry or take short cuts – the stable door should be open wide and the horse led straight and slowly so that the hip does not catch. If there is a danger of the gate or door swinging closed on the horse, it should be fastened back or held by a helper; horses that have had a door or gate swing shut on them may rush, increasing the risk of banging themselves or slipping. Once the horse is in the stable, carefully turn it to face the door making sure that it does not slip and then close the door, release the horse and leave the stable.

The horse should be led from the near (left) side with the right hand holding the rope close to the headcollar and the remaining rope coiled in the left hand. The horse should walk freely forwards with the handler at the horse's shoulder. Do not pull on the rope or look back at the horse. If it hangs back either get a helper to encourage or carry a long whip in the left hand which can be used to tap the hindquarters.

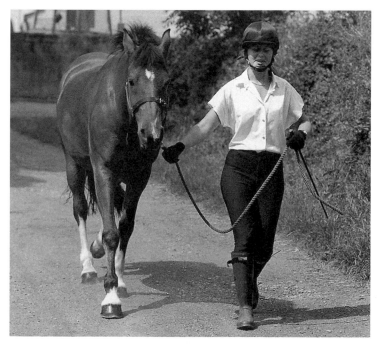

Figure 18.4. A quiet horse being led safely.

Presenting a horse for inspection

At some time in its life the horse will have to trot up in hand – it may be for the vet to check soundness or to show the horse off to a potential purchaser – and it is important for both horse and handler to know what they are doing. Ideally, there will be a level, straight stretch of hard surface about 40 m (120 ft) long so that there is enough room for the horse to trot forward freely, pull up and turn.

First, the horse should be made to stand up straight, square and with its weight equally balanced on all four feet, with the handler standing in front. If the horse is wearing a bridle, the reins should be taken over the head and each rein held a little below the bit either side of the head to keep the horse straight and still. When asked, the handler should move to the horse's near side and walk the horse in a straight line away from the examiner until asked to turn. The horse should then be turned to the right, away from the handler, and walked back straight towards the examiner. This is then repeated in trot allowing the horse a few walk strides to balance itself and get straight after turning, before being asked to trot. The horse should not be pulled, held too tight or have his head turned towards the handler as this will prevent the head 'nodding' – the sign of lameness the vet will be looking for.

Turning out into a field

Horses can become quite excited in anticipation of being turned out into a field and the handler must be suitably equipped with gloves, stout shoes and, possibly, a hard hat. The horse should also be suitably restrained. If a normally quiet horse becomes excited and is only wearing a headcollar it can give more control if the rope is placed over the horse's nose from the off side and secured through the noseband of the headcollar. The field gate should be opened wide enough to avoid any risk of the horse banging itself. If there are other horses barging at the gate, help should be sought rather than struggling to squeeze the led horse through and risking injury to horse and handler.

Once in the field, turn the horse, close the gate and release the horse. Horses should never be chased once released. If several horses are being turned out at the same time they should all be led well into the field, turned to face the fence, well apart from each other and released at the same time. The last person in the field closes the gate and tells everybody else when ready to let their horse go. Horses often have a buck and a kick, so turning them to the fence means that they have to turn around to gallop off, giving the handlers a chance to step back out of the way.

Every time a horse is turned out into the field a quick check should be made for hazards such as litter, broken fencing and poisonous plants, and action taken as necessary – either clearing up the problem or reporting it to the person in charge.

Catching a horse in the field

Depending on the horse's temperament, catching one horse in a field containing several horses can either be easy or a very frustrating, not to say dangerous, exercise. Go prepared with a suitable headcollar and rope and a few nuts in a bucket if necessary – if there are several horses a bucket can be liability as they all crowd around to get a mouthful. In this situation the reward may be better hidden in your pocket and just offered to the horse you are trying to catch; this is one situation where giving a horse a titbit is justified.

Having shut the gate, approach the horse's shoulder slowly and quietly with the headcollar discreetly held over your arm or shoulder; do not march straight up to the horse; almost pretend it is not that horse you are after. Avoid staring at the horse. When you are close, speak and offer the food, give the horse a couple of nuts, a pat and place the rope around the neck before fitting the headcollar. This way you can discourage the horse from moving before you have got the headcollar on.

Quietly lead the horse to the gate, avoiding the other horses, open the gate, lead the horse through, turn the horse and close the gate. Assistance may be needed at this point if all the horses decide they want to come with you. Squeezing your horse past may result in it getting caught in the gate or the other horses escaping. If you are on your own, scatter some feed on the ground away from the gate to distract the other horses while you lead the caught horse out of the field.

Catching a difficult horse

Some horses are always difficult to catch, while others may become upset by other horses galloping about or by wild, windy weather. Some may let you catch them and then pull away from you; again be prepared and use a headcollar and lunge line or bridle to lead the naughty horse. If possible get help and quietly aim to confine the horse in the corner of the field, with one person either side. Each should carry a headcollar and have some feed for the horse. Never try to herd or chase the horse as it will only make it worse, and be very careful that the cornered horse does not spin round and kick out or gallop over the top of you.

Occasionally, leaving the horse, giving it time to settle down and coming back later will work; horses do not like to be ignored. Talking to other horses in the field or catching another horse may excite curiosity and make the horse more amenable to being caught because it thinks it is missing out on something! Always assume that youngsters are going to be difficult to catch; this way they are unlikely to get into bad habits.

Simple methods of restraint

It is always safer to have an assistant when treating a horse, trimming or clipping, and it is important that the helper is not nervous and is alert, aware and knows what to do. Always start off quietly; a small feed may be enough to distract a horse, or it may respond to being held in the bridle. Do not just put a twitch on the horse without any regard for the horse's temperament.

A simple and gentle restraint is to hold up a horse's front leg; the helper should always be on the same side as the person treating the horse as the horse is more likely to jump away from the treatment than towards it. The horse should be untied and the foot picked up as if the helper is about to pick out the foot and then held by the toe so that the helper can stand upright. Care should be taken that the horse does not snatch the foot away and get a leg over the rope that the helper is holding. If the helper feels about to let go of the foot the other person must be warned so that they can stop what they are doing; remember the other person is relying on the helper for safety.

Grasping a large fold of skin in the middle of the horse's neck frequently is enough to make the horse lower its head and be submissive, and is a useful emergency restraint (Figure 18.5).

Some horses will need more severe restraint and here a twitch is used. A twitch can be made from a piece of broom handle 75–150 cm (2.5–5 ft) long with a piece of stout cord or plaited baling twine looped through a hole drilled near

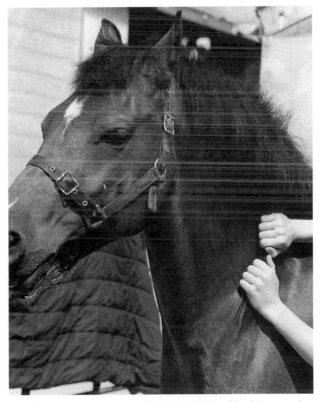

Figure 18.5. Grasping the skin on the neck can provide effective restraint.

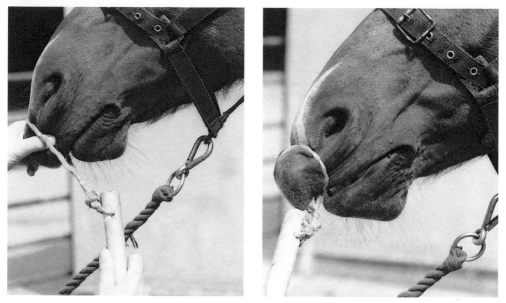

Figure 18.6. Applying a twitch.

the end of the stick. The loop of the twitch is passed over the hand and put on the horse by grasping the upper lip, sliding the loop onto the lip and twisting it tight, adjusting the tension according to the horse's response (Figure 18.6). The twitch must be put on and taken off quickly or horses will learn to fight it. Most horses react well to the twitch, becoming quiet and amenable. However, a few may try to avoid it, becoming quite dangerous. A sedative or tranquilliser prescribed by the vet may be used for these horses. The horse's ears or tongue should never be twitched and the twitch must not be left on for prolonged periods of time.

Another humane twitch is shaped like a large nutcracker that is passed round the horse's upper lip and then fastened at the open end by a piece of cord. This twitch can be used without an assistant, but this is not recommended because if the horse panics it may be difficult to catch the horse and take the twitch off.

Chapter 19
The daily routine

Yard routine

Routine is as important to those working in the yard as it is to the equine inhabitants; an efficient, yet flexible, routine ensures that all the necessary tasks are complete and gives the horses peace of mind. The routine to be followed will vary from yard to yard depending on the type of horse and the priorities of the yard manager. The following routine is rather old-fashioned and would be suitable for hunters or competition horses. Many livery yards would not start until 8 am while racing yards tend to start earlier.

7.00 am	*Morning stables*
	Check the horses and refill water buckets
	Tie up, adjust rugs and give haynets
	Muck out
	Quarter
8.00 am	Feed horses, sweep yard and have breakfast
9.00 am	Skip out stables
	Tack up and exercise (perhaps ride and lead)
	On return allow to drink and stale
11.30 am	Groom and replace rugs. (If there is a second group of horses to exercise, grooming may be done at evening stables)
12.30 pm	Water, hay and give lunchtime feed
	Set fair stable and yard
1.00 pm	Break for lunch
2.00 pm	Carry out daily or weekly chores
	Clean and put away tack
4.00 pm	*Evening stables*
	Tie up, skip out, pick out feet, water and rug up
	Set fair stable, give hay and sweep yard
4.30 pm	Give teatime feed
7.00 pm	*Late-night check*
	Give last feed, water and hay if necessary
	Adjust rugs
	Skip out stables

This routine ensures that the horse's health is checked before being fed and leaves the horse in peace and quiet to eat its breakfast. However, in many yards the first job of the day is feeding; this is often carried out by a senior member of staff 30 minutes before the rest of the staff arrive. It is important to note and report back whether the horse has eaten all the previous night's feed and if there are any signs of ill-health (the signs of health that should be monitored in an early morning inspection are detailed later in this chapter). Mucking out, tidying the muck heap and sweeping the yard are normally done before breakfast, helping to work up a healthy appetite!

Over breakfast it will be decided which person is to ride which horse and how much exercise the horse needs. Once the horse returns from exercise it is cared for promptly and rugged up again. Many yards try to get all horses ridden in the morning. The horses are then given hay and fed, and staff have their lunch break.

The afternoon may be needed for tasks such as clipping and trimming. After the weekly chores any horses not yet fully groomed are attended to and all of the horses are 'done up' for the night. Droppings are picked up from the stables (skipping or skepping out), the banks and the bed are tidied up (setting fair), rugs are changed or straightened, the horses given hay and water, and the yard swept. Finally, the horses are fed and the yard is locked up for the night. Where possible the horses are given a late-night check, water buckets are topped up, rugs straightened, and hay and a late feed given if it is in the ration.

On top of the routine outlined above there are other jobs that need to be done. Every day the water buckets and feed mangers must be scrubbed out and automatic drinkers cleaned. Once a week the horses' shoes must be checked so that a shoeing list can be drawn up, the grooming kits should be washed and each horse's rugs shaken out. Yard maintenance routines are described in Chapter 20.

Housing

Although horses are hardy creatures and may be kept at grass all year round, it is often desirable that they should be housed in stables. Stabling provides protection for the horse and convenience for its owner. A horse that is fit has lost its protective fat; a groomed horse no longer has the natural protective oils in its coat. Such horses need protection from the elements. Where the horse is clipped out, as is the case with many working horses, it has lost its coat. Stables protect the horse from the cold, wet and wind during the winter months, and from heat, flies and sun during the summer.

From the owner's point of view, having a stabled horse is a convenience. The horse is at hand, is clean and dry, and is easier to feed and water. Even where adequate pasture is available, stabling the horse saves the grass. Indeed, it is possible to keep a horse without pasture at all, provided it is adequately housed. This is done at some racing stables by choice, and of necessity by some horse-owners in towns. Stabling also provides security and safety. This is especially so where the stables are near the house.

There are many other advantages of stabling. Obviously, it is easier to monitor and control the horse's food and water intake when it is inside. The stabled horse is easier to control, both as regards exercise and, where necessary, restraint. Stabling is, indeed, essential in cases of ill-health or sickness when isolation is desirable.

Requirements of a stable

Sound stabling is a good investment from every point of view. Stabling need not necessarily be grand, but ideally it should be purpose built. Although this represents a substantial capital investment, in most cases a stable block adds to the value of the property. Brick- or block-built stables are the best, but are very expensive, and most private owners today are content with stabling of the sectional wooden type. This is available from a number of manufacturers and varies considerably in both quality and price.

Whatever type of stabling is used, there are certain essentials to be borne in mind. Stables should:

- Be warm and dry.
- Have dry foundations.
- Have free drainage.
- Have good ventilation with adequate fresh air yet free from draughts.
- Have good light, both natural and artificial.
- Have a water and electricity supply.
- Be accessible.
- Be arranged to minimise on labour.
- Be *safe* – no projections, and with all electric wiring and lighting protected.
- Be able to be thoroughly disinfected.
- Have adequate fire precautions.

Wood, brick and blocks create a better environment than galvanised iron sheets or asbestos. Galvanised iron, in particular, has no insulation value and buildings constructed wholly or partly of this material are prone to condensation and overheating. This to some extent can be overcome by providing adequate insulation and boarding over the interior of the stable.

Siting the stables

The ideal site probably does not exist. However, the site should be level and well drained and, if starting from scratch, a concrete base should be installed with a good drainage system. The best ground to build on has a sub-soil of gravel or deep sand which gives a firm base and is dry and free-draining. Rocky soil such as limestone, chalk and granite is next best while clay, peat or marshy soils are the worst and need extensive drainage surrounding the stable yard. Buildings require proper foundations, and in the case of new buildings, planning permission is needed. Approval by the local authority under the Building Regulations is always necessary. The stables should be protected from the prevailing wind, particularly from the north and east. Too many surrounding trees and buildings can prevent the free circulation of air, which is essential to health. If the stabling is to be erected near a dwelling house, the stable block should be sited downwind of the house. Consideration must also be given to ease of access, not only for people, but also for routine and emergency vehicles.

The stable block

Today, most private owners prefer loose boxes (see Figure 19.1) as opposed to stalls where the horse is tied up. However, if converting an existing range of outbuildings not designed as stabling, the arrangement may dictate that the buildings are better converted to stalls.

The stable block itself, large or small, consists not only of loose boxes or stalls, but also of ancillary accommodation. Provision must be made for the storage of feed in the form of concentrates, and of hay and straw or alternative litter. A secure tack room is needed, and there must be somewhere to dry rugs and so on.

In a commercial stable there are additional requirements, e.g. an office and possibly a staff restroom or lounge. In every case, various items need to be stored: tools, wheelbarrows, horse-box or trailer, etc., and there must always be somewhere to dispose of manure.

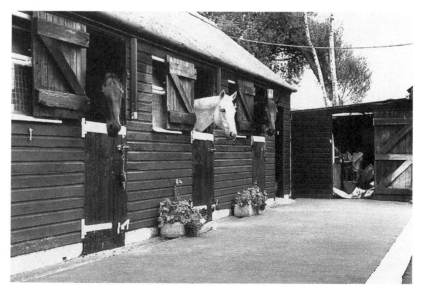

Figure 19.1. Individual loose boxes.

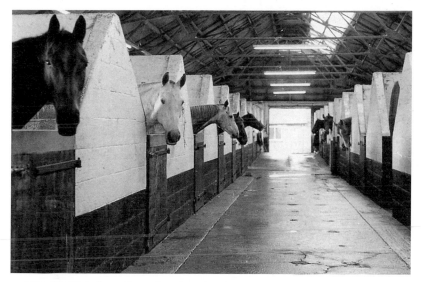

Figure 19.2. Stabling in an 'American barn' system.

A variety of housing systems, modern (see Figure 19.2) and traditional, are in use. Stalls are traditional, but still have their place; however, in modern practice, loose boxes with ancillary accommodation are generally the answer.

Choosing a loose box

Size

The first requirement for a loose box is that there should be adequate head room with a minimum of 3 m (10 ft). The recommended dimensions for loose boxes are:

- large hunter: 3.7 m × 4.3 m (12 ft × 14 ft)
- pony: 3.7 m × 3.0 m (12 ft × 10 ft)
- foaling box: 4.6 m × 4.6 m (15 ft × 15 ft).

The single box should give not less than 42 m³ (1500 ft³) space per horse.

Stalls should be 1.8 m (6 ft) wide by 2.7 m (9 ft) long, with a passage behind with a minimum width of 1.8 m (6 ft). Dividing partitions should be 2 m (6.5 ft) high at the front and 1.5 m (5 ft) high at the rear.

The aim is to provide a minimum of 28 m³ (1000 ft³) of air for each horse housed in the building.

Roof

The stable and its roof should be designed to keep the temperature below 15°C (60°F), even in the hottest weather. Horses tolerate cold, but high temperatures cause them distress. A sloping roof provides a large air space with light and good ventilation. Flat roofs are used if there are lofts or living quarters overhead, but this may reduce ventilation. The roofing material used should be durable, quiet, non-flammable and insulating. The ceiling inside the box should be non-conductive or moisture in the warm air coming off the horse will condense as it hits the cold surface and drip onto the horse. There must be an adequate air outlet at the highest point of each stable.

Floor

Floors should be laid on a solid foundation and raised above the outside ground. They should be non-slip, smooth, durable and insulating so that they do not strike cold to the horse. Concrete is the most commonly used material today, but possible alternatives are brick, tarmac, slats or chalk. Floors should be level from side to side but slope front to rear or vice versa to allow for drainage; slopes are usually 1 in 60 in the loose box and 1 in 40 in any gutters. There should not be an open drain in the stable; instead, there should be a trapped drain at the front or back. The drain should be free of sharp angles and closed; underground drains must be checked regularly.

Stable doors

The stable door should be 2.4 m (8 ft) high for horses and a minimum of 1.2 m (4 ft) wide. It should open outwards or sideways. The door should be divided in two, the top part being hinged outwards and left fastened against the wall so that the horse can look out. The bottom half of the door should be about 1.4 m (4.5 ft) high for horses with a metal covering along the top edge to prevent the horse chewing the wood. Weaving grids or grilles can be attached to the bottom door if necessary. Weaving grids usefully limit horses chewing the door and its surrounds so are fitted as standard in some yards. Door latches should be horse-proof, strong and easy to use, and should not project on the edge of the door when it is open. Proper stable bolts are best, with a kick bolt at the bottom.

Windows

Each loose box should have an opening window protected by a grille or mesh. The best is the hopper type 'Sheringham window' which directs cold air upwards so that it mixes with the warm air in the stable. Windows on the wall opposite the door greatly improve light in the stable; the also enable a pleasant breeze to be available in summer.

Kicking boards

The walls of the boxes should have strong kicking boards up to 1.2 m (4 ft) high. These give the horse protection and can have ridges along them to help prevent the horse getting cast.

Stable fittings

Generally speaking, the fewer stable fittings the better – considerable care is needed to make them accident-proof.

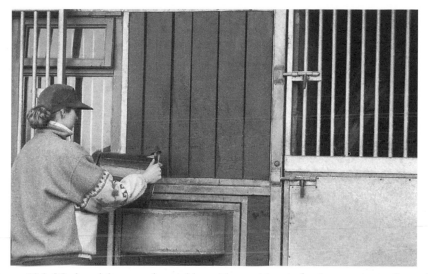

Figure 19.3. Modern labour-saving stables with provision to feed concentrates from the outside.

There should be securely fitted tie rings – one at chest height and one at eye level. Feed mangers should be placed in the corner 1.1 m (3.5 ft) from the ground. The manger should be large, with a rim too broad for crib-biting, smooth and with rounded corners. Some boxes are designed so that there is access to the manger without going in to the stable, thus saving time and increasing efficiency and safety.

Hay may be fed from a rack at horse's eye level but this is an unnatural position for the horse and hay seeds can fall into the eyes; they are, however, more labour-saving than hay nets. An alternative is a large deep hay manger but there must be suitable provision for removing debris that would otherwise accumulate below it. Many people prefer to feed hay on the floor. Again, labour economy requires that hay be fed without having to open stable doors (see Figure 19.3).

Automatic drinkers are efficient and labour saving although costly to install – they must each have a cut-off tap and the whole system must cope with frost. The amount the horse is drinking usually cannot be monitored with drinkers. They should be placed away from the manger and hayrack. Strong plastic buckets are an adequate alternative where labour is cheap: they should have the handle removed and be placed in the corner near the door. Alternatively, the bucket handle can be clipped to a ring. Empty bucket-holding brackets are potentially dangerous.

Lighting
Artificial lighting in each box is important as there must be adequate light to work both early and late during the winter months. Electric light fittings should

be protected by a wire grille or be of the self-contained type. All fittings should be tamper-proof, and switches and power points are better outside the box protected from rain.

Stalls

Stalls are individually partitioned areas in which the horse is tied up with hay, feed and water placed in front of it. Stalls are also useful as day standings for horses brought in from the field, such as in riding schools. Stalls allow more horses to be housed in a smaller space and are warm, labour saving, inexpensive and require less bedding material. Mares are particularly easy to muck out in stalls.

Yards

Young horses or riding-school ponies may be yarded, in other words several are housed together in a large pen inside a barn. Yards are usually deep littered with straw. Providing that they are watched for bullying at feeding time and no single horse is being 'picked on' this is a natural way to keep horses inside as they are herd animals. In some yards the horses are tethered apart at feeding times.

The stable environment

The horse's respiratory system must be kept healthy if the horse is to perform at its best. All stabled horses face a constant challenge to their lungs due to dust, mould spores, mites, viruses, bacteria, humidity and noxious gases (including ammonia) present in the stable environment. This challenge can be reduced using 'dust-extracted' bedding, paper and shavings, and by feeding soaked hay and semi-wilted forages.

Arguably, the single most important factor in reducing this respiratory challenge is to ensure that the stable is adequately ventilated. Many stables are poorly ventilated due to the widely held misconception that good ventilation leads to cold and draughty boxes where horses 'don't do well'. With the correct positioning and size of air inlets and outlets and the use of air-baffling techniques, there is no reason why a well-ventilated box cannot provide a 'comfortable' environment. Cold, fresh stables are better than warm, stuffy ones – the horse can always wear an extra rug. The only temperature change likely to be harmful results in chills caused by hot, tired horses standing in a draught. Essential for good stable environment are:

• Generous air movement, free from draughts.
• A dry atmosphere with no condensation.
• A reasonably uniform temperature.
• Dry flooring with good drainage.

Ventilation

Good ventilation provides a constant supply of fresh air, removing airborne microorganisms, noxious gases and excess moisture. Natural ventilation relies on three forces to provide air movement:

- the stack effect: warm air rises and is replaced by cool air
- aspiration: as wind passes over the roof air is sucked out
- perflation: air movement from side to side and end to end of a building.

The stack effect is the key to natural ventilation – air warmed by the horse's body rises creating a flow of air through the stable.

Air inlets should be designed so that fresh air is evenly distributed to all parts of the stable without creating low-level draughts, with a generous air change rate above the horse and gentle currents at horse level. Inlets may be at the top half of the stable door, hopper and louvre vents and windows. Hopper windows should open inwards with side cheeks to reduce down-draughts. The aim is to direct incoming air above the horse, with secondary currents providing ventilation at horse level.

Air outlets should be at the highest point of the stable roof – in a pitched roof building the air outlet should be a ridge vent. A pitch of 15° or more is recommended; a lower roof pitch will inhibit air movement and may limit the available air capacity.

There has been much debate about correct ventilation rates for stables, often quoted as the number of air changes per hour or as cubic metres per hour per kilogram body weight. The aim is to avoid stagnant air or draughts. The optimum ventilation rate is determined by the percentage of dust and mould spores in the air. As a general rule, a stable with a high air volume per horse will have a lower requirement for air changes and vice versa. Where horses occupy shared air space in American barn-type stabling, a higher air change rate is needed. If the natural ventilation is not adequate electric fans may have to be installed; such a system must meet minimum ventilation rates, avoid creating draughts and easily be controlled manually.

Beds and bedding

One important aspect of stable management is to provide a clean and safe environment for the horse. This involves 'mucking out', the one job that all grooms are determined not to spend the rest of their lives doing. Mucking out is much like doing the housework – a boring, menial task that is repeated every day while being taken completely for granted by the inhabitants of the house! Yet providing and maintaining suitable bedding is essential to the horse's health and fitness.

A bed is necessary to:

- prevent injury and encourage the horse to lie down
- prevent draughts and keep the horse's lower leg warm

- encourage staling and absorb or drain fluid
- cushion the feet
- keep the horse clean.

Types of bedding material

Ideally, the bed should be economical, dry, soft, absorbent of fluid and gases, clean to use, easily obtainable, good quality, not harmful if eaten, light in colour and readily disposable. Few materials can satisfy all these criteria.

Straw

There are three common types of straw that can be used for bedding horses: wheat, barley and oat straw. Generally, wheat straw is considered to be the best as it is less palatable to horses and they are less likely to eat it. It is also said to be harder and shorter than the other straws making it easier to handle. However, the horse owner is not always in a position to choose which sort of straw to buy and it is more important that the straw is free from dust and mould. Straw is less absorbent than some other beddings and is best suited to a stable that drains well. Wastage also tends to be greater as it is more difficult to separate clean and dirty straw than, say, clean and dirty shavings.

Straw will rot down and can be spread onto fields as a fertiliser. However, disposal of straw muck heaps is becoming more difficult and European regulations look set to escalate the problem. Although cheap and easily available, straw is not a suitable bedding for horses with a respiratory problem and an alternative should be sought. Dust-extracted chopped straw packed into plastic bags is available; this is more expensive than ordinary straw and may still be eaten by the horse. Hemp straw can also be used; it is highly absorbent.

Wood shavings

Increasing numbers of horses appear to be suffering from respiratory disorders and in an attempt to make the horse's environment as dust-free as possible shavings have become a very popular bedding material. Shavings are compressed and packed into plastic bales and can be bought singly or stored outside, an advantage for the one-horse owner who does not have much storage space. Alternatively, the shavings can be bought loose. Shavings are highly absorbent, suiting a poorly drained stable or a deep litter system. Horses are also unlikely to eat shavings making it a very popular bedding for competition horses. One minor disadvantage is that it does tend to get everywhere; rugs need to be shaken out thoroughly and shavings are not a suitable bed for a foaling box. Shavings take a long time to rot down so disposal can be a problem.

Paper

Shredded paper is another dust-free bedding which is highly absorbent. Its use is not so widespread for several reasons: it is expensive, unappealing to the eye and difficult to get rid of. The shreds of paper are very light and tend to blow in the wind so it is useful to put a muck sack over the barrow on the way to the muck heap.

Peat moss

Shavings have largely replaced peat moss which is a dark, dusty and highly absorbent bedding. The dark colour gives the stable a dull look and makes mucking out more of a chore as the droppings and wet patches soon become lost in the bed and regular skipping out is essential. It is very expensive and is sold in plastic-wrapped bales which can be stored outside. It is inedible.

Other materials

The search for economical dust-free bedding continues, with one of the least conventional alternatives being rubber matting covering the stable floor; the matting allows urine to drain away and appears to be comfortable and warm for the horse to lie on as well as being non-slip. As muck disposal becomes more difficult it may be that rubber stable floorings become more popular.

Mucking out equipment

Forks, rakes, shovels and barrows are all potential hazards in a busy stable yard. Observe these guidelines for safety's sake:

* Never leave tools where a horse can reach them and do not put barrows in the stable doorway if the horse is not tied up.
* Store tools out of the way of passing people and animals.
* Do not use tools in need of repair and make sure repairs are safe – string holding something together is not safe.
* During mucking out, prop up outside the stable those tools not in use.
* Move the horse out of the way so that you never have to use the fork close to it.
* Stout footwear is essential as it is only too easy to stab one's foot with the sharp prongs of the fork. Many people wear gloves for protection and hygiene.
* String or plastic from forage or bedding must be disposed of safely in a special bin and not left lying round the yard to cause a hazard.
* Wheelbarrows should be rinsed daily and the remaining tools washed weekly to prevent the muck and urine causing them to rot prematurely.

A three- or four-pronged fork is needed to muck out straw, while a special many-pronged fork is used for shavings. Straw beds can be laid with a two-pronged fork. A brush and shovel are needed to tidy up, while all waste is put into a wheelbarrow or muck sack. A skip or skep is a small container used for removing droppings during the day; plastic laundry baskets make an inexpensive skip.

Caring for a straw bed

Ideally, the horse should be placed in a separate box while mucking out takes place; this is better for his wind, avoiding the dust that is shaken up during mucking out, and allows more efficient and safe mucking out. If this is not possible use a headcollar, tie the horse to a loop of string on the tie ring and move the horse to one side of the box so that all obvious piles of droppings can be picked up. Remove water buckets and then, starting at the door, use a fork to throw clean straw to the back or one side of the stable. As the straw is shaken the heavier, soiled material falls through the prongs and can be collected on a muck sack in a wheelbarrow.

Once a week clear and sweep the floor, disinfect it and allow it to dry. The horse should never be asked to stand on bare floor as this is slippery. If the horse has to stay in the box put a thin layer of straw down to stop slipping and yet allow the floor to dry. Regularly turn the banks of straw at the sides of the stable to prevent mould forming; thus throw the bedding to a different side every day.

Then replace the bedding, shaking it well. First, build the banks. Banks are useful in preventing draughts and helping to prevent the horse getting cast. Throw the straw up against the wall and then pack it firmly using the back of the fork so that the bank stands above the bed a minimum of 30 cm (12 in) high. Lay the bed so deep that the fork does not strike through to the floor; straw is easily displaced as the horse moves round the box so the bed must be deep enough to ensure that the floor is not exposed – a layer of 23–30 cm (9–12 in) should be adequate. Depending on the horse – some are much cleaner than others – allow half a bale of straw per day to keep the bed deep and clean. Large horses in small boxes or broodmares with foals at foot may use as much as a bale a day.

Place the soiled straw on a muck heap, which should be close-packed and neatly squared off. The saying goes that if you want to know if a yard is well run go and look at the muck heap!

Scrub out the water buckets, refill and put back in the stable; do not place them in the doorway or under the haynet or manger, but in a corner where they are visible from the door. If the stable has a fitted manger or drinker check this to make sure that no straw was fallen into it and if necessary clean it out. Both mangers and drinkers should be cleaned daily.

Caring for a shavings bed

The initial cost of laying a shavings bed can be quite high with a 3.7 m^2 (12 ft^2) loose box needing five or six shaving bales to start it off. As before, when mucking out, the horse should be taken out of the box or tied up and moved to one side of the box. The piles of droppings can then be picked by hand (wearing rubber gloves) into a skip and then transferred to the barrow. A shavings fork can be used, but, although quicker, this tends to be more wasteful as some clean shavings will be removed. Working from the door the bed can then be thrown up. As the forkful of shavings is thrown against the wall droppings will fall to the bottom of the bank to lie on the floor and can be forked up. As shavings are highly absorbent the wet patches tend to be consolidated like cat litter, not spreading to the rest of the bed. Clean shavings can be scraped off to uncover the wet patches which should then be forked into the barrow.

Once the floor is uncovered it can be swept and, as with straw, either left to dry or have the shavings replaced and new shavings scattered on top. Many shavings are very dusty when fresh and if possible it is better to wait until the horse is out of the box before mucking out. Some people like to put down some clean shavings every day while others put them down a bale at a time when needed. On average, two bales of shavings a week should keep the bed topped up adequately, providing that the bed was thick enough in the first place; a foundation of 15 cm (6 in) is the minimum to encourage the horse to lie down and prevent injury.

Deep litter system

Both straw and shavings can be used on a deep litter system. The bed is laid as normal, but no droppings or wet patches are taken out. Clean bedding is added whenever necessary. This system is particularly useful when young horses or ponies are yarded together or the stable floor is very uneven or poorly drained. The advantages of the system are that it tends to be economical, less bedding is used on a day-to-day basis, it is labour-saving and provides a solid bed which does not move when the horse rolls.

The system does have some disadvantages: at the end of the winter the bed must be completely removed, often a job for a tractor as it is very heavy work to do by hand, the horse's feet must be regularly picked out; and if the bed is not cared for properly it will become unhygienic and unsightly with the horses covered in muck like cattle. Some yards use a similar system in loose boxes, just taking out the droppings but leaving the wet patches, as outlined in the next section.

Semi-deep litter system

The semi-deep litter system is a useful compromise between a thorough daily mucking out and leaving all the waste in. The way in which yards manage a semi-deep litter system varies from leaving in all the wet material and removing only the droppings daily to removing the wet material and droppings daily, but not moving the banks. The latter is a useful way of managing a shavings bed which has very high banks. The banks are left untouched to become quite solid while the middle of the bed is mucked out and the floor swept as normal.

Skipping out

Skipping out involves removing droppings without taking out any bedding. A heavy-duty pair of rubber gloves can be used, particularly in shavings beds.

Alternatively a fork can be inserted beneath the dropping and, with the skip tipped towards the dropping, it can be flipped into the skip. The stable should be skipped out every time you go in; this is hygienic and saves bedding from becoming soiled. In any case, the stable should be skipped out at lunchtime and evening stables. As long as the stable door is secured and the horse is placid enough it is not necessary to tie the horse up in order to skip out the stable.

Disinfecting boxes

Any stable that has been occupied by a horse suffering from an infectious disease should be thoroughly disinfected before being used by another horse.

- All bedding and leftover hay should be removed and burnt.
- Any salt lick should be thrown away.
- The walls, door, manger and other fittings should first be thoroughly cleaned, possibly with a pressure washer, and then scrubbed with a suitable disinfectant.
- The stable can later be rinsed and left to dry.
- If necessary the walls can then be repainted and the woodwork creosoted.
- Any equipment used on the infected horse or in its stable should also be treated; this includes haynets, grooming kit, buckets, rugs, blankets and tack.

The early morning and late-night check

Two important yard routines are the early morning check made before feeding the horses and the late-night check made in the evening. The checks are made to ensure that the horse has eaten up its food and looks healthy. In addition, the late-night check must include a check on the security – everything should be locked and the stable doors secured.

Prompt recognition of the stable signs of ill-health allows rapid treatment and, consequently, speedy recovery. In order to identify the sick horse the horsemaster must be able to recognise the everyday signs that indicate that the horse is healthy. This should be second nature, a subconscious routine, every time the horse is handled.

Chapter 20
Yard work and riding out

Yard maintenance

Safety is paramount; horses are large creatures that evolved to take flight
or lash out when threatened. It is essential that anybody involved with
horses realises the potential danger. The yard routine and layout should be
organised in such a way as to minimise any risk to the health and safety of
both horse and handler. One of the most simple and yet important things
is to keep the yard tidy during and after the daily chores are carried out.
For example, during mucking out, tools and barrows should be placed
where they will not interfere with the movement of horses and humans,
and after use should be stored in a convenient place that is out of the way
(Figure 20.1).

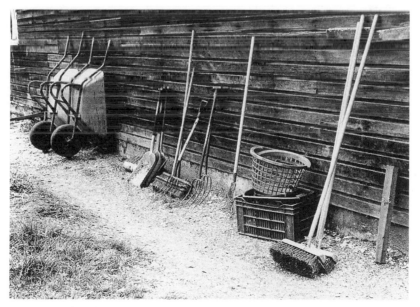

Figure 20.1. Yard tools and barrows safely out of the way.

Disposal of manure

Siting the muck heap

The muck heap should be sited within easy reach of the yard to save too much time spent wheeling barrows back and forth, yet it should be out of sight of the car park and yard entrance. The road or track leading to the muck heap should allow access for the tractor and trailer or lorry that will remove the manure. The base of the area that is going to contain the muck should be concreted and surrounded on three sides by railway sleepers set in steel joists up to a height of 1.8 m (6 ft). An alternative and time-saving method of muck disposal is to have a trailer parked below a ramp and to empty the wheelbarrows at the top of the ramp directly into the trailer which is emptied when full.

Building the muck heap

The muck heap needs daily attention if it is to be kept under control. The heap should be built in steps with a flat top and vertical sides that should be raked down to prevent loose pieces of straw blowing around the yard (Figure 20.2). The surrounding area must be swept and kept clean. The secret of success is to pack the soiled straw down as firmly as possible by stamping it into place; any straw that falls to the ground is thrown up onto the heap and trampled down again. A muck heap built in this way can store more muck in the same area and rots down better because it heats up throughout.

Removing the muck heap

Disposal of manure is a problem for many yards. Straw muck may be regularly collected by firms supplying market gardens and mushroom growers or local farmers may be prepared to spread either shavings or straw muck on their fields.

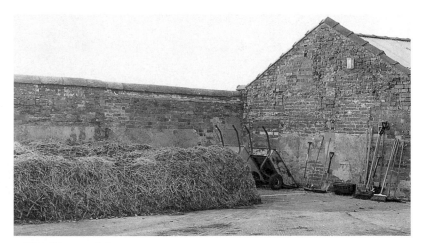

Figure 20.2. The muck heap.

Providing the horses have been regularly and effectively wormed and that the manure is well rotted, then the muck may be spread on fields belonging to the yard once or twice a year.

A muck heap can be burned, but the fire may smoulder for days and sometimes weeks. It can be a fire hazard and may cause considerable nuisance to neighbours.

Weekly chores

As well as keeping the yard and stable area neat and tidy on a day-to-day basis (Figure 20.3) there are yard maintenance jobs that need to be done on a weekly or seasonal basis. These include:

- cleaning stable windows and removing cobwebs
- clearing out drains
- checking first-aid kits and fire-fighting equipment
- replacing light bulbs
- cleaning stored tack
- brushing out rugs
- cleaning out the feed room, hay and straw shed
- scrubbing out feed and water containers
- checking feed stocks
- ordering and collecting feed
- disinfecting stable floors.

Unfortunately, many of these jobs are often neglected with staff having more than enough to do caring for the horses. This is short sighted as maintenance is important for appearance, safety and the long life of equipment and fittings.

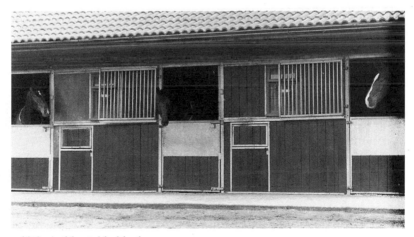

Figure 20.3. A tidy stable block.

Clearing drains

Once a week drains and sinks should be flushed with cold water to ensure that they are working properly and then disinfected. Occasionally, drains will become blocked and have to be cleared; this unpleasant job should be done with care as there is a health risk involved. Heavy-duty rubber gloves are essential and drainage rods should be used where possible to loosen the material clogging the drain. To prevent some drains blocking they can be fitted with a removable grid or trap that catches solid material and can be cleared regularly. In cold weather drains may freeze over and should be melted with liberal applications of salt.

Disinfecting stable floors

Although desirable, it is unlikely to be feasible to take up the bed once a week, scrub the floor with disinfectant and allow it to dry before putting the bed back down. Thus, many yards only do this twice a year and in the meantime sprinkle powdered disinfectant on the swept stable floor once a week. This is a useful compromise that keeps the stable sweet-smelling and is not time consuming.

Personal hygiene

There is little point in maintaining a high standard of stable management if this is not reflected by the staff. Working with horses is a grubby job and yet effort should be made to maintain personal hygiene: clothing should be clean, hair tied back, fingernails kept short and easy to scrub, and no dangling scarves or jewellery worn which may be unsafe.

Lifting heavy objects

Back pain is the major reason for people being off work, yet lifting heavy and often awkward objects is unavoidable in stable work. Safe procedure will help avoid accidents that often result from careless short cuts (Figure 20.4). Whenever possible, bales and sacks should be moved on a wheelbarrow, but they still have to be lifted onto the barrow. To minimise the risk of back injury, any weight should be picked up from the ground by standing in front of it and bending the knees. Avoiding lifting a bale or muck sack, swinging it onto your shoulder and turning at the same time; lift it straight up to rest on something and turn before taking hold of it again and carrying it on your shoulder.

Load a barrow with the weight towards the front, over the wheels. Although the temptation is great, avoid overloading barrows, trying to carry too much or moving things single-handed. Full water buckets are easier to carry if the weight is equally distributed so carry one in each hand.

- *Assess the situation:*
  Dress – boots, gloves, etc.
  Equipment – pitch fork, bale hook, pulley, trolley, jack, lever, etc.
  Assistance – machine, team, mate, etc.
  Reconnoitre – safe object, safe route, safe landing zone, safe weight.

- *Stance:*
  Feet apart – balanced; one foot forward.
  As close as possible to the object.
  Back straight, chin in.
  Legs bent.

- *Grip (lifting from floor):*
  Hand close and under weight or object clutched close to body.

- *Vision:*
  Do not block your view.

- *Lift:*
  Up and forwards – use leg muscles (calves, thighs, buttocks) but *not* back muscles.
  Do *not* twist or bend your spine.
  Keep weight close to body.

- *Carry:*
  Do not hurry, easy breathing, short steps.

- *Deposit:*
  Reverse of lift.

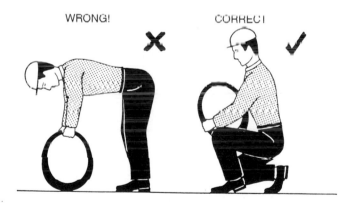

WRONG! CORRECT

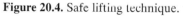

Figure 20.4. Safe lifting technique.

Bales and muck sacks are not the only heavy objects that need to be moved; bags of feed have to moved and stored. Small bags which can be lifted high and held against the chest can generally be carried comfortably, but if you need to lean back to support the weight, the bag is too heavy and should be put on a barrow.

The feed room

The feed room should be sited conveniently to avoid wasting too much time going back and forth to it. It is best constructed of brick or concrete blocks to discourage vermin. It should also be secure so that there is no possibility that a loose horse could stray into the feed room. Large yards may have a feed room and a separate feed shed to allow storage of large quantities of fodder. If this is not the case, the feed room should be accessible for door-to-door delivery of feed.

Ideally, the room will have a tap, sink and draining board, to allow regular washing of feed bowls and utensils. An electric socket for boiling a kettle should be well away from the wet area.

All types of feed will deteriorate if kept in poor conditions; ideally, the feed room should be built and designed so that it is always cool with little variation in temperature. It should be well ventilated, dry and light but protected from direct sunlight and free from vermin such as rats, mice, birds, insects and mites.

It is almost impossible to make a feed room vermin-proof and so open bags of feed should be stored in galvanised feed bins, raised off the floor on small wooden blocks, or in plastic dustbins with well-fitting lids. These should be cleaned out regularly and always emptied before a new bag of feed is emptied on top. Unopened bags of feed should be stored on pallets to raise them off the ground and prevent dampness. Damp food soon becomes stale, mouldy and unappetising to horses.

The feed room floor should be swept daily; a commercial type of vacuum cleaner with a long tube will help to keep awkward areas clean. There should be room around the bins for a terrier or cat to patrol and discourage vermin. Empty feed sacks and other rubbish must be collected in a dustbin that should be emptied once a week and any leftover feed should be buried in the muck heap. Simple housekeeping measures like this may not be enough to keep rats and mice away in which case a pest control programme will be needed. Rats are a constant health hazard, eating food, making it unpalatable to horses and possibly passing on the disease leptospirosis to horses, dogs and sometimes humans. Rats are not the only problem; mice and birds can also rip bags and leave droppings on the floor and in the food.

The feed room may also be fitted with a shelf for supplements, a lockable cupboard for medicines and a feed board.

The hay barn and plastic-packed forage

Hay may be stored for daily use in a store in the yard, but large stocks are usually kept in a barn, sited away from the stable because of the fire risk, yet easily accessible to staff. The barn should also be accessible to a tractor for the delivery of hay and straw, and there should be no overhead wires that could be damaged by high loads. Even well-made hay loses nutritional quality with age, but good storage conditions will help keep it palatable for longer. Hay must be protected from the weather and from damp rising up from the ground. Also, air should be able to circulate through the stack so the stack should be raised on pallets or bales of straw and there should be small gaps between the bales. Storing hay in a barn is better than covering it with plastic sheeting as that traps in moisture and allows fungi and mould to grow – ventilation is very important.

The safety regulations apply to the hay barn as well as the stable yard. String should be knotted and put in a waste bin or bag, any loose hay should be used or cleared up immediately and the bales should not just be taken from the front but removed layer by layer from the top.

Plastic-packed forage will only stay palatable if the bags are not punctured. The bags must be protected from rats and mice that chew the bags and from sharp edges that may rip them. Careful handling is also very important. Protecting the bags from direct sunlight will prolong their life.

Monitoring feed stocks

Every week feed stocks should be checked and, if necessary, ordered or bought. Small yards may visit the local supplier and collect what they require; larger yards may have a weekly or fortnightly delivery. Delivered goods should be checked off against the delivery slip as they are unloaded. This slip should then be checked against the subsequent invoice before paying the bill. It is wise to have an agreement with the feed merchant that if any bags are not up to standard they will be replaced free of charge.

Riding out

When riding out, responsible people know and follow two codes: the Country Code and the Equine Road Users Code (Figure 20.5).

The Country Code

- Enjoy the countryside and respect its life and work.
- Guard against all risk of fire.
- Fasten all gates.
- Keep dogs under close control.
- Keep to public paths across farm land.
- Use gates to cross fences, hedges and walls.
- Take litter home.
- Help to keep all water clean.
- Protect wildlife, plants and trees.
- Make no unnecessary noise.

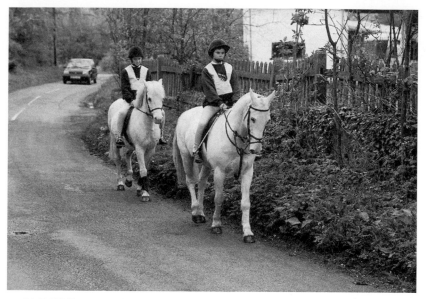

Figure 20.5. Riding out safely dressed and equipped.

Remember that you have a responsibility to yourself, your horse, the land, farmers and other path users. Behaviour that spoils other people's pleasure, causes accidents, damages crops or stock, or inconveniences landowners leads to barred gates and a 'horses not welcome' attitude.

The Equine Road Users Code

- Untrained horses or inexperienced riders may not go on the road alone, nor may they go on busy highways until the rider is experienced and the horse well behaved on quieter roads.
- Riders and drivers must be familiar with the Highway Code and the British Horse Society publication *Riding Safely on the Roads*.
- Horses must stay on the left. Led horses should be on the left of their leader.
- Horses may not go on pavements.
- Riders must wear fitted, property secured hats to current safety specifications.
- Footwear must have heels, soles should not have heavy cleats and stirrups must be wide enough.
- Tack must be in good order and properly fitted.
- Bright wear is advisable and in poor light it is essential on both horse and rider. After sunset a lamp (white – front, red – rear) is required.
- Respect other road users and adjacent pedestrians.

Chapter 21
Staff and the law

Unsurprisingly, there has been a tendency for people involved in working with horses and yard management to concentrate on the horses. Staff need attention, and staff who are content and happy with their jobs are more likely to be reliable and have a rapport with horses and other members of staff. It is important for all equestrian establishments to invest in people.

Yard staff

Good workers have the following attributes:

- responsible
- reliable
- efficient
- skilled
- realistic
- resourceful
- caring
- loyal.

Working relationships

For most stable staff it is important that they have good relationships with others. Single-handed jobs need a special, strongly motivated person who can take pleasure from working alone. But, most stable yards rely on a team approach and that needs some extra qualities to those already listed.

Everyone in a yard needs to 'pull their weight'. If one person is a slacker, then everyone else has to work harder or else standards fall. Also, each person must contribute positively to a team approach; some people take the attitude that it is always someone else's job to greet a stranger, pick up litter, change a light bulb or do any other task. The other crucial ingredient for a good team worker is that they promote good relationships and have a good effect on the rest of the team. Everyone has off days when workmates find the person grumpy or difficult; there is generally a good reason. On these days the rest of the team will make allowances. Similarly, there will be times when one is relied on by workmates.

Maintaining good working relationships with others is important and should not be taken for granted. Working as a team is enjoyable and, if well done, aids efficiency. It is important to be able to take orders and deal with requests; some people all too easily take offence when none is intended. If it is something which cannot be done now then it is helpful to clearly and politely say so. If a problem crops up between one person and another it is important to try and talk it through and resolve it; if necessary a senior person may be brought in to help. The great thing is that the team should be strong and harmonious.

Supervisory skills

The job of the head girl, senior lad, supervisor, or whatever title is used, is crucial to the atmosphere of the yard, the level of horse care, tidiness and much else besides.

A good supervisor is easily identified by two particular aspects of the yard:

- Good practice: for every yard there must be selected and agreed safe, effective and efficient ways of doing all routine tasks. All staff including trainees must adopt and stick to these practices. The supervisor is the arbiter of good practice.
- High standards: standards of quality, tidiness and, where appropriate, of work rate are consistently high. The supervisor leads from the front with a forthright cheery example.

A good supervisor has particular attributes:

- Reliability: reliability is not just necessary from the employer's point of view, it is also sought by all team members. A good supervisor will always do their best, both for the employer and for the staff; where their needs conflict the supervisor may seek a compromise, but ultimately has to enforce the employer's requirements with tact, loyalty and authority – it is sometimes a tough job.
- Skill: change must be brought in with understanding, clarity and ongoing enforcement. The supervisor should use their authority without giving rise to resentment. Problems should be dealt with clearly, but pleasantly, be they problems with jobs, people or horses. The supervisor advises, demonstrates, refers and helps both individuals and teams in order to achieve high performance. Yet after listening to, and discussing, others' ideas, the supervisor should always be willing to accept improvements. This person should be a good communicator; they should accept that a good relationship with the team is a two-way process, and show authority and sensitivity in making it good.
- A particularly difficult skill is that of counselling. Staff have problems and may seek help. The skill lies in listening and then helping the person to reflect wisely on possible alternative scenarios. The mistake is to give pat solutions or trite advice for others' problems. Where appropriate it may be best to tactfully encourage staff towards suitable help from specialists.

Staff training

The yard supervisor together with the employer will design the staff training programme, basing it on an assessment of each person's needs and ambitions. As training proceeds each individual will be given the opportunity to report on their own perception of their progress and how this affects their training plan. The supervisor will review the effectiveness of the training methods being used.

Often the supervisor is the trainer, so they will plan and deliver the training. Staff will need encouragement and will want to know how well they are progressing. The employer will also want to know how beneficial the training is proving to be.

In many cases National Vocational Qualifications (NVQs) will be used which means that staff will have plenty of ongoing feedback on their level of skills and on their progress. British Horse Society qualifications, or those of other organisations, may also be used in parallel with NVQs.

The supervisor has to develop as an effective trainer and so will need training themselves to be skilled and up-to-date on qualifications, training techniques and resources.

Staff contracts

All staff should be given a contract within 13 weeks of beginning work. Among other things the contract should include:

- date of commencement of work
- hours of work
- days off
- holiday arrangements
- pay details
- sick pay arrangements
- termination of employment details
- special arrangements including free livery, lodgings, etc.

The law

There are several acts of law concerning horses and stables. These include:

- Riding Establishments Act 1964 and 1970
- Animals Act 1971
- Protection of Animals Act 1911 and 1912
- Protection Against Cruel Tethering Act 1988
- Reporting of Injuries, Diseases and Dangerous Occurrences Regulations (RIDDOR) 1985
- Control of Substances Hazardous to Health (COSHH) regulations
- Health and Safety at Work Act 1974 (see also Chapter 22).

Riding Establishments Act 1964 and 1970

Any equestrian establishment that hires out horses or gives riding lessons by way of business falls under this legislation, even if part time. A licence must be obtained from the local authority and the applicant needs to meet specific requirements:

- Must be a body corporate or at least 18 years of age.
- Must not be disqualified from keeping a riding stable, a dog, pet shop, boarding kennels or from having custody of animals.
- Must satisfy the local authority of his/her suitability and qualifications by examinations or experience to run a riding establishment.

Licences are granted on a provisional (3 months) and annual basis. Before the licence is granted there will be an inspection of the premises.

The Act clearly states that the licence holder must hold current public liability insurance. If staff are employed, compulsory insurance is required under the following:

- Employers' Liability (Compulsory Insurance) Act 1969
- Employers' Liability (Defective Equipment) Act 1969.

Animals Act 1971

This Act is not applicable in Northern Ireland or Scotland. This law is based on strict liability. People who own and control animals are under a duty of care. This Act deals with any damage or injury caused by horses straying or injury caused by horses *per se*. Strict liability means there is liability without proof that the person against whom the claim is made was negligent, if they were responsible for the animal causing injury or damage.

Protection of Animals Act 1911 and 1912

Both Acts are similar in content and relate to cruelty to domestic and captive animals. This Act includes sections relevant to horses, such as:

- cruelty and unnecessary suffering
- order of destruction of horses that are suffering
- power of confiscation of horses considered to be suffering
- proper care of impounded horses
- disqualification from future care and ownership (1954 amendment of the Act) following conviction for cruelty to an animal
- diseased and injured horses may be dealt with by the police and veterinary profession where the owners cannot be found.

Protection Against Cruel Tethering Act 1988

It is an offence to tether any horses under such conditions or in such a manner as to cause that animal unnecessary suffering.

Reporting of Injuries, Diseases and Dangerous Occurrences Regulations (RIDDOR) 1985

Certain accidents must be reported to the enforcement authority (Health & Safety Executive or the local authority) immediately or within 7 days.

Accidents, which result in absence from work for more than 3 days, must be reported. Fatal accidents must be reported immediately. Records of reportable injuries must be kept for at least 3 years and include:

- date and time of accident
- name and address of person affected
- place of accident, nature and description
- additional information such as witnesses.

Control of Substances Hazardous to Health (COSHH) 1989

Employers must be responsible for risks associated with the use of hazardous substances and take necessary steps to eliminate or control the risks. This relates to:

- disinfectants
- creosote
- liniments
- insecticides
- mouse and rat poison
- veterinary products.

The regulations also cover exposure to harmful microorganisms, such as those that cause tetanus, and to dust from feed, bedding, forage and arenas.

Health and Safety at Work Act 1974

This applies to people not premises. It applies to employers and employees engaged in keeping and managing livestock. Although riding schools, livery yards and trekking centres are not specified, they still come under the Act.

Employers must be responsible to themselves and their staff to see that the conditions for work are as safe and healthy as possible.

Any business employing more than five people, including casual workers, must issue a safety policy statement.

In December 1986, Her Majesty's Agricultural Inspectorate of Health and Safety published further requirements to the 1974 Act. This gives strict regulations including for:

- food preparation
- first aid
- sanitation
- responsibility for staff training
- instruction
- suitability of horses
- dress.

People who are going to set up a yard should obtain a copy of *Horse Riding Establishments Guidance on Promoting Safe Working Conditions* by the Health & Safety Executive.

The general obligations cover both employers and employees to maintain safe working practices, premises and equipment. Risk assessment should be undertaken; specific areas should be given special attention with precautions taken.

The main risk factors include:

- electrical equipment and machinery (all equipment must be regularly serviced and maintained)
- combustible materials: stables, barns, oil/diesel, electric or gas heaters and bonfires
- barley boilers
- tractors and all field equipment/machinery
- vehicles, trailers, horses boxes
- horse walkers
- steps and stairs
- ladders and stepladders
- lifting loads
- wheelbarrows
- baling string
- yard surfaces, ice
- narrow doors, gateways
- fields, fences and gates
- trees
- yard entrances, car parks.

For further practical information on health and safety see Chapter 22.

Chapter 22
Health and safety

Information regarding the Health and Safety at Work Act 1974 may be found in Chapter 21. Practical applications of the Act are discussed in this chapter.

The law requires that records are kept, staff are trained, safety equipment is tested, accidents and incidents are recorded, safety clothing used where necessary and dangerous substances properly stored and used.

Duties of employers

The employer must make reasonably sure that the workplace, all machinery and systems of work are safe. All the kit and anything used must be safe and handled, stored and moved about safely. The employer must make sure that all staff are taught how to do jobs safely and that they are supervised so that they adhere to safe practices. There must also be provision for welfare, such as a first-aid kit, lavatories, hand-washing facilities and somewhere to get warm after working outside in winter.

Duties of staff

Staff, including trainees, must co-operate on health and safety matters. Staff must also take reasonable care for themselves, their workmates and anyone else who may be affected by what they do or fail to do. Those who are self-employed are both employer and staff all rolled into one and so must take on the responsibilities of both.

Safety policy and records

If there are five or more staff the employer has to write a safety policy which staff must be familiar with and obey.

Reporting incidents

Staff should always report incidents when things go wrong. The person in charge can then decide if the matter should be entered into the accident or incident book. Such a book is compulsory for British Horse Society (BHS) and Association of British Riding Schools (ABRS) approved riding schools; it is also required by the 1981 First Aid Regulations. The entry must show the time, date and place of the incident; it must include the names and addresses of witnesses; it must give a clear account of what happened; it must include the names of the horses and people involved and state who was in charge and who was hurt, with added details of any injury sustained and treatment given; it should include a plan or diagram of the accident, plus informative notes, clearly written, and be signed by both the person in charge and, if possible, the person who suffered the incident. If a loose-leaf form is used it should be kept in a file with an index of contents.

Reporting hazards

Any machinery or equipment that is faulty or anything hazardous must be reported to the person in charge as soon as it is noticed. That person has a duty to act straight away. A simple notice stating 'Faulty – do not use' could be the first step, or 'Slippery surface – take care'; then further steps must be taken to put the matter right.

Reporting injuries, diseases and dangerous occurrences

Certain matters have to be reported to the local environmental health department; this is enforced by the Reporting of Injuries, Diseases and Dangerous Occurrences Regulations (RIDDOR) 1985. These matters have to be reported immediately by telephone and then confirmed in writing; the yard has to keep its own record for at least 3 years.

Examples of injuries that must be reported include:

- death in an accident at work
- when a member of staff is off work for more than 3 days following an accident at work
- most broken bones (but not fingers and toes)
- eye wounds
- amputations
- injury or unconsciousness from electric shock or lack of oxygen or due to absorption of a substance through breathing, eating or drinking it or from having it spilt on the skin
- acute illness from bacteria or fungi or other infected material
- any injury which results in the person being admitted to hospital for more than 24 hours; this includes clients at riding establishments.

'Dangerous occurrences' that have to be reported are more likely to occur in factories or on building sites.

Reportable diseases include:

- asthma caused by working in consistently dusty conditions
- 'farmer's lung' which is a breathing difficulty caused by regularly handling mouldy hay or straw
- leptospirosis (Weil's disease) which can be contracted when working in places infested by rats.

First aid

Under the Health and Safety (First Aid) Regulations 1981 the yard must have first-aid provision. This means that someone must always be in charge and take responsibility for calling an ambulance if it is needed. Ideally, this person should have first-aid training. First-aid boxes and kits should be kept at the stables, in vehicles and taken on expeditions.

Accident procedures (when a person is badly hurt)

Accidents can, and will, occur. Frequently, they involve a rider falling from a horse on the road, in the school or in a field. Whatever the cause the procedure to follow is much the same. Most importantly remember to *keep calm* and use your *common sense*. The telephone number of your local doctor and vet should be beside the telephone or carried with you on a hack. Remember that a telephone is no good locked in the house; yard staff must always have access to one. A small emergency first-aid pack must be taken with you on a hack, along with money, a phone card or a mobile phone.

Immediately after the accident has happened, secure the scene in order to minimise the risk to yourself and any others in the vicinity. Do this standing guard over the hurt person while sending others to catch the loose horse and to summon the police and/or ambulance if appropriate. The first priority is the casualty who should be reassured and examined. Be sure to take no unnecessary risks. The next thing is to remember the accident ABC.

- *A is approach and airway*. Approach the hurt person being careful not to get hurt yourself, and once you have reached them ensure that their mouth and windpipe are free of obstruction.
- *B is for breathing* Mouth-to-mouth resuscitation may be necessary.
- *C is for circulation*. If the person is bleeding, pressure must be applied to the area to stop the bleeding as rapidly as possible.

Check for consciousness

Speak loudly and clearly to the casualty, watching the eyes to see if they flicker or open. If the person is conscious they should be asked if they have any pain in the back or neck and if the answer is 'yes' they must not be moved and you should stay with them until help arrives.

Open the airway

The unconscious casualty's airway may be blocked making breathing difficult or impossible. It is vital to first remove any obvious obstruction from the mouth and, secondly, to open the airway. This is done by placing two fingers under the chin to lift the jaw. At the same time the head should be tilted well back. If a head or neck injury is suspected the head should only be tilted just enough to open the airway.

Check for breathing and a pulse

Look for chest movements, listen for the sound of breathing and feel for breath on your cheek. The pulse can be felt on the neck, between the Adam's apple and the strap muscle that runs across the neck to the breastbone.

The recovery position and mouth-to-mouth resuscitation

If skilled help is not going to arrive quickly the casualty can be put in the recovery position. This prevents the tongue from blocking the throat and allows the unconscious casualty to be left if necessary. It involves turning the casualty with minimum movement of the head, neck and spine. In order to turn an injured person without help:

- Open the airway.
- Straighten the legs.
- Kneeling at the person's side, bring the arm nearest you out at right-angles to their body, with the elbow bent and the hand palm uppermost.
- Bring the other arm across the chest and hold the hand, palm outwards, against the casualty's cheek.
- With the other hand grasp the thigh furthest away and pull the knee up, keeping the foot flat on the ground.
- Keeping the hand pressed against the cheek, pull at the thigh to roll the person gently towards you, supporting the head all the time.
- Once the person is turned, tilt the head to make sure the airway is open and adjust the hand under the cheek to ensure that it stays open.
- Bend and bring forward the upper knee to prevent further movement.

In serious cases the casualty may be unconscious and not breathing. Immediate action must be taken:

- Undo the chin strap of the hat, but leave it on.
- Press back on the person's forehead and lift the jaw up and forwards to open the air passage to the lungs.
- If this does not start their breathing support the jaw, pinch the nose and blow a normal breath into their mouth, repeating every 5 seconds.
- Watch to see if the chest begins to rise and fall; if not check that the airway is not still obstructed.
- A Laerdal pocket mask is available to avoid the risk of transmission of disease from mouth-to-mouth resuscitation.

Even if the fallen rider appears to be unhurt, if there is any doubt call for medical assistance or send the person to hospital for a check-up and remember to fill in an accident report no matter how minor the incident. Anyone who has, or might have, been concussed must not ride or drive again that day.

Accident prevention

Good housekeeping reduces trips and falls. Pot holes, broken steps, defective gates, projecting nails, items left in passages, tools lying about and any obstruction can cause an accident. Children and animals should not roam unsupervised around work areas.

Those riding or leading horses on the road should keep to the left and the horse should be on the handler's left. Both horse and handler should be properly trained and equipped; inexperienced or overfresh horses should be escorted by a car.

Approved hard hats must be properly fitted and fastened before mounting and remain so until dismounting. Footwear for riding must have a sharp-edged heel (trainers or Wellington boots must never be worn). Footwear for stable work should be robust and, when handling young horses, toe protection is advisable. Gloves should be worn for lungeing and leading young and fresh horses. Bridles give greater restraint than a headcollar.

All electrical appliances and extension cables should be connected using a safety cut-out [residual current device (RCD)]. Tractors, and even lawn mowers, must only be used by trained staff, as should chaff cutters and oat rollers which must be guarded. Horse walkers should be in a fenced-off area and staff trained before using them. Pressure washers combine water and electricity so require special care. The use of ladders requires caution: the base must not slip so it may need securing on a shiny floor; the top must be at least 1.05 m (3.5 ft) above the landing place. If a ladder is left in place, a board must be tied to it so children cannot climb up. Agreed procedures must be implemented when entering riding schools. Finally, it is best to keep visitors and traffic away from horses. Wandering visitors should always be greeted and escorted to a safe place. Safety is everyone's responsibility.

Part 5
Horse care

Chapter 23
Horse clothing

Apart from the tack in which the horse is ridden, clothing for the horse includes rugs, blankets and sheets, and boots.

Care of tack

The majority of a horse's tack is made of leather and both leather and stitching will rot if exposed to sweat, water and heat and then neglected. Thus, it is important for appearance, safety and durability that tack is kept clean and supple. It is also an ideal time to check the stitching and leather for signs of wear and damage. Unsafe tack should be put to one side and not used again until it is repaired, otherwise it may break and cause an accident. The stitching on stirrup leathers tends to wear relatively quickly. To check it, grasp the sewn-down end and pull firmly; if the stitching is weak it will be possible to tear the end away. Remember, tack that has broken and been repaired, for example, reins, is weakened and should not be used for competition or other strong work.

Many yards only clean the bit and wipe the tack over on a daily basis, just removing straps from their keepers to clean and soap underneath. If this is the case, the tack should be taken apart and cleaned thoroughly once a week. If the tack is exposed to much mud and rain then it should be treated with a leather dressing such as neat's-foot oil on a monthly basis. Over-oiling will make reins difficult to hold and may rot the stitching. The stirrup leathers and surface of the saddle should be treated with care or the leather dressing will come off onto the rider's clothing. Similarly, if a saddle is used without a numnah, leather dressing used on the lining of the saddle may stain the horse's back or cause a reaction on a sensitive horse.

Leatherwork should be rubbed clean with a damp cloth or sponge that is regularly rinsed in warm water. Saddle soap should then be rubbed well into the leather, particularly the fleshy or rough side, using a slightly damp sponge. Saddle soap comes in many forms: glycerine, tins, tubes and liquid. Read the instructions and remember not to use too much or to make the sponge too damp.

Only if the tack is caked with mud is it necessary to use more water and get the tack really wet. Wet leather should be dried with a chamois leather or dry cloth. If the leather has been soaked with rain it should be wiped clean and left to dry naturally. A suitable leather dressing or oil should be used before the leather is soaped to replace the oils lost and to prevent the leather drying out and becoming brittle.

Leather may become mouldy or dry during storage. This can be prevented by dismantling the piece of tack, treating it with a leather dressing, wrapping it in newspaper and then putting it in a plastic bag.

Cleaning saddles

The saddle should be placed on a saddle horse and the girth, leathers, irons and numnah removed. If the irons and stirrup treads are very dirty they can be taken off the leathers, separated and washed in warm water in a bucket. First, the underneath of the saddle should be wiped with a damp cloth or sponge, a clean stable rubber put on the saddle horse and the saddle replaced.

The rest of the saddle should be cleaned, removing any lumps of accumulated grease (jockeys) with a pad of horsehair. The seat of the saddle may not need wiping if it is clean. The leathers, girth, irons and treads should be washed, paying particular attention to any folded areas. All the leather should then be soaped, taking care to do both sides of buckle guards and girth straps. The seat and saddle flaps should be wiped with a dry cloth to remove excess soap which may stain the rider's breeches. Irons and treads should be dried with a towel and polished if necessary. Any suede, serge or linen surfaces should not be soaped but brushed clean. After cleaning the leathers, the irons should be replaced, run up and the leathers put through and under the irons. The girth can be laid on top of the saddle and the saddle covered with a cloth or cover before being returned to its rack.

Cleaning girths

Leather girths should be cleaned carefully after use or they will become hard and rub the horse. The inner felt lining of three-fold girths should be removed, oiled and replaced regularly.

Nylon, string, lampwick and webbing girths should be brushed off every time they are used. If they are muddy or stained they should be soaked in a non-biological detergent, scrubbed and thoroughly rinsed. Care must be taken not to soak any leather parts, and if they are hung up by both buckle ends to dry this will prevent the buckles rusting. Finally, any leather parts should be soaped or oiled.

Cleaning numnahs

Quilted cotton, linen-covered foam and synthetic sheepskin numnahs should be shaken or brushed after every use and washed by hand or machine when necessary. Some horses have sensitive skin in which case soap flakes or suitable washing powder should be used. Sheepskin numnahs must be washed by hand in soap flakes, rinsed and have oil applied to the skin side to prevent hardening.

Cleaning bridles

Hang the bridle up and remove the bit or bits which should be soaked in warm water, hang the reins up and take the rest of the bridle apart, remembering which holes the pieces were done up on. All the leather should be cleaned and soaped as described above and the bit washed, dried and the rings polished. If oiling is necessary this is the time to do it and to check stitching and the condition of the leather where it is folded or bent. The bridle should then be put back together again in the following order (Figure 23.1):

- The headpiece should be threaded through the browband, ensuring that the throatlash is to the rear.
- The headpiece should be hung on a hook – for a double bridle the bridoon headpiece (sliphead) should be threaded through the near side of the browband, first under the main headpiece and buckled on the off side.
- The noseband headpiece should be threaded through the browband from the off side to buckle on the near side. It should lie under the headpiece.
- The two cheekpieces should now be attached. A double bridle will have two buckles on each side.

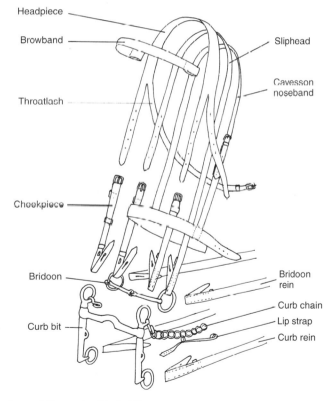

Figure 23.1. Assembling a double bridle.

- The bit or bits should be attached the right way up and the lip strap if fitted put on. The lip strap should be pushed through the 'D's on the bit from the inner side to the outer side and buckled on the near side.
- All straps should be placed in their runners and keepers and the noseband placed around the bridle and secured by a runner and keeper.
- The reins should be replaced; on a double bridle the wider rein attaches to the bridoon while the narrower rein goes on the curb bit.
- The curb chain should be hooked on with the lip strap ring hanging down and the lip strap then fastened through the ring to prevent the chain being lost.
- The bridle can then be 'put up' by passing the throatlash around the bridle in a figure of eight, through the reins and securing by a keeper and runner.

Remember, buckle fastening always goes to the outside while billets (fixed hooks) go on the inside. The rough or flesh side of the leather goes against the horse's skin.

Rugs

Rugs are worn in winter to keep the horse warm and dry and in summer to protect from flies and keep the horse clean. Rugs generally fasten at the front with cross-over surcingles and leg straps often attached. Leather rollers or webbing surcingles may also be used to hold the rug in place.

Modern textile materials are now used that are breathable and lightweight while remaining waterproof and warm.

It is important to buy a rug that is well made and fits well. Clipped horses will need a minimum of a stable or night rug, New Zealand rug, sweat sheet and a summer sheet. Some traditional yards still use old-fashioned jute rugs with additional blankets as and when required with a roller to keep them in place.

Types of rug include:

- stable or night rug
- day rug
- sweat rug/sheet or cooler
- summer sheet
- exercise or quarter sheet
- hood, cap, neck cover, vest
- New Zealand rug.

Stable or night rugs (Figure 23.2)

This is a more heavy-duty rug for use in winter and cooler summer nights.

- Synthetic rugs: made from artificial fibres such a polyester. They are lightweight, warm and easy to wash. They are often quilted to provide improved insulation and warmth. They come in different weights to suit different times

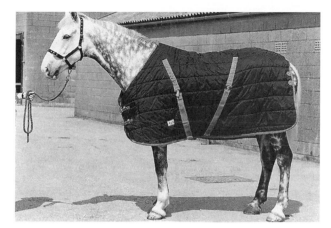

Figure 23.2. Quilted stable rug with cross-over surcingles.

of the year. They tend to have cross-surcingles, removing the need for an additional roller or surcingle.
- Canvas or jute rugs: traditional blanket-lined rug, heavy duty and recommended for large horses.
- Hemp rugs: lightweight and often half-lined with blanket. Not as tough as canvas or jute rugs.

Day rug (Figure 23.3)

Woollen rug with contrasting binding often used for special occasions such as shows and competitions. This fastens at the front, often with a matching surcingle. It often has the initials of the owner or stable embroidered on the bottom corner.

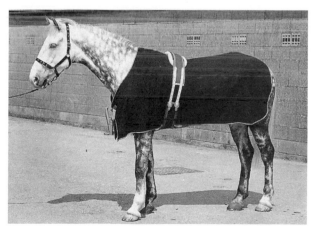

Figure 23.3. Day rug.

Sweat rug/sheet or cooler (Figure 23.4)

There are several types available and these are used to cool off and dry horses after exercise. The open-mesh type works on the same principle as a string vest, trapping pockets of air to insulate and dry the horse. To work effectively a top rug or sheet is often placed over the top of the sweat rug although this is not necessary when the weather is very warm.

Coolers are rugs made from material with special properties, the moisture from the horse's body is not soaked up, but taken from the skin through the rug to condense on top of the rug, leaving the horse warm and dry underneath. These make very useful rugs for travelling.

Summer sheet

Made in a variety of patterns, colours and checks, this lightweight rug is designed to keep the flies off the horse in the summer and keep the coat clean. In warm weather it is also used as a lightweight travelling sheet. Fillet strings attached to the back, lie under the horse's tail and prevent the sheet blowing up and frightening the horse. Summer sheets are useful and are often used beneath stable rugs to help keep the coat flat and clean (see Figure 23.4).

Exercise or quarter sheet

This may be used under the saddle on cold days or on horses that have been tacked up prior to exercise such as racehorses being led round the paddock. The sheet runs from the withers to the top of the dock. It is also kept in place by a fillet string. When used under the saddle, the front corners are folded back under the saddle flap, or held in place by loops through which the girth runs.

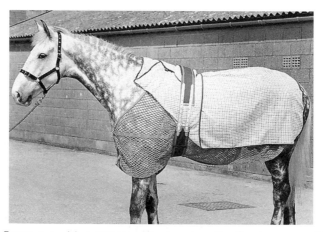

Figure 23.4. Sweat rug with a summer sheet on top; the front corners of the summer sheet have been folded back and secured with a roller.

Hood, cap, neck cover, vest

A cloth hood may be used in the stable or during exercise to keep the horse warm and prevent the coat on the head and neck growing too thick. Stretch or waterproof hoods may also be used with a New Zealand rug to keep the horse clean and dry in the field. A cap is a shortened version of the hood. They are available in a variety of colours and materials but are mostly lightweight and durable.

Vests are close fitting and usually slightly elasticated and are worn under the rug particularly around the chest area to prevent rubbing.

New Zealand rug (Figure 23.5)

This is used for out-wintered horses and stabled horses that are turned out in the day.

The rug is made from lined waterproof canvas or synthetic material. Canvas rugs are self-righting when the horse rolls. Canvas types are tougher and withstand heavier use, whereas synthetic rugs are less likely to rub at the front. Most New Zealand rugs have cross-over leg straps or surcingles. New lightweight, waterproof materials are arriving on the market all the time.

Ideally, horses should have two rugs so that when one gets excessively wet or dirty it may be replaced with the second one while the first is cleaned and dried.

New Zealand rugs should be deep and reach the top of the tail, if they are slipping backwards they do not fit. Leg straps should be oiled and cleaned to prevent them rubbing the horse's hind legs (see Figure 23.6).

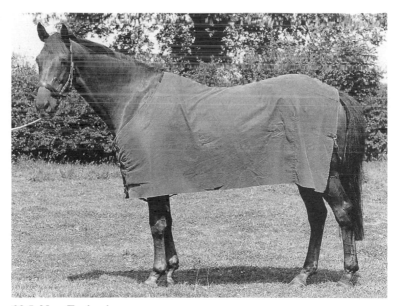

Figure 23.5. New Zealand rug.

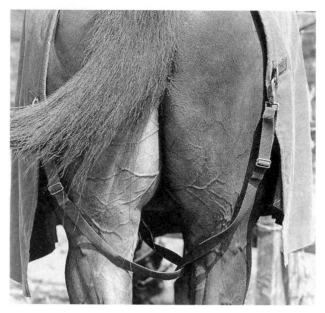

Figure 23.6. Correctly fitted leg straps.

Care should be taken when fitting a horse with a rug for the first time and this should preferably be done in the stable with an assistant to hold the horse quietly while the rug is put on.

Out-wintered horses should have their rugs removed and replaced daily, this is important so that the horse's condition underneath the rug may be closely monitored. It is difficult to keep an eye on weight loss or gain underneath a rug.

Keeping rugs in place

Rugs are kept in place by use of:

- rollers
- breast girths
- surcingles
- belly straps
- leg straps.

Rollers

Rollers are made of leather or webbing and are fastened around the horse's girth to keep rugs in place. Leather rollers are long-lasting, but expensive. Webbing or jute rollers are a less expensive alternative, but make sure they are wide enough for the size of horse or they will soon concertina into a narrow band under the horse's girth. A roller has padding either side of the spine, but it may still be advisable to use a thick pad under the roller to minimise pressure on the spine (see Figures 23.3 and 23.4).

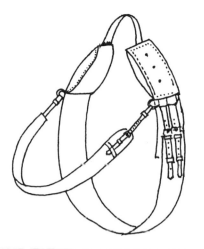

Figure 23.7. Anti-cast roller with breast girth.

An anti-cast roller has a metal arch over the withers designed to stop the horse getting cast. Unless this arch is large it is unlikely to work as it merely gets buried in the stable bed (see Figure 23.7). A thick pad is needed under the roller as it tends to concentrate pressure either side of the horse's withers. There should be buckles on both sides so that it can be undone if the horse does get cast.

Specialist leather rollers can be used for breaking in horse. These have 'D's for side reins, a crupper and a breast girth.

Breast girths
The breast girth is a leather or webbing strap that is fastened to a strap attached to the front 'D's either side of the roller (Figure 23.7). It is designed to stop the roller sliding back. It should fit closely around the chest just above the point of the horse's shoulder. A similar strap can be used with a saddle, in racing for example.

Surcingles
Surcingles are narrow unpadded straps that hold rugs in place. They are usually stitched into place and care must be taken that pressure is not put on the horse's back.

Cross-over surcingles are stitched at an angle on the off side of the rug, passed under the horse's belly, crossed over and fastened on the near side. These hold the rug in place effectively and with little pressure on the back (Figure 23.2).

Belly straps
Some quilted rugs have broad bands of matching material that pass from one side of the rug, under the horse's belly and fasten on the other side. Some designs of rug have bands of material that also pass between the front legs in a nappy-type arrangement.

Leg straps

Some night rugs are held in place by leg straps in the same way as a New Zealand rug. Some designs also fasten around the front legs.

Measuring for rugs

Rugs are generally sold with reference to the length of the horse from point of shoulder to point of buttock, for example, a 16 hands horse will need a 1.8 or 1.9 m (6 or 6 ft 3 in) rug depending on its build.

The horse should be measured from just in front of the withers to the top of the tail and from the centre of the horse's breastbone to the point of buttock to ensure that the rug will be long enough.

Putting on the rug and blanket

See Figures 23.8–23.12. Rugs should fit snugly. To put on a rug or blanket:

- Tie up the horse.
- Collect up the blanket, left side in left hand and right side in right hand. It may be folded in half.
- Gently talk to the horse as you throw it on the horse's neck and withers. Do not slide it up against the horse's coat if in the wrong position, take it off an start again.
- If folded in half, place over the horse's neck and withers and then slowly unfold over the horses back.
- Fold the front corners of the blanket up to the withers to form a triangle shape.
- Collect up the rug and gently place over the blanket.
- The front buckle may then be fastened.
- The front part of the blanket should then be drawn back over the top of the rug and secured in place with a roller or surcingle.
- Alternatively, fasten the cross-surcingles, making sure they are not twisted on the blind side.

Removing the rug and/or blanket

- Tie up the horse.
- Unfasten the front buckle on the rug and the roller or surcingles.
- Fold both rugs back and gently slide off over the quarters and tail.
- Fold the rugs and put neatly away.

Storing rugs

In spring, winter rugs should be mended, cleaned and stored ready for the next winter. Rugs may either be washed at home or sent to a specialist cleaner. Follow washing instructions on labels where attached. Any leather attachments should be oiled prior to washing. Leather rollers and fittings should be washed and treated with a suitable dressing. Clothing may then be stored in trunks or in bags on racks away from mice and moths.

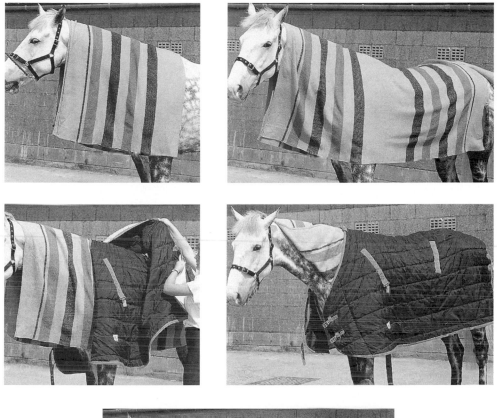

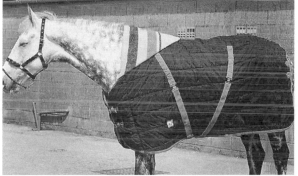

Figures 23.8–23.12. Putting on a rug under a blanket.

Bandages

Bandages are placed around the horse's lower leg to give protection, warmth and support during exercise, travelling or after injury. They must be properly applied as they can cause serious damage if incorrectly put on.

Putting bandages on

Regardless of the type of bandage to be applied there are a few golden rules which will help make the job easier and more efficient:

- The bandage must have been correctly and firmly rolled up. The tapes must be flat and the bandage rolled towards where the tapes or Velcro are fastened.
- The bandage must not be too tight; there should be room to insert a finger in the top and bottom of a support or exercise bandage.
- The tension throughout the bandage should be even with no wrinkles and the tapes tied no tighter than the bandage itself.
- The bandage is ideally applied from front to back to avoid pulling too much on the tendons at the back of the leg.
- The padding underneath the bandage must always run in the same direction as the bandage and the edge of the padding must not lie on the tendons as this will cause a pressure point and possible damage.
- The tapes must be tied on the outside of the leg, not on the bone at the front or on tendons at the back.
- The tapes should be tied neatly in a knot or bow and the ends tucked in to the tape and secured by sewing, insulating tape or pulling one of the folds of the bandage over the tape. It is very important that if insulating tape is used it is not pulled tighter than the rest of the bandage.

Taking bandages off

Untie the tapes and unwind the bandage, moving quickly, passing the unwound bandage from one hand to the other. Once the bandage is off, feel the leg carefully to check all is well. The bandage should then be shaken out, brushed or washed as necessary. Reroll the bandage and store them in twos or fours.

Padding under bandages

Nearly all bandages are applied with some form of padding underneath. The exceptions are Sandown and some thermal bandages which will be discussed later.

- *Gamgee* is cotton wool in gauze cover. Fresh from the packet it is clean and gives good protection, especially wrapped round twice. However, it is easily soiled and expensive. Its life can be prolonged by blanket stitching the edges so that it can be washed and reused. Gamgee is very popular for use over the top of wounds that require bandaging and is frequently an important item of the first-aid kit.
- *Fibagee* is felt-covered foam. It is easy to wash and durable, making it popular for use under exercise and travelling bandages.
- *Leg wraps* are commonly used in the USA. They are thick padded squares that are durable and give good protection, but they are not suitable for use under exercise bandages.

- *Hay or straw* can be used for thatching legs to dry horses and keep them warm.
- *Shaped tendon-protector shells* in a firm synthetic material may be used under exercise bandages.

Fastening bandages

Bandages can be fastened by tapes sewn to the bandage. The tapes should be wide and flat; smoothing them while they are wet will save having to iron them later. A more modern alternative commonly found on stable bandages is Velcro. This must be kept clear of hay and straw or it will not fasten effectively. Two pieces of Velcro must also be long enough to allow sufficient overlap to fasten securely.

Types of bandages

Stable bandages

Stable bandages have several uses and it is important to be able to put them on quickly and correctly. They are used for:

- warmth
- drying off wet legs
- protection, for example, travelling bandages
- support for a sound leg
- keeping a dressing in place.

They may be made of wool or synthetic material and are 10–12 cm (4–5 in) wide and 2–2.5 m (7–8 ft) long. Except for special thermal or Sandown bandages they are always fitted with padding underneath.

If the bandage is being used for keeping a poultice in place or for supporting an injured leg, elastic bandages may be used with double gamgee. If the bandage is being used to protect the legs during travelling ensure that the gamgee extends well over the knee and coronet.

The procedure for fitting a stable bandage (Figures 23.13–23.17) is as follows:

- Place the padding round the leg. It should extend about 2 cm ($^3/_4$ in) over the knee and below the coronet.
- If the bandage is long enough start just below the knee or hock.
- If the bandage is short, start just above the fetlock so that you are bandaging upwards towards the heart.
- Initially leave a vertical flap of bandage 10 cm (4 in) long. Then the first few horizontal turns secure the bandage.
- Each turn of the bandage should overlap half the width of the bandage.
- Complete the bandage.
- Tie the tapes in a neat bow and tuck the ends in.
- If the bandage is for support, for example, for a tendon injury, use a stretch bandage.

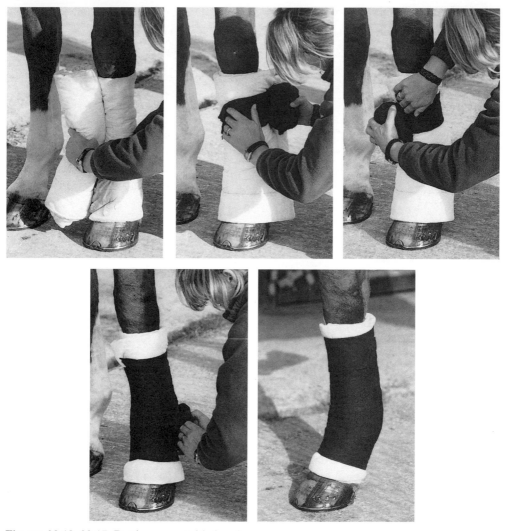

Figures 23.13–23.17. Putting on a stable bandage.

Exercise bandages

Exercise bandages may be fitted on the horse that is working to protect the leg in much the same way as a boot and to support the tendon. It is debatable how much help bandages are in actually preventing tendon strain, but they may help the leg cope with twists and turns.

Exercise bandages have considerable stretch and can be made of elastic, crêpe or self-adhesive material. They should be 8–10 cm (3–4 in) wide and about 2 m (6–7 ft) long. It is essential that adequate padding is used under the bandage, for example, gamgee or a tendon-protector shell.

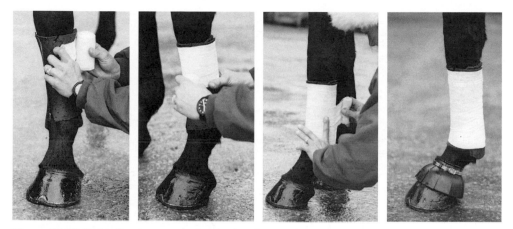

Figure 23.18–23.21. Putting on an exercise bandage.

The principles of fitting an exercise bandage (Figures 23.18–23.21) are the same as for fitting any other bandage except:

- they are applied more firmly
- a longer flap is left initially, for security
- they extend from below the knee to the fetlock joint (ergot)
- for competition purposes they are sewn or taped
- they should not be left on for long periods
- overlap two-thirds of the bandage
- do not remove from a tired horse until it has stopped blowing.

Tail bandages

Tail bandages are made of stretch elastic or crêpe material and are a little narrower and shorter than exercise bandages. They can be used on a pulled tail to improve the horse's appearance, in which case the tail hairs are damped with a water brush before the bandage is put on. The bandage should not be left on any longer than 4 hours; otherwise the pressure may cause the tail hairs to turn white or fall out. The bandage should be applied firmly, but not too tightly.

Tail bandages can also be used to protect the tail during short journeys. However, if the horse is travelling for longer than 4 hours a tail guard should be used instead. Bandages can also be used to keep the tail hairs safely tucked away during clipping or when mares are being covered.

To put on a tail bandage (Figures 23.22–23.24):

- If the tail is not plaited, damp it at the top.
- Stand behind the horse and hold up the tail or put the dock over your shoulder.
- Put the bandage under the tail leaving a 10 cm (4 in) flap.
- Secure the end of the bandage and then make one or two turns as high as possible.

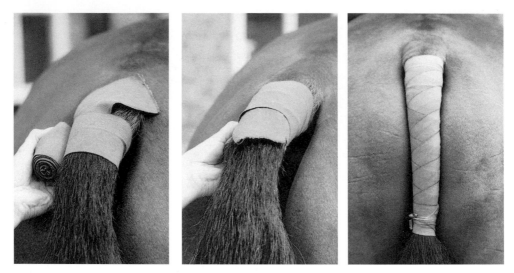

Figures 23.22–23.24. Putting on a tail bandage.

- Bandage down the tail, overlapping about half the bandage at each turn.
- The bandage should reach the end of the dock.
- Wrap the tapes around the tail and tie to the side so that the horse cannot lean on the knot during travelling.

To remove a tail bandage undo the tapes and pull the bandage off with both hands. However, if the tail is plaited the bandage must be carefully unwound.

Boots

Boots are used to protect the horse's lower limbs from injury. Usually the injury is self-inflicted; the horse knocks or treads on itself with another foot. This knock may be due to the horse's conformation, action or shoeing, but could also be caused by fatigue, weakness, immaturity, thoughtless riding, stumbling on landing after a fence ('pecking'), deep going or a change in the ground under foot.

Types of boot

Brushing boots

Brushing boots are designed to protect the inside of the leg below the knee or hock, primarily the fetlock region that can be hit by the other foot at slower paces. The boots should be fitted slightly high to allow for them slipping while the horse is working and should be fastened from the top to the bottom, easing them gently into position. Synthetic boots with Velcro fastenings are very

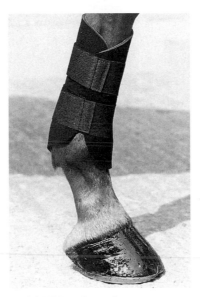

Figure 23.25. Exercise boot with Velcro fastenings.

popular as inexpensive exercise boots (Figure 23.25), while leather boots with buckle fastenings are more suitable for fast work. The boot may be shaped to protect the underside of the fetlock.

Speedicut boots
Speedicut boots protect against high brushing wounds, just below the knee or hock, which can be sustained when the horse is galloping or being driven.

Over-reach boots
Horses are said to over-reach when a front foot stays on the ground too long and is struck by the inside edge of the hind shoe. This can occur when the horse is jumping and there is an extra effort on take-off or the horse lands in deep going and cannot get its front feet out of the way in time. A low over-reach results in a cut or bruise on the heel while a high over-reach or 'strike' may damage the tendons at the back of the leg.

Low over-reaches may be avoided by using over-reach boots; bell boots are synthetic boots which pull over the hoof or fasten round the pastern to protect the heel and coronet (Figure 23.26). The boot must not be too long or the horse may tread on it and this type easily turns up in heavy going. A similar boot consisting of petals does not turn up and individual petals can be replaced if they get torn. A tough leather or fabric coronet boot is often used in polo to give added protection to the coronet. Over-reach boots can also be used to protect the horse from tread wounds caused by other horses during travelling or hunting. High over-reaches may be avoided by using brushing boots.

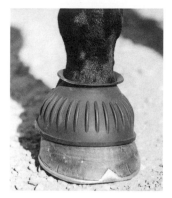

Figure 23.26. Over-reach boot.

Yorkshire boots

Yorkshire boots are usually used to protect the hind fetlock from low brushing wounds, but their use has been largely replaced by the use of synthetic fetlock boots. They consist of a rectangle of thick material with a tape or Velcro two-thirds of the way down. The boot is wrapped round the leg, tied, eased over the fetlock and the top of the boot turned down.

Rubber rings

A rubber ring with leather or a chain running through it can be fitted either above or below the fetlock (Figure 23.27). Round the pastern it acts to stop the horse knocking the coronet while above the pastern it prevents brushing wounds. The ring is fastened by a buckle on the strap or chain running through the ring.

Sausage boots

A sausage boot is a large leather-covered padded ring that is fitted round the horse's front pastern to stop the horse bruising or capping the elbow while lying down with its feet tucked under the elbow.

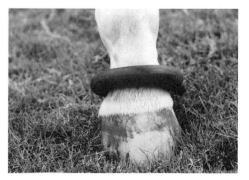

Figure 23.27. Rubber ring.

Tendon boots

Tendon boots are similar in design to brushing boots, but they have added padding down the back of the leg to protect the tendons from injury should the horse strike into itself; they are used for fast work or jumping. Open-fronted tendon boots are often used for show jumping; the boot is left open at the front so that the horse is not encouraged to hit fences (Figure 23.28).

Polo boots

Polo boots are similar to brushing boots, but they are made of heavy felt and extend down over the fetlock and may strap around the pastern. They are designed to protect the fetlock and pastern from brushing by stick or ball.

Travelling boots

Travelling boots are an alternative to travelling bandages and are long padded boots designed to protect the horse from knee/hock to coronet. They are frequently shaped to fit over the joints of the leg (Figure 23.29). They usually have Velcro fastening and care should be taken when they are first fitted to a horse as the restricted feeling may alarm the horse as it is asked to walk.

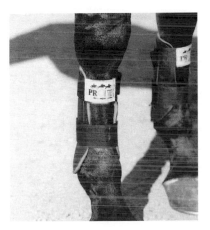

Figure 23.28. Open-fronted tendon boot.

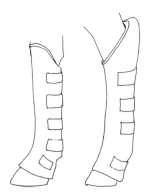

Figure 23.29. Travelling boots.

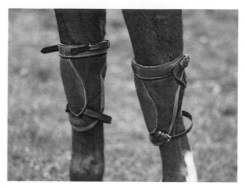

Figure 23.30. Knee boots.

Knee boots

Knee boots are designed to protect the horse's knees when exercising on the roads or during travelling when they are used in conjunction with travelling bandages. They may be made of leather, heavy cloth or synthetic material and fasten well above the knee with the buckle on the outside. The top strap usually has a strong elastic insert to allow the boot to be fastened tightly enough to prevent it slipping without damaging the leg (Figure 23.30). Once the top strap is done up the boot should be eased down to the top of the knee to check that it will not slip over the joint and then the lower strap should be fastened very loosely to allow the knee to flex without interference. The buckle fastens from back to front, which goes against the normal 'rules'.

Skeleton kneecaps or pads are sometimes used for road work and a horse may jump in kneepads which do not have a bottom strap.

Hock boots

Hock boots protect the point of the hock during travelling. There is a top strap with an elastic insert that holds the boot in place and a bottom strap that is fastened more loosely (Figure 23.31).

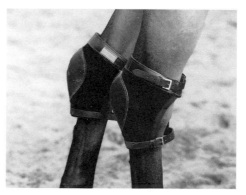

Figure 23.31. Hock boots.

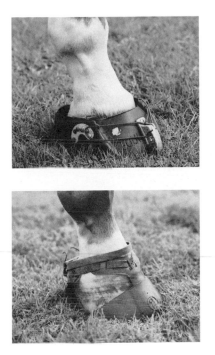

Figure 23.32. Equiboot.

Figure 23.33. Shoof.

Overboots

The overboot is a plastic galosh-type boot designed to fit over the horse's hoof (Figures 23.32 and 23.33). It can be used on the unshod horse to protect the foot from wear or it can be used as an alternative to a poultice boot to keep a foot dressing in place. It is also useful for exercising horses during recovery from pus in the foot where the horse may have a tender place on the sole that the boot protects.

Poultice boots

A poultice boot is designed and shaped to accommodate the horse's hoof and lower leg, and it is used for keeping foot poultices in place (Figure 23.34).

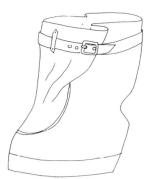

Figure 23.34. Poultice boot.

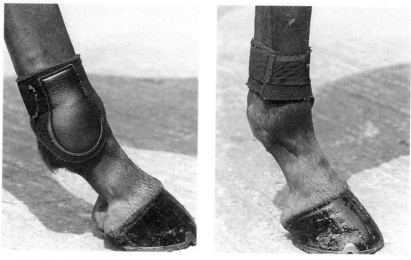

Figures 23.35 and 23.36. Fetlock boot.

Fetlock boots

This boot protects the inside of the fetlock and is sometimes used on the hind legs when show jumping to protect from injury while also discouraging the horse from hitting the fence (Figures 23.35 and 23.36).

Jacuzzi boots

This big rubber boot resembles an equine Wellington boot. When on, it has a hose attached and water circulates inside the boot to cool the horse's lower leg. It is used after strenuous exercise.

Chapter 24
Saddlery and tack

Horses are fitted with saddles, bridles and martingales to enable the rider to have control of the horse. It is important to know how to fit a saddle and bridle and have knowledge of bits and their applications.

Bridles and bits

Bridles can be classified into five families:

- the snaffle
- the double bridle
- the Pelham
- the gag
- the bitless bridle.

Under different competition rules, some bits or bridling arrangements may not be allowed, particularly in dressage and Pony Club show jumping.

The leather of the bridle should be of a suitable size and weight for the horse; for example, for showing and dressage lightweight leather may be used while for hunting and eventing heavier leather would be advisable.

Parts of the bridle

The parts of the bridle are basically the same for all types of bridle (Figure 24.1) and consist of:

- *Headpiece and throatlash.* The throatlash should be fitted to allow a hand's-width between it and the horse's jaw; if too tight it will be uncomfortable when the horse flexes at the poll.
- *Browband.* This prevents the headpiece slipping back.
- *Cheekpieces.* These attach to the headpiece and hold the bit in place.
- *Noseband.* A simple snaffle bridle has a cavesson noseband that is fitted so that it lies about 2.5 cm (1 in) below the projecting facial crest running down the side of the horse's head. It may be fastened so that two fingers can be inserted between the noseband and the horse's nose or it may be tightened to prevent the horse opening the mouth.
- *Reins.* These attach to the bit and allow the rider to control the horse. Reins may be plain leather, rubber-covered, laced, plaited or made of web with

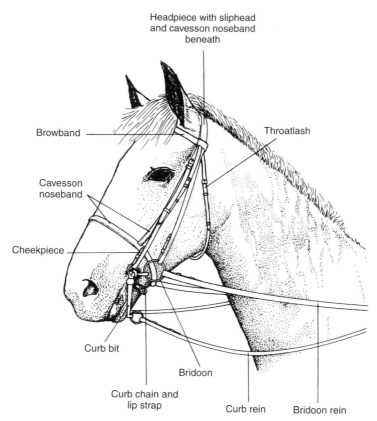

Headpiece with sliphead
and cavesson noseband
beneath

Browband

Throatlash

Cavesson
noseband

Cheekpiece

Curb bit

Bridoon

Curb chain and
lip strap

Curb rein   Bridoon rein

Figure 24.1. Parts of the bridle.

finger slots of leather placed at intervals (Continental reins). Reins measure from 1.3 m (4 ft 3 in) long for ponies to 1.5 m (5 ft) long for horses and the width varies according to use.

- *Bit*. This is discussed in more detail below.
- *Bridoon sliphead*. In the case of a double bridle the bridoon bit has it own support; its off-side cheekpiece attaches to a strap which passes through the browband and becomes the cheekpiece on the near side.
- *Bridoon rein*. This rein attaches to the bridoon bit and is thicker and sometimes slightly shorter than the curb rein.
- *Curb rein*.
- *Curb chain*. The curb chain attaches to the curb bit and may be made of metal, leather or elastic.
- *Lip strap*. The lip strap is a narrow leather strap used to keep the curb chain in place. It prevents the curb chain from being lost.

The action of bits

Bits act on one or more of seven parts of the horse's head (Figure 24.2):

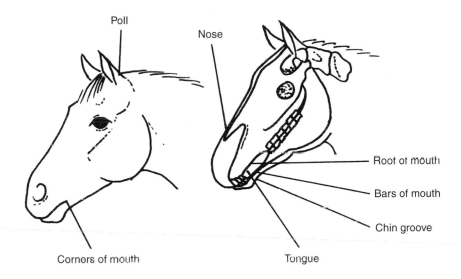

Figure 24.2. Points of action of a bridle.

- corners of the mouth
- bars of the mouth
- tongue
- poll
- chain groove
- nose
- roof of the mouth.

The action of the bit is affected by:

- the shape of the bit
- the shape of the horse's mouth
- how the horse carries his head and how the rider carriers their hands
- martingales, nosebands and other devices.

The snaffle

The snaffle is the most straightforward bit with either a jointed or straight mouthpiece. It acts on the corners of the mouth with an upwards action thus raising the horse's head. The jointed mouthpiece has a more direct squeezing action while the mullen or half-moon mouthpiece has more action on the tongue. However, as the horse learns to accept the bit and flexes at the poll the snaffle acts increasingly on the lower jaw; a drop noseband can accentuate this action.

There are many types of snaffle varying in action and severity (Figures 24.3–24.5). A loose-ring snaffle encourages the horse to mouth the bit and

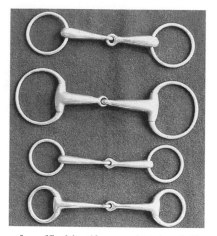

Figure 24.3. A selection of snaffle bits (*from top*): jointed German loose ring; jointed German eggbutt; loose ring bridoon; eggbutt bridoon.

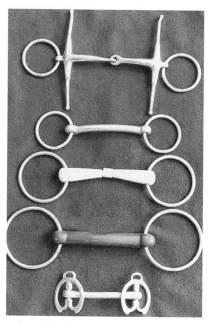

Figure 24.4. A selection of snaffle bits (*from top*): Fulmer (or Australian) loose ring; mullen mouth (metal): jointed nathe; rubber mullen mouth; horseshoe cheek mullen mouth stallion show bit.

salivate, resulting in a softer contact. A fixed-ring or eggbutt snaffle has a more direct action, but may encourage the horse to lean on the bit and constant pressure will reduce the blood supply to the horse's mouth resulting in poor contact. A horse that is reluctant to take the bit or one that moves the bit too much may go well in a Fulmer snaffle which has cheeks secured to the cheek-

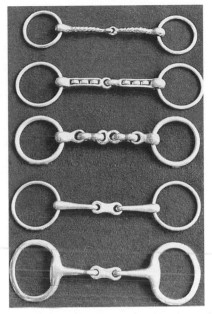

Figure 24.5. A selection of snaffle bits (*from top*): wire ring twisted bridoon; Magenis; Waterford; loose ring French link; eggbutt French link.

pieces by short straps called check retainers. The French link has a curved spatula in the centre which allows more room for the tongue. Jointed rubber and nylon bits (Figure 24.4) are useful for young horses which may resent a metal mouthpiece, while mullen mouth snaffles are mild, allowing room for the tongue for horses that cannot cope with a jointed bit.

Generally speaking, a bit with a thick mouthpiece, such as the German snaffle, is mild as it spreads the pressure over a larger area while thin mouthpieces are more severe. Snaffles can also be made more severe by twisting the mouthpiece, as in a twisted snaffle, by having rollers on the mouthpiece, as in the Cherry roller (Figure 24.6) or the Magenis, or by having extra joints, as in the Waterford or the W-mouth (Figure 24.7).

Snaffle bits are measured between the rings when laid flat. In the horse's mouth they should fit snugly with about 0.5 cm ($^1/_4$ in) projecting either side. If the bit is too narrow it will pinch the horse's lips; if too wide it will slide across the horse's mouth and the joint lying low on the tongue will encourage the horse to try and put its tongue over the bit. An approximate guide to the size of jointed snaffle needed for different horses is:

14.4–15 cm ($5^3/_4$–6 in)	hunter
13.1–13.75 cm ($5^1/_4$–$5^1/_2$ in)	14.2–15 hands and Thoroughbreds
11.9–12.5 cm ($4^3/_4$–5 in)	less than 14.2 hands (ponies).

Mullen mouthpieces need to be about 0.75–1.25 cm ($^1/_4$–$^1/_2$ in) narrower to fit correctly.

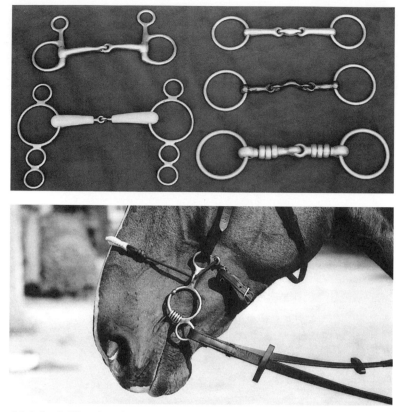

Figure 24.6. (*top*): Hanging cheek snaffle; KK bit; bubble bit; sweet iron bit; cherry roller. (*bottom*): Myler bit.

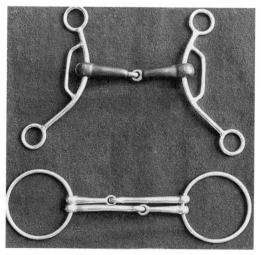

Figure 24.7. (*top*): American gag; (*bottom*): W-mouth snaffle.

Hanging cheek snaffle (see Figure 24.6)

The hanging cheek snaffle is suspended in the horse's mouth giving more room for the tongue. It can be useful for horses that put out their tongues over the bit.

KK bit (see Figure 24.6)

The KK range of bits is made out of an alloy, rather than stainless steel. This is said to encourage salivation and thus to be more comfortable for the horse. This particular bit has a lozenge that joins the two parts of the snaffle, removing the nutcracker action. Many horses, particularly those that set their jaw against the bit, relax in this bit.

Bubble bit (see Figure 24.6)

This bit, also known as a continental snaffle or Dutch gag, has three rings. Attaching the rein to the lowest ring gives greatest leverage and action on the poll, while the top ring gives a direct snaffle action.

Sweet iron bit (see Figure 24.6)

Originating from American Western bits, this type of metal encourages the horse to 'make a mouth', in other word to salivate and accept the bit.

Myler bit

The Myler concept ranges from mild simple snaffles to more severe long shank bits. The bit in Figure 24.6 is a short Myler bit that also acts on the nose and the jaw as a contact is taken on the rein. The principle of this type of bitting is to encourage the horse to place its head and work in the comfort zone.

The double bridle

The double bridle consists of a curb bit used in conjunction with a snaffle or bridoon (Figure 24.8). This sophisticated arrangement works on many areas of the horse's head giving a fine degree of control. This means that a double bridle should only be used by trained riders on horses that work correctly in a snaffle bridle.

The bridoon is normally jointed and is thinner and lighter than a snaffle (Figure 24.3). The curb bit is unjointed with an upward curve called a port that accommodates the tongue so that the bit can work directly on the bars of the mouth. A long-cheeked curb bit is more severe than one with short cheeks as the amount of leverage is much increased. The bridoon acts on the lips and corners of the mouth to raise the horse's head while the curb acts on the bars of the mouth, the poll and the chin groove to flex the poll.

The Weymouth, or curb bit, may have fixed cheeks, used in conjunction with an eggbutt bridoon, or a slide mouth, used with a loose-ring bridoon. The curb chain should be adjusted so that it comes into play when the bit is at a 45° angle to the mouth.

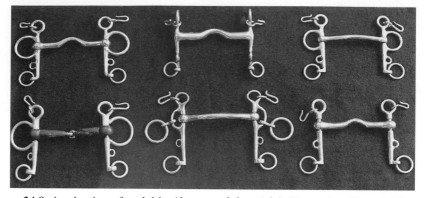

Figure 24.8. A selection of curb bits (*from top, left to right*): Hartwell pelham (with port); fixed cheek Weymouth; mullen mouth pelham: jointed rubber pelham; Rugby pelham; slide cheek Weymouth.

The pelham

The pelham (Figure 24.9) is a compromise between the snaffle and the double bridle being a curb bit with one mouthpiece and a top snaffle rein and a bottom curb rein. The action is on the corners of the mouth (snaffle rein), poll and chin groove (curb rein), but the action tends to be indistinct, particularly when roundings are used to allow the use of one rein. (A rounding is a loop of leather running between the two rings of the bit.) The mouthpiece may be straight or jointed, and a vulcanite pelham with its mild mouthpiece and curb action is often useful for horses with good mouths that are strong, for example, over cross-country.

The curb chain should be adjusted so that it lies comfortably in the chin groove and comes into play when the tension on the curb rein increases and pulls the cheeks of the curb bit to an angle of 45°. The curb chain then tightens and has a downward and backward pressure on the lower jaw. Attaching the curb chain through the top rings of the bit allows the curb to have a more direct action and helps stop the curb chain rising up out of the chin groove.

Curb chains are made of a series of linked metal rings that may be single or double (Figure 24.10). Double-linked chains spread the pressure over a larger area and are probably preferable to the more severe single-link chains. Curb chains may also be made of elastic or leather. Provided that the leather is kept soft and supple the pelham is less likely to cause rubbing than metal curb chains.

An important member of the pelham group is the Kimblewick that uses a single rein and frequently is seen on strong ponies. However, horses can learn to lean on this bit and it should not be overused.

The gag

The gag is a type of snaffle, but the rings of the bit have holes in them allowing an extended cheekpiece to pass through and attach to the rein (Figure 24.11).

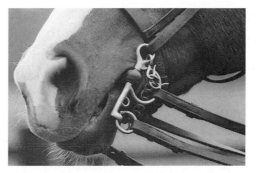

Figure 24.10. Pelham.

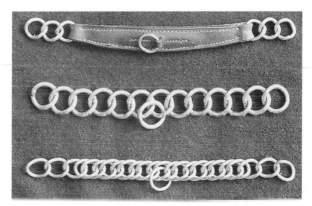

Figure 24.9. A selection of curb chains. From top: leather; single link; double link.

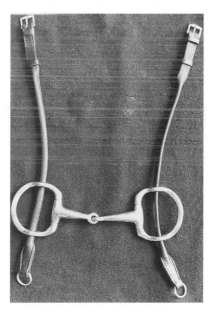

Figure 24.11. Gag.

This means that when the reins are pulled the bit is pulled up the horse's mouth encouraging the head to be raised. The gag usually has a second rein attached to the bit ring in normal fashion so that the gag rein need only be used when necessary. The gag can be severe and is best used by those who are skilled.

The American gag is useful for strong horses (Figure 24.7). The rein is attached to the bottom ring and when tightened can exert a very powerful pressure on the poll which acts to lower the head. The leverage is increased by the length of the cheekpiece above the mouthpiece.

The bitless bridle

A bitless bridle acts on the horse's nose and chin groove and is useful for horses with mouth problems (Figure 24.12). However, it can be severe and should be used with care. The nose and curb pieces must be well padded to avoid rubbing.

Fitting a snaffle bridle

- The browband should fit snugly round the horse's forehead without pinching the base of the ears.
- The buckles of the cheekpieces onto the headpiece should be an even height on both sides and preferably just above eye level.
- The bit should just wrinkle the corners of the mouth with 0.5 cm ($^1/_4$ in) showing either side – the bit should be pulled straight in the horse's mouth to check its width. The mouth should be opened to check that the bit clears the tushes (the canine teeth found in geldings and stallions lying between the incisors and molars).
- It should be possible to fit a hand between the throatlash and the jaw (Figure 24.13).
- A cavesson noseband should lie two fingers' width [2.5 cm (1 in)] below the cheekbone (Figure 24.14) and allow two fingers between it and the jaw when tightened.

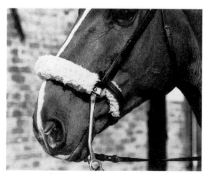

Figure 24.12. A simple type of bitless bridle.

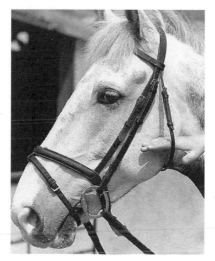

Figure 24.13. Fitting a snaffle bridle: throatlash.

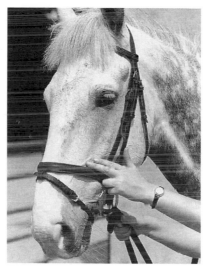

Figure 24.14. Fitting a snaffle bridle: noseband.

Fitting a double bridle (Figure 24.15)

A double bridle is fitted as a snaffle bridle except:

- The bridoon has a separate headpiece which buckles on the off side a little below the buckle of the main headpiece. The bridoon should slightly wrinkle the lips.
- The curb bit is fitted to lie below the bridoon so that it can work separately, but it must not be so low as to interfere with the tushes.

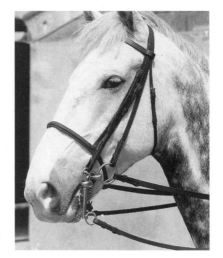

Figure 24.15. A double bridle correctly fitted.

- The curb chain is hooked on the off side and twisted clockwise so that the lip strap ring hangs down. The flat ring of the curb chain is put on the near side hook and the selected link is picked up, maintaining the twist to the right and placing it on the hook. If the curb chain is shortened more than three links, an equal numbers of links should be taken on each side. The chain must lie flat in the chin groove and remain flat when the curb is used. Double-link chains or ones made of leather are most satisfactory.
- The lip strap is buckled on the near side having been passed through the loose ring on the curb chain.

Fitting a pelham

The bit should lie close to the lips without causing them to wrinkle (Figure 24.8). The curb chain should lie in the chin groove and can be placed through the top rings of the bit to prevent chafing. Note that the curb chain hooks should open outwards away from the horse's face to avoid injury.

Nosebands

Drop noseband (Figure 24.16)

This noseband fits around the nose below the bit and is designed to prevent the horse opening the mouth and thus evading the bit. It should be fitted so that the front lies on the bony part of the nose; if too low it will interfere with breathing. The noseband should be attached to its cheekpieces so as to prevent it flopping downwards onto the horse's nostrils. It must not be fitted too tightly and must allow flexion and movement of the jaw.

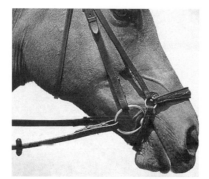

Figure 24.16. Drop noseband.

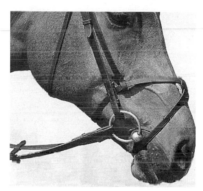

Figure 24.17. Grakle noseband.

Grakle noseband (Figure 24.17)

This has two straps that cross over the nose and below the bit in a figure of eight. It is designed to prevent the horse crossing the jaw and it is less likely to affect breathing than the drop noseband. It is fitted so that the headpiece ends just above the facial crest running down the side of the horse's head. The two straps are stitched together or pass through a leather pad.

Flash noseband (Figure 24.18)

This consists of a cavesson plus a strap that passes through a loop on the front of the noseband and does up under the bit. Again, it is less likely to affect breathing than a drop noseband and it also allows the use of a standing martingale.

Kineton noseband (Figure 24.19)

This noseband transfers the bit pressure to the nose and is used on strong horses. It consists of two metal loops attached to each other by an adjustable strap. Each loop fits around the bit ring next to the horse's face so that the centre strap rests on the bony part of the nose. When the reins are pulled the pull is transferred via the bit to the nose.

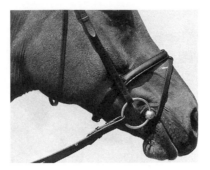

Figure 24.18. Flash noseband.

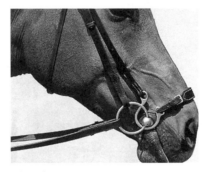

Figure 24.19. Kineton noseband.

Combination noseband (Figure 24.20)

This noseband acts as a combination of a cavesson and a drop noseband. The front part of the noseband sits higher on the nose than a drop noseband while the rear part sits below the bit in the chin groove. The two pieces of the noseband are connected by a strip of metal. The noseband has a fairly strong action and prevents the horse opening its mouth and also helps keep the horse straight.

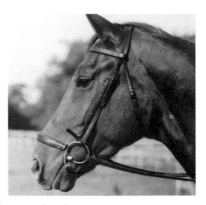

Figure 24.20. Combination noseband.

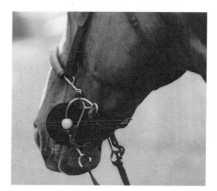

Figure 24.21. A combination bridle.

Combination bridle (Figure 24.21)

This is a combination of a bit and a noseband. The bit has an integral front noseband and a rear strap acting as a curb. Thus, taking a contact on the rein exerts pressure on the horse's poll, nose and chin. It is used on strong horses that have sensitive mouths and would resent the action of a gag or curb bit.

Martingales

Competition rules frequently limit the use of martingales as schooling aids. These rules often apply at the venue as well as during the competition.

Standing martingale (Figure 24.22)

A standing martingale has a neck strap through which passes a leather strap with a loop at either end; one end attaches to the girth, the other to a cavesson

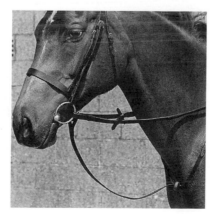

Figure 24.22. Standing martingale.

noseband. The martingale holds downwards on the horse's nose so that the horse does not lift its head beyond the point of control. The martingale should be adjusted so that it does not interfere with the horse when its head is carried in an acceptable fashion, nor should it tie the horse down and prevent it jumping spread fences effectively. When standing in a relaxed position it should be possible to push the martingale up into the horse's gullet.

Running martingale (Figure 24.23)

A running martingale has the reins passing through the rings of the martingale thus helping to keep the pressure on the bars of the horse's mouth when the head is raised. Correctly fitted, the martingale should only come into play when the horse raises its head above a permitted level. The rings of the martingale should nearly be able to reach the withers. A bib martingale has a centre-piece of leather to prevent the horse getting caught up in the branches of the martingale. Rein stops must be fitted on the reins to prevent the martingale rings getting caught on the rein fastening to the bit.

Irish martingale (Figure 24.24)

An Irish martingale or rings is a short strap with rings like a pair of spectacles, designed to prevent the reins coming over the head in the event of a fall.

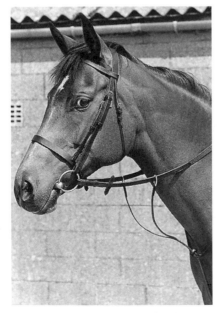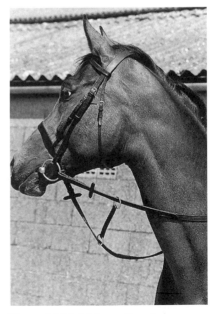

Figure 24.23. Running martingale.   **Figure 24.24.** Irish martingale.

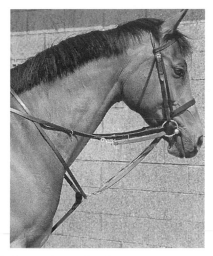

Figure 24.25. Market Harborough martingale.

Market Harborough martingale (Figure 24.25)

This has a normal martingale body that splits in two, passes through the bit rings and fastens onto the rein. Its action exerts a strong downward pull on the bit when the horse throws its head up.

Breastplate (Figure 24.26)

Breastplates are used to stop the saddle slipping back. A hunting breastplate is similar to a martingale with straps running back to fasten to the saddle 'D's'. Care must be taken not to fit them too tightly as they can cut into the horse's

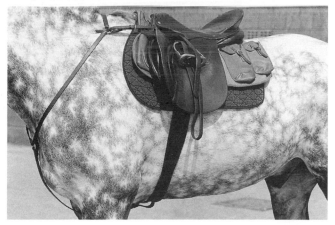

Figure 24.26. Breastplate. (The saddle is also fitted with a weightcloth.)

chest when jumping. Standing and running martingale attachments can be fitted to the breastplate. An Aintree breastplate is used for racing; this fastens around the chest and is kept in place by a strap over the withers.

Schooling aids

Most schooling aids are designed to teach the horse to lower and stretch the head and neck, thus stretching the muscles of the back and allowing the horse to engage the hindquarters. Schooling aids are common throughout much of Europe and elsewhere in the world. However, if misused they can cause accidents and so must only be employed properly by those trained and skilled in their use.

Draw reins (Figure 24.27)

Draw reins start at the girth, pass between the front legs, through the bit rings and back to the rider's hands. Each rein passes from the inside to the outside of the bit ring. Draw reins should be used with a normal rein placed above the draw rein. The draw rein may also be fitted so that it runs from the girth straps of the saddle, through the bit rings and back to the rider's hands.

Chambon (Figure 24.28)

The Chambon runs from the girth, between the horse's front legs to the poll and then down to the bit to put pressure on the poll and induce a lowered head carriage. It is used on the lunge with a mild snaffle bit.

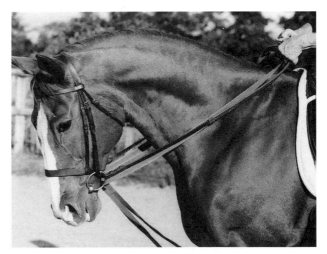

Figure 24.27. Draw reins.

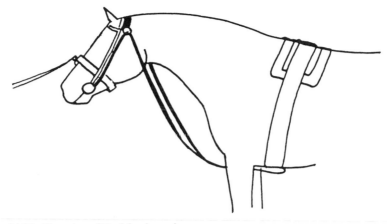

Figure 24.28. Chambon fitted for lungeing.

De Gogue (Figure 24.29)

The De Gogue is more advanced than the Chambon and can be used for ridden work as well as on the lunge. On the lunge, the De Gogue has a strap running from the martingale body to the poll, to the bit and back to the martingale or saddle 'D', forming a triangle. For riding, instead of passing from the bit back to a fixed position, a rein is attached.

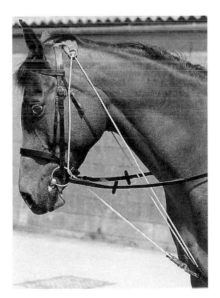

Figure 24.29. De Gogue.

Saddles

Structure of the saddle

The parts of the saddle (see Figure 24.30) are listed below:

- tree
- stirrup bars
- seat
- saddle flaps

- panels
- lining
- girth straps.

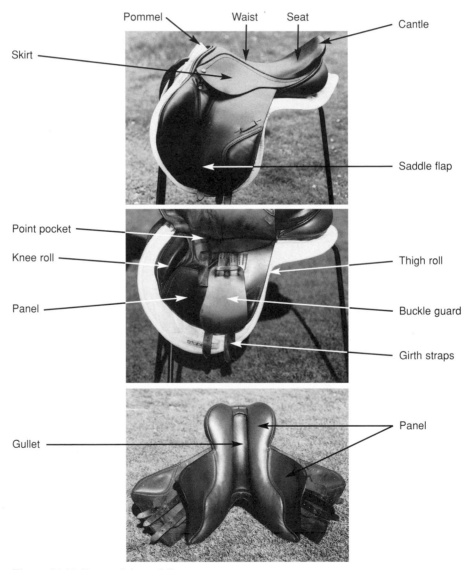

Figure 24.30. Parts of the saddle.

Tree

This is the framework of the saddle, and its size and shape depends on what the saddle is to be used for. Traditionally, it is made of beech-wood, but now tends to be made of laminated wood, bonded and moulded, giving a lighter and stronger tree. Racing saddles may have light, fibreglass tress.

The tree may be either rigid or spring: a rigid tree gives strength and solidity; a spring tree (Figure 24.31) has two flat panels of steel from the pommel to the cantle and allows the rider more direct communication with the horse underneath them. However, it may tend to concentrate the rider's weight onto a small area and is generally used with a numnah.

Stirrup bars

These are made of forged steel that is riveted to the points of the tree. A hinged safety catch is usually fitted and must never be used in the up position. The bars are placed forward in jumping saddles and further back in dressage saddles.

Seat

Initially, webbing is fixed from pommel to cantle and then covered in stretched canvas or linen to form the seat shape. Wool or foam is placed on top as a padding and finally the whole is covered in leather with skirts to cover the stirrup bars.

Saddle flaps

Saddle flaps and girth straps are then added. If the first two straps are fitted to the same webbing piece and the third is independent then the girth should be attached to the first and third straps. Dressage saddles may have long girth straps.

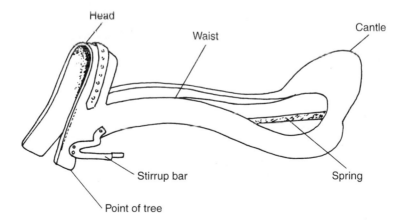

Figure 24.31. Part of the spring tree.

Panels

A full panel gives a greater weight-bearing surface and, combined with a wider-waisted saddle, is better for the horse. Thigh and knee rolls are also added to some saddles to help the rider's position. Short or half panels tend to be used on some pony saddles or on show or polo saddles.

Lining

Most modern saddles are leather lined and with careful treatment will give many years of use.

Serge and linen linings may be still found on sidesaddles, although they are rarely seen on new saddles today. Linen is more easily cleaned and harder wearing than serge.

Types of saddle

These include:

- jumping
- dressage
- working hunter
- general purpose
- showing
- long distance
- racing
- polo
- close-contact
- competition saddles.

Jumping (Figure 24.32)

The jumping saddle has forward-cut flaps and knee and thigh rolls to help the rider stay in balance in a forward position. A show jumping saddle may have a deep seat while a cross-country saddle may have a flatter seat to allow a greater range of movement by the rider.

Dressage (Figure 24.33)

This saddle helps the rider to achieve a deep seat and a long leg and is straighter cut with a long saddle flap. It may have large thigh rolls.

Working hunter

The working hunter saddle is a straight cut show saddle but with knee rolls for showing in working hunter classes.

General purpose

This is more forward cut than a dressage saddle, but still allows the rider to ride with longer stirrup. It is designed to suit all disciplines, and is also called an event saddle.

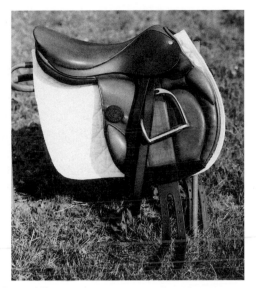

Figure 24.32. Jumping saddle.

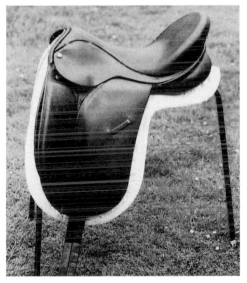

Figure 24.33. Dressage saddle.

Showing

This saddle is designed to show off a horse's shoulder and is only slightly forward cut with a half panel and a relatively flat seat. It is worn without a numnah. Some showing saddles also have a plain flap, no knee roll and a full panel.

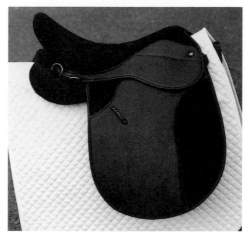

Figure 24.34. Long-distance saddle.

Long distance (Figure 24.34)
This saddle is designed like cavalry and Western saddles to spread the rider's weight over a greater area.

Racing
This is a lightweight saddle with a sloping head and very forward-cut tree. The design varies from the flat race saddle weighing a couple of kilos, or even less, to the more substantial National Hunt saddle.

Polo
This has a reinforced pommel with short panels and long sweat flaps. There are no knee or thigh rolls so that the player can move freely in the saddle.

Close-contact
Many eventers and show jumpers now favour this. They have a flat seat with a minimum of padding between the horse and rider to give maximum contact between the two.

Competition saddles
Many top-class professional riders now have saddles specifically manufactured to their specification for their competition horses.

Accessories

Several types of girth are available and include:

- Leather girths.
- Lonsdale or short girth: to fit on dressage saddles, may be leather or artificial.
- Synthetic: popular type.

- String or nylon: easily washed and commonly used.
- Lampwick: soft and comfortable, not suitable for hard work.
- Webbing: preferred for racing and by some eventers, it is less restricting than leather. Two girths should be used.

Leather girths (Figure 24.35) may be one of four designs:

- three-fold
- Balding
- Atherstone
- stud (Figure 24.36).

The shape of the latter two allows the horse's elbows to move while reducing the risk of rubbing. The three-fold girth has a material insert between the folds, which should be kept well oiled. All four may have elastic insets at the ends of the girth before the buckles to allow some stretch as the horse's chest expands when galloping.

The stud girth is shaped to prevent the horse injuring itself with its studs, when jumping.

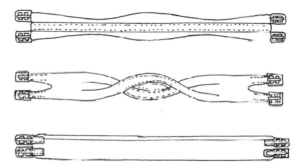

Figure 24.35. Girths (*from left*): three-fold; Balding; Atherstone.

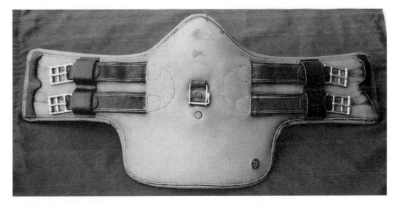

Figure 24.36. Stud girth for close-contact jumping saddle.

Stirrup leathers

These must be of the best quality and regularly checked for safety. The length and weight of leather will depend on the rider, with buffalo or rawhide being the strongest but also the most prone to stretching.

Stirrup irons

These should be made of stainless steel; nickel is soft and potentially dangerous. The size and weight of the iron must be suitable for the weight of the rider and the discipline, with clearance either side of the foot. Too big an iron is as dangerous as one that is too small. The bent leg (Simple) safety stirrup is designed for riders who like to have their foot well forward in the iron. Children often use a safety iron that has a thick rubber band replacing the outside of the iron. If the child falls off the rubber band pops off so there is no risk of being dragged. This stirrup is essential with the child's felt-pad saddle with 'D's instead of bars. Racing irons are made of lightweight stainless steel or aluminium. Rubber treads are often fitted to the stirrup iron to help the rider keep his or her foot in the stirrup.

Buying and fitting saddles

The importance of a well-fitting saddle for the comfort, well-being and performance of both horse and rider is now recognised. As a general rule it is wise to buy the best you can afford. For the large majority of saddle purchasers the services of a competent and experienced saddle fitter should be sought to ensure that a really good fit is obtained.

Saddle fit very much depends on the horse's breeding. For example, a Thoroughbred nearly always has high narrow withers thus requiring a narrow fitting saddle to avoid the saddle resting on the withers. Cobs and hunters generally require a fairly straightforward wide fit, but breeds such as Arabs and the New Forest ponies have problems all of their own, to the extent that 'Arab' and 'Forester' saddles have now been developed to cope with their shape.

Remember that the horse's shape changes as it matures and becomes fitter. The shape of the saddle also changes as the padding flattens.

Examining saddles

The following procedure should be used to examine a saddle:

- Test the tree for breakage and damage.
- Place the hands on either side of the pommel and try to widen and move the arch or hold the cantle and grip the pommel between the knees. Any movement or sounds may indicate damage.
- Up-end the saddle and view the underside for signs of ridges or uneven surface.

- Place the saddle on the horse to check it sits evenly with no tilt towards the pommel or cantle.
- Check the width of the gullet so there is no pressure on the horse's spine.
- Weight should be evenly distributed over the lumbar muscles not the loins.
- The saddle should not interfere with movement of the shoulder.
- When the rider is on the saddle it should be possible to place three fingers under the pommel (four fingers under a new saddle to allow it to drop).
- There should be ample clearance under the cantle and along the gullet.
- When viewed from behind, it should be possible to see a clear channel of daylight, even when the rider leans forwards or backwards.
- Take particular care when fitting second-hand saddles.

Measuring a horse for a new saddle

- Use flexible wire such as a coat hanger approximately 45 cm (18 in) long.
- Place this at right angles over, and just behind the withers, where the saddle should rest.
- Shape into the required outline and trace onto a piece of paper.
- Take the next measurement about 23 cm (9 in) further back and trace.
- Take a third outline from the top of the withers along the spine.
- Give details of the rider to the manufacturer.

Horses with conformational problems

Horses often do not conform to the ideal shape and may need special attention when having a saddle fitted:

- high, overly pronounced withers
- straight shoulders
- overweight horses with low withers.

High withers

A narrow tree will be required which may have to be cut back at the pommel to give room for the withers.

Straight shoulders

This saddle may slip forwards, particularly if the horse or pony has a large belly, for example, from eating grass. The saddle should be padded carefully.

Overweight horses with low withers

This is common in fat ponies and a crupper may be used which attaches to the back of the saddle and fits round the horse's dock, preventing the saddle slipping forwards.

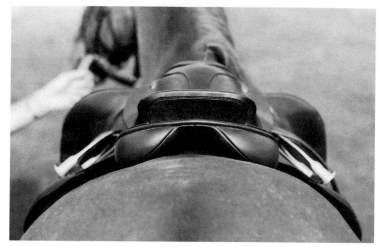

Figure 24.37. A correctly fitting saddle.

Common problems associated with a poor-fitting saddle

An ill-fitting saddle may be quite restrictive and could be responsible for any of the following problems:

- inability or reluctance to engage the hind quarters
- inability or reluctance to bend
- shortened stride
- reluctance to go forward
- hollow outline
- apprehension and general nervousness.

A correctly fitted saddle is shown in Figure 24.37.

Tacking up

- Collect the saddle, bridle, martingale and boots (if worn). Check that the throatlash and noseband of the bridle are undone and carry the bridle so that the reins are clear of the ground. Check that the saddle has a girth and numnah attached and carry it over your lower arm with the pommel towards the elbow.
- Put the equipment in a safe place outside the stable and catch and tie up the horse. Remove any rugs, groom the horse as necessary and pick the feet out.
- Put on the boots if appropriate.
- If a martingale is used, fit it before the saddle; untie the horse and pass the neckstrap over its head from the near side. Then tie the horse up again and put on the saddle, remembering to put the girth through the loop of the martingale.
- Put on the saddle before the bridle in order to allow the horse's back to warm up. With the saddle usually on the left arm, approach the horse from the near

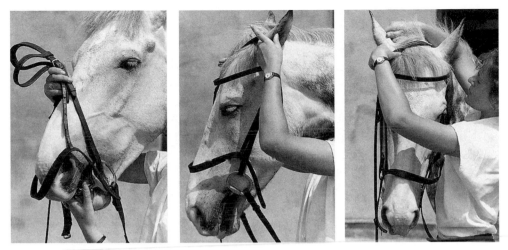

Figure 24.38. Putting on a bridle.

side and pat its back. Then using both hands place the saddle on the withers and slide it back into position. Straighten the numnah, pull it up into the arch of the saddle; ensure its straps are attached to the same girth straps on both sides. Check that the girth hangs straight on the far side before fastening it at the near side, checking that the skin is not wrinkled. Ensure that the stirrup bars are down for safety's sake.

- If the weather is cold replace the rug. If the horse is restless, fasten the buckles and roller.
- Put on the bridle (Figure 24.38). Carry the bridle and reins over the left arm with the browband nearest the elbow. Hold the bridle up against the horse's head to ensure that the fit is approximately correct. Then standing on the near side behind the horse's eye, reassure, untie the horse and unfasten the headcollar, perhaps placing it round the horse's neck. Pass the reins over the head and, holding the headpiece with the right hand, place the left hand under the bit, guiding it to the horse's mouth. Gently open the mouth by placing the first finger in the gap between the horse's incisors and molars. As the horse opens its mouth, slip the bit in and simultaneously lift the bridle with the right hand. Use both hands to put the bridle over the ears and to tidy the mane and forelock. Adjust the fit as necessary and then fasten the throatlash and noseband and replace the keepers. Put the headcollar back on over the bridle. If it is a double bridle ensure that the bridoon is on top and in front of the Weymouth.

Leaving a saddled horse

The horse should be tied up with the reins made safe; they may be doubled round the horse's neck, twisted and looped through the throatlash or slipped under a stirrup leather.

Untacking

On dismounting, run up the stirrup irons and loosen the girth. Take the reins over the horse's head and lead the horse into the stable, making sure to turn the horse round and close the stable door. Some stable yards insist that a headcollar is then placed round the horse's neck leaving the rope untied. Then unfasten the noseband and throatlash and release the martingale from the girth. Ease the bridle over the head, steadying the nose and allowing the horse to drop the bit in its own time. Put the bridle over your left arm, put on the headcollar and tie the horse up. Unfasten the girths and lift the saddle over the horse's shoulder, putting it on your left arm. Turn muddy girths before placing them over the saddle. Then place the saddle on the stable door or on the ground with the pommel towards the ground and the cantle, protected by the girth, against the wall. Finally remove the boots.

Care of the horse after untacking

After the horse has been untacked pick out the feet and, if necessary, wash off the hooves and heels. Check the legs for heat and swelling. Sponge the saddle and bridle areas to remove sweat marks, at the same time checking for rubs. Then brush the horse and replace the rugs.

Other saddlery

Numnah

Large protective pads made from a variety of materials aimed at protecting the horse's back underneath the saddle. They add comfort to the fitted saddle and also keep the underside of the saddle clean.

Saddle pad

Made from a variety of artificial materials, these include polypads, riser pads and gel pads. These are used under the saddle.

Headcollar

Leather headcollars can be expensive, but are safer to use than the Nylon version. This is because the Nylon headcollar will not break if the horse catches the headcollar on an object in the field or stable.

A well-fitted headcollar should have a noseband that lies about 5 cm (2 in) below the cheekbone. It should be possible to place a hand underneath the leather and jawbone.

Great care should be taken with foal slips as they grow out of them very quickly. Owners have been caught out with the foal's skin growing over the tightly fitted slip as the head increases in size. Foal slips must be checked and adjusted if necessary on a daily basis.

Care of tack and horse clothing

This is an important aspect of stable management, as poorly maintained tack is more likely to break and possibly cause an accident. Leather equipment and stitching will rot if exposed to the horse's sweat, heat and water.

Tack should be soft and pliable, not hard and brittle. It is important to clean tack for the following reasons:

- maintains it in good order, making it safer as less likely to break
- ensures pliability and softness reducing the chance of injury to the horse's skin
- allows the tack to be inspected for faults and breakages
- faulty tack should be removed and repaired before further use.

Many yards simply wipe over the tack and wash the bits on a daily basis. The tack is then taken apart once per week and given a thorough cleaning.

It is also important to keep tack in a dry environment that is not too warm. An overheated environment will result in the leather drying out.

Equipment required for cleaning tack

The following is a list of equipment required for tack cleaning:

- saddle horse
- bridle hook
- bucket containing warm water
- sponge for washing
- sponge for soaping
- brush for applying leather dressing or neatsfoot oil
- saddle soap (tin or bar)
- metal polish and cloth
- duster for polishing
- chamois or dry cloth for drying.

Cleaning leather

- Rub clean using a damp cloth or sponge.
- Muddy tack may need washing down with warm water.
- If excessively wet, dry off with a dry cloth or chamois.
- Rub in saddle soap with a slightly damp sponge.

- For leather that has been very wet apply a good leather dressing to replace the lost oil, before thoroughly applying saddle soap.
- The surface of the saddle should not be oiled as it may stain the rider's breeches.

Leather may become mouldy or dry during storage. This can be prevented by dismantling the tack, treating it with a leather dressing, wrapping it in newspaper and then placing in a plastic bag.

Cleaning bridles

- Hang the bridle up and remove the bit.
- Soak the bits in clean warm water.
- Take the rest of the bridle to pieces.
- Clean all the leather parts.
- Rub in saddle soap.
- Wash and dry the bit.
- Check stitching.

The bridle may then be put together again in the following order (see Figure 23.1 in the previous chapter):

- The headpiece should be threaded through the browband, ensuring that the throatlash is to the rear.
- The headpiece should be hung on a hook – for a double bridle the bridoon headpiece (sliphead) should be threaded through the near side of the browband, first under the main headpiece and buckled on the off side.
- The noseband headpiece should be threaded through the browband from the off side to buckle on the near side. It should lie under the headpiece.
- The two cheekpieces should now be attached. A double bridle will have two buckles on each side.
- The bit or bits should be attached the right way up and the lip strap if fitted put on. The lip strap should be pushed through the 'D's on the bit from the inner side to the outer side and buckled on the near side.
- All straps should be placed in their runners and keepers and the noseband placed around the bridle and secured by a runner and keeper.
- The reins should be replaced; on a double bridle the wider rein attaches to the bridoon while the narrower rein goes on the curb bit.
- The curb chain should be hooked on with the lip strap ring hanging down and the lip strap then fastened through the ring to prevent the chain being lost.
- The bridle can then be 'put up' by passing the throatlash around the bridle in a figure of eight, through the reins and securing by a keeper and runner.

Remember, buckle fastening always goes to the outside while billets (fixed hooks) go on the inside. The rough or flesh side of the leather goes against the horse's skin.

Cleaning saddles

- Place the saddle on the saddle horse.
- Remove the girth, stirrup leathers and irons and place on a hook.
- Turn the saddle over and wash the underside with a damp cloth.
- Clean the girth, stirrup leathers and irons with a damp cloth.
- Wash the girth.
- Apply saddle soap with a dampened sponge to all parts of the saddle, flaps, etc.
- Wipe the top surface with a dry cloth to prevent staining to the rider's clothes.
- Clean stirrup irons with metal polish if necessary.
- Check stitching particularly girths and stirrup leathers.

Top surfaces of suede or reversed cowhide should not be treated with saddle soap or leather dressing. Use a soft clothes brush to remove dry mud and dirt.

Cleaning and storage of clothing

Cleaning and storage of horse clothing takes place throughout the calendar year, e.g. heavy-duty winter stable rugs will be stored over the summer months as will summer sheets over the winter months:

- before storage, wash and dry
- if necessary carry out repairs
- brush woollen day rugs and blankets
- wash badly stained blankets
- send stable rugs to a specialist cleaner or wash at home
- wash webbing rollers and surcingles at home, taking care to oil any leather-work prior to washing
- clean leather rollers as per cleaning leather instructions above.

Storage

Rugs need to be stored correctively to prevent damage occurring from mice and moths. Rugs should be placed on shelves in rug boxes in a dry airy room.

Chapter 25
Preparing horses for use

Grooming

Stabled horses need regular grooming to help maintain their health. Grooming is important for several reasons:

- promotes health by stimulating the blood supply to the skin and helping tone surface muscles
- removes dirt and waste products from the skin
- improves the horse's appearance, keeping the coat clean and tidy
- promotes gloss and shine by spreading oils through the coat
- allows inspection for early signs of disease or ill health
- develops the horse–owner relationship.

Grooming kit

The grooming kit consists of several items, each having a specific use (see Figure 25.1):

- box to keep the kit in
- dandy brush
- body brush
- curry comb – rubber or plastic/metal
- water brush
- sponge
- wisp
- mane comb
- stable rubber
- hoof pick
- sweat scraper
- hoof oil and brush.

Dandy brush
This brush has coarse, stiff bristles and is used for removing mud and dried sweat from the body and limbs. It should not be used on any horse's head and only with discretion on the body of a thin-skinned horse or clipped horse. The

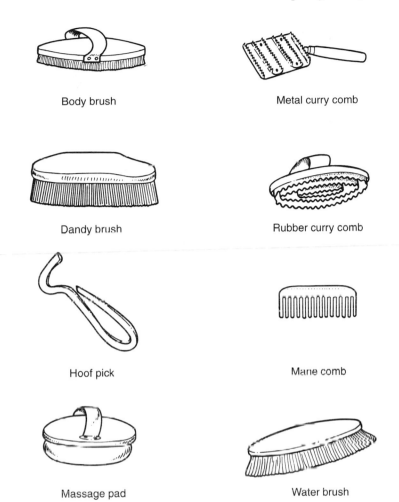

Body brush

Metal curry comb

Dandy brush

Rubber curry comb

Hoof pick

Mane comb

Massage pad

Water brush

Figure 25.1. Items of the grooming kit.

hairs of the tail should not be brushed out with a dandy brush or the tail will become thin. It is very useful for grass-kept horses and is the brush used for the first stage of grooming.

Body brush
The bristles of the body brush are shorter and softer than the dandy brush. It is used to remove grease and dirt from the coat (see Figure 25.2). The brush is held in the left hand when grooming the near side of the horse and changed into the right hand for the off side. It is used with a circular action to get deep into the coat and loosen the grease, followed by a long stroke to remove the dirt. The body brush is used to clean the horse's head.

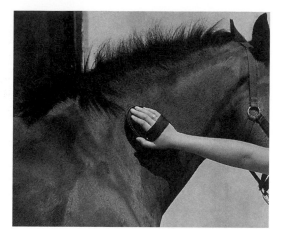

Figure 25.2. Using the body brush.

Curry comb

The curry comb is held in the other hand and used to clean the body brush; the body brush is swept over the curry comb every four or five strokes. The accumulated dirt is tapped out the curry comb at regular intervals. The metal curry comb with rows of teeth is only ever used to clean the body brush; using it on the horse's body would cause considerable discomfort. However, the rubber or plastic curry comb can be very useful for removing dirt and hair when the horse is shedding its coat.

Water brush

The water brush has fairly long soft bristles and is used to dampen or 'lay' the mane and tail before plaiting or to encourage the mane to lie flat or before applying a tail bandage. It can also be used to scrub the legs or feet clean.

Sponge

Several sponges will be needed: one for the eyes, nose and lips, one for the dock and sheath (these should be marked so that they are not mixed up), and a large sponge for washing the horse down or removing stable stains. These sponges should be kept for use on the horse not find their way into the tack cleaning kit!

Wisp

A thorough grooming may include the horse being strapped or wisped. This consists of stimulating the blood flow to the muscles and thus increasing muscle tone, by gently banging the muscles of the neck, shoulders and quarters (see Figure 25.3). It is similar to patting the horse, but a steady rhythm is established using more weight behind the 'bang', and as the horse anticipates the next blow its muscles tense. The wisp may be a stuffed leather pad or a traditional wisp made form a length of twisted hay or straw. If the horse is not accustomed to the process, it should be introduced very gently.

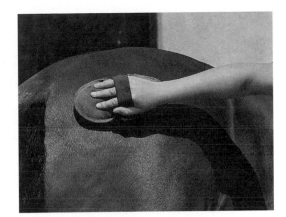

Figure 25.3. 'Strapping' or 'wisping' a horse.

Mane comb
A metal or plastic comb is used to comb out the mane, for pulling the mane and tail, and for preparing the mane and tail for plaiting.

Stable rubber
This is a linen cloth similar to the type of tea-towel used for drying glasses. It is used slightly damp to wipe over the horse at the end of grooming to remove any dust. It can also be used when strapping the horse to wipe the coat flat in between 'bangs' or used instead of the wisp as a folded pad.

Hoof pick
The hoof pick is perhaps the most important item of the grooming kit and yet the one most likely to disappear! It is used to remove mud and stones from the foot and may have a brush on one end to thoroughly clean the underside of the hoof. It should be used from heel to toe, following the contours of the frog (see Chapter 5 and Figure 5.2).

Sweat scraper
The sweat scraper is used to remove excess sweat or water from the horse's coat after exercise or washing the horse (see Figure 25.4).

Hoof oil and brush
These are used for oiling the feet after they have been thoroughly cleaned.

Grooming

There are several methods of grooming including:

- Quartering
- Strapping
- Full grooming.

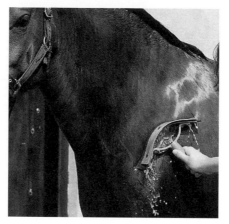

Figure 25.4. Using a sweat scraper.

Quartering

Done first thing in the morning, usually before exercise. The procedure is as follows:

- after feed and haynet, tie the horse up
- pick out feet
- turn back the rug
- brush or wash off and dry stable stains
- replace rugs to keep horse warm
- sponge eyes nose and dock
- brush mane and remove bedding from the tail.

Strapping

A full grooming is given first followed by a thorough strapping and wisping for quarter of an hour to stimulate muscle tone. This is not often undertaken today, but can be very useful for older horses prone to stiffening up.

Full grooming

This thorough grooming is best carried out following exercise when the horse is warm and the skin pores are open.

On competition days it may take place in the morning instead of quartering. The procedure should take approximately half an hour and may be carried out as follows:

- Tie up the horse, either in the stable or outside in a safe place. Tie the rope to a piece of string attached to a ring, and not directly to the ring.
- If warm enough, remove the rugs, if not fold them back over the quarters.
- Pick out feet using a hoof pick, starting at the frog and check the hoof health and shoes for signs of wear. Horses that are used to this procedure will let you pick all four feet out from the near side.

- If hooves are dirty, scrub them and allow to dry before applying dressing.
- Using a rubber curry comb remove any dried mud and sweat.
- Use the body brush to remove dirt and grease from the coat. Start on the near side just behind the ears and place the body brush in your left hand with the curry comb in the right. Brush the coat down in long sweeping strokes, periodically cleaning the brush against the curry comb.
- Put the curry comb down in a safe place.
- Brush the front leg by crouching beside it and holding it steady with your free hand.
- Brush the hind leg and hold the tail at the same time to prevent the horse raising it and possible kicking out.
- After brushing the body and legs, brush the mane with the body brush.
- Lay the mane over using a damp water brush.
- Untie the horse and remove the headcollar before gently brushing the head with the body brush as the horse may pull back.
- Replace headcollar and tie up the horse.
- Wipe the horse over with a damp stable rubber.
- Replace the rugs.
- Use a clean sponge to wipe the eyes, ears, muzzle and nostrils.
- Use a second sponge to clean under the dock.
- Brush with a body brush or finger the tail through.
- If the tail has been pulled, put a tail bandage on for half an hour.

Grooming the grass-kept horse

Care should be taken not to remove valuable oil and grease from the coat as this acts as a waterproof layer. Clean off the mud and sweat but do not thoroughly groom. The procedure is as follows:

- bring in from the field
- tie up in a safe place
- pick out and wash the feet
- remove mud from the coat with a dandy brush
- brush head with a body brush after untying the horse
- sticky sweat marks and wet muddy legs should be sponged off
- sponge the eyes, ears and nose
- use a second sponge to clean the dock area
- clean the mane with a dandy brush
- finger out the tail or use a body brush; if excessively dirty, wash the tail.

Cleaning the sheath
Greasy dirt naturally accumulates inside the horse's sheath and some geldings need to have this area regularly washed to prevent excessive build up. The sheath should be washed using warm water and very mild soap with the hands protected by rubber gloves.

Preparing the horse for competition

Horses should be well turned out and as clean as possible prior to competition. This should begin with bathing of the horse.

Washing the mane (Figure 25.5)

As always, it is important to be organised and the first thing is to gather all the equipment needed: warm water, horse shampoo, a large sponge, towel and sweat scraper. The horse should wear a headcollar, but should not be tied up in case it pulls back. The mane should be wetted with the sponge and a small amount of shampoo worked into the forelock. To prevent the shampoo going in the horse's eyes it may be useful to pull the forelock back between the ears. Gradually work down the mane using the fingers to thoroughly clean the crest. The mane should then be rinsed using the sponge until all the shampoo has been removed. Sweat scrape both sides of the neck and towel dry the ears before brushing out the mane and leaving to dry.

Washing the tail

Collect the washing equipment as before, put on a headcollar and tie the horse up. You may need an assistant for a young or nervous horse. The top of the tail should be soaked using the sponge and the end of the tail immersed in the bucket of water; if the end of the dock goes into the water the horse may drop its hindquarters suddenly. Shampoo should be worked into the tail and rinsed out as before. Excess water can be removed by gently swinging the end of the tail in a circle; stand to one side of the horse when doing this. The tail can then be brushed or fingered through. Spray preparations to prevent tangling can be applied at this stage.

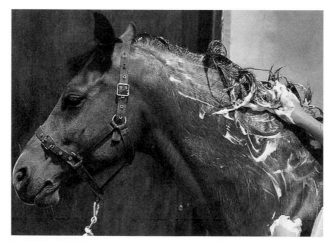

Figure 25.5. Washing the mane.

Bathing the horse

Light-coloured or muddy horses may have to be bathed prior to a competition. To prevent the horse becoming chilled choose a fine day, work quickly and dry the horse off rapidly. If the weather is chilly use warm water; a hose can be used on warm days. Hosing should be introduced carefully as the horse may be alarmed; trickle a gentle stream of water on the horse's front foot, gradually working up the leg until the horse accepts the feel of the water. Wash and dry the head first with the horse untied. Tie the horse up for washing, shampooing and rinsing. Then scrape dry and towel off, paying particular attention to the lower legs and heels. The legs may be bandaged to help them dry and, depending on the weather, the horse lunged or walked, with or without rugs, to dry off and keep warm.

Washing the legs

Many people wash their horses legs on return from exercise or if they are muddy after being turned out in the field. Care must be taken as constant washing removes protective grease from the skin resulting in cracked heels and mud fever. If the legs are to be washed use plenty of water and either let the legs 'drip-dry' in a deep clean bed or towel dry and apply stable bandages. The motto is – do it properly or not at all! Barrier cream on the heels and underside of the pastern can help keep the skin soft.

Care of the horse after exercise

The hot and sweaty horse needs prompt attention to prevent it getting chilled and help the body systems to recover.

- After the rider has dismounted, loosen the girth and noseband, and run up the stirrups.
- The horse should be walked until it stops blowing.
- Remove tack, including boots and bandages, and put the headcollar on.
- If cold, stand the horse in a sheltered area and sponge down the sweaty and muddy areas with warm water, paying particular attention to the bridle and saddle areas.
- In warm weather, stand the horse in the shade and use cold water or hose the horse down.
- Remove surplus water with a sweat scraper.
- Apply a sweat sheet with a stable rug on top and folded back and secured by a roller if the weather is cool. If warm, use a summer cotton sheet.
- Pick out the feet, wash them and remove studs if necessary.
- Put the horse back in its stable.
- Check after 30 minutes and remove sweat sheet if dry and replace stable rug if necessary.

Improving the horse's appearance

Not content with rearranging the horse's way of life, we also alter the way the horse looks, tidying the mane, tail, feathers and coat to suit fashion and the job the horse has to do. Thus, the competition horse and hunter has its mane and tail pulled, feathers and whiskers trimmed, and coat clipped.

Pulling the mane (Figures 25.6–25.9)

The horse's mane is pulled for several reasons:

- to improve appearance
- to thin and shorten the mane
- to make the mane easier to plait
- encourage the mane to lie flat.

However, Arabs and Mountain and Moorland ponies do not have their manes or tails pulled.

If possible pull the mane after exercise or on a warm day; the pores of the skin will be open, making it less painful for the horse when the hairs are pulled out. Some horses object quite strongly to the process and a handler may be necessary to restrain them. Thoroughbred-type horses tend to have fine manes that are easy to pull, while part-bred horses can have very thick manes that are tough to pull. Do not wash the mane first, as the hairs become too slippery to hold on to the pull effectively. The mane should be pulled so that it lies on the right (off) side of the neck. If it is reluctant to do so, loose stable plaits left in for a day or two followed by regular brushing and damping down will help train the mane.

Method

- Comb the mane thoroughly to remove all tangles.
- Separate out a few hairs from the underneath of the mane and run the comb up to the roots and remove them with a sharp pull.
- Repeat this process until the mane is of the desired thickness and length. Any remaining long hairs from the top of the mane can be shortened by breaking off the ends with the fingers. The forelock is pulled last.
- Remove the underneath hairs to ensure that the mane lies flat and grows evenly.

Plaiting the mane (Figures 25.10–25.14)

The horse's mane is plaited to make the horse look smart for competitions, to show the horse off in the show ring or to prospective buyers, or to make the mane lie tidily on the correct side.

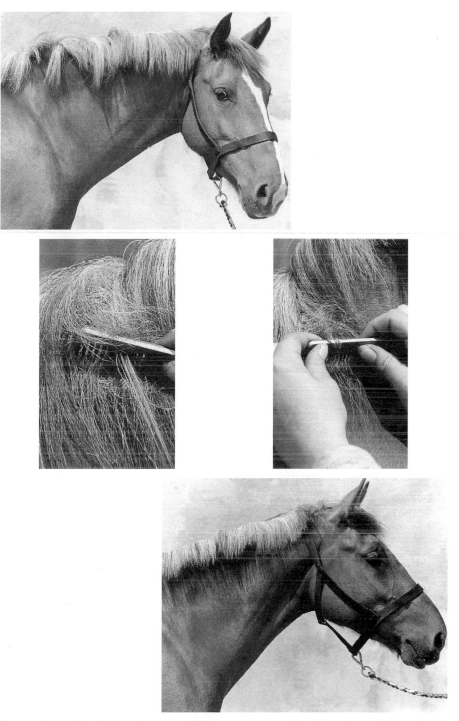

Figures 25.6–25.9. Pulling the mane. This mane now needs to be put into stable plaits to make it lie evenly.

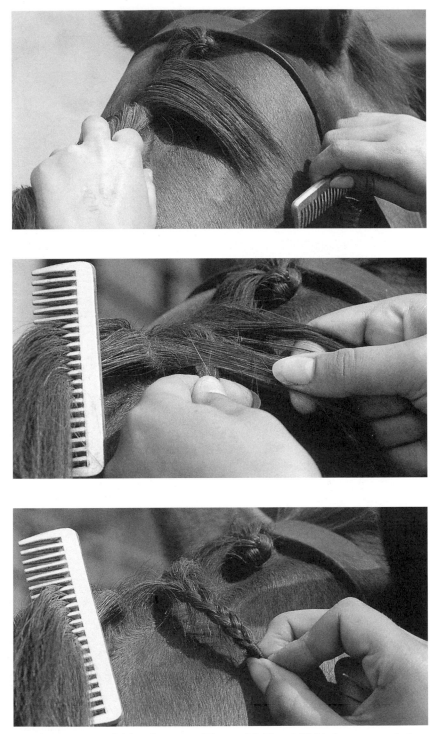

Figures 25.10–25.12. Plaiting the mane (Figures 25.13 and 25.14 shown opposite).

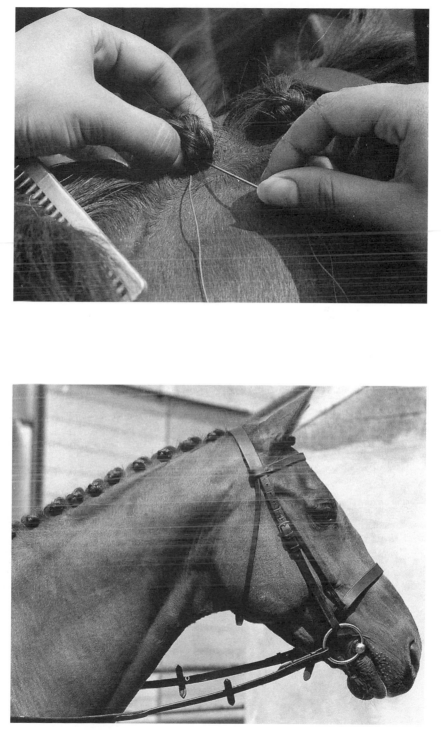

Figures 25.13 and 25.14. Plaiting the mane (*contd.*).

Equipment

Before starting to plait, the necessary equipment should be collected together. This includes a mane comb, water brush, water and something to stand on. The mane can be secured with thread of a suitable colour, traditionally the preferred method, or with rubber bands. If using thread, a pair of scissors and several needles will also be required. The needle should be of the thick, blunt-ended type used for sewing with wool.

Before starting

It is advisable not to plait the horse in a bedded stable in case a needle is dropped and lost. If this happens, the bedding in the area should be removed, the floor swept and fresh bedding put down. Before starting, it is a good idea to thread several needles with enough thread to do two plaits to save having to rethread the same needle and to place them securely in a piece of thick fabric within easy reach. Plaiting aprons with large front pockets are useful.

Method

- Comb out the whole mane and dampen it down using the water brush.
- Starting at the poll, divide the mane into as many plaits as required. Tradition used to demand seven or nine plaits, but the modern trend is for many small plaits. A thin neck benefits from larger plaits placed high on the crest while a fat neck can be disguised by smaller tight plaits.
- Using the mane comb to keep the remaining mane out of the way, divide the section nearest the poll into three equal bunches and plait down to the end. Pull the hair tightly at the beginning of the plait or the finished plait will look loose and fluffy.
- Once the end of the mane is reached, secure by wrapping the thread around it. There are various ways of making the actual plait. One way is to turn the end of the plait under, rolling the plait up towards the neck. Each turn may have to be stitched to keep the plait tight and secure. The plait can then be finished by pushing the needle through the whole plait from underneath and snipping off the thread. This way no thread will be seen. Alternatively, once the ends of the mane are secured the plait can be folded under to bring the end up to the roots of the mane, sewn and then folded again. If the mane is the correct length this will result in a tight ball at the top of the neck. If extra security is needed, the needle can be pushed up through the middle of the plait and the thread taken around the plait alternately to the left and right before cutting the thread as close to the plait as possible.
- Work down the mane until it is all plaited.
- The forelock is done last and can be plaited as the mane or in a similar way to a tail plait. If the horse is restless or head-shy, untie it and get a helper to keep the horse still.

Removing plaits

Take care when removing plaits; it is all too easy to cut the mane. Use small scissors or an unpicking tool working in the direction of the hair. In time you will be able to use very little thread and remove the plaits with two or three snips. Undo the plait with your fingers and damp down the mane to remove the curl.

Pulling the tail (Figures 25.15 and 25.16)

The horse's tail is pulled for several reasons:

- to improve appearance
- to show off the quarters
- to avoid having to plait the tail.

If possible, as when pulling the mane, pull the tail after exercise or on a warm day when the pores of the skin are open, making it less painful for the horse when the hairs are pulled out. Some horses object violently to the process and it may be necessary to restrain them. It is likely that the horse will bleed where each hair is pulled out and it may be better to spread the process out over several days.

Method

- Brush the tail thoroughly to remove all tangles and comb out the top.
- Separate out a few hairs from the side of the dock, run the comb up to the roots and remove them with a sharp pull.
- Repeat this process down each side of the dock until the tail is neat and tidy. Any long hair in the middle of the dock can be shortened or pulled to match the sides.
- Side hairs should lie flat and neatly against the dock.

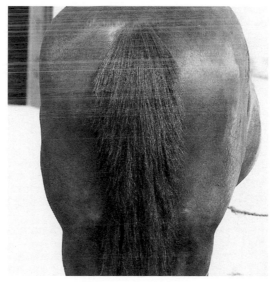

Figure 25.15. Unpulled tail.

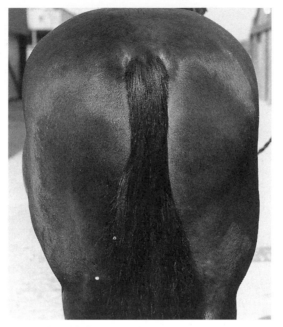

Figure 25.16. The same tail pulled.

Once the tail has been pulled it can be kept tidy by regular damping and bandaging. As the hairs grow they can be removed on a regular basis – tweaking out a few every day keeps the tail smart without making the horse resentful.

Plaiting the tail (Figures 25.17–25.21)

A full tail may be plaited for competition or hunting. The equipment needed is the same as for mane plaiting.

Method
• Wash and brush out the tail.
• Separate out a few hairs from either side of the dock and some from the middle of the dock to make the third strand of the plait.
• Plait down the tail incorporating a few hairs from the side of the tail each time. Make sure that the hairs are pulled as tight as possible.
• Continue the plait two-thirds of the way down the dock and then continue plaiting without taking any more hair.
• When the end of the hair is reached, sew it, loop it up underneath and stitch it firmly into place.

A bandage can be put on top of the plait to keep it tidy or for travelling. However, the bandage must not be pulled off, but unrolled carefully.

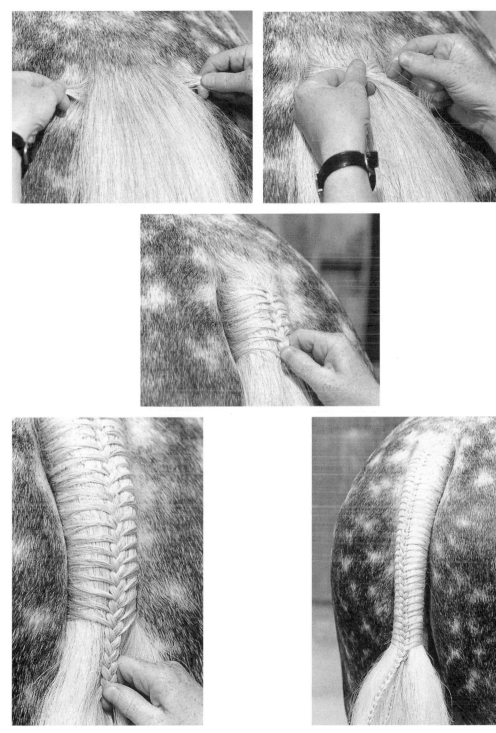

Figures 25.17–25.21. Plaiting the tail.

Putting up a tail

Tails may be put up for cross-country, hunting and polo to keep them out of the way. Plait the tail all the way down to the end and secure with a band or thread. Then turn up the plait to just below the dock, double it over and tape or stitch it into place.

Quarter marks

These are patterns of hair, set at angles to the normal lie of the coat. For example, the hair on the quarters can be brushed horizontally towards the tail to make the quarters look longer, while the hair on the barrel can be brushed vertically downwards to make the back look shorter and the girth deeper. A short comb, a pattern sheet or a brush can be used to create the patterns.

Clipping

Horses are clipped to remove excess coat; this usually means the thick winter coat that grows in October and lasts until about March.

Reasons for clipping

- To avoid heavy sweating and loss of condition.
- So that the horse can work longer and faster without distress.
- To make the horse easier to clean.
- To dry the horse off quicker thus avoiding chills.
- To improve appearance.

When to clip

The first clip is done usually after the horse's winter coat has established in early October. After this the horse may need reclipping as often as every 3 weeks until Christmas. Horses are not usually clipped after the end of January, once the summer coat has started to grow, as this may spoil the growth of the summer coat. However, performance horses may be clipped in summer to prevent overheating.

Types of clip

Full clip
With a full clip the whole coat is removed. A full clip is used for horses that grow a thick coat or for performance horses, for example, show jumpers, in the summer. A triangle is left at the top of the tail to avoid clipping the tail hairs.

Hunter clip (Figure 25.22)
With a hunter clip all the hair except that on the legs and saddle patch is removed; the hair on the legs gives protection from thorns, mud fever and cracked heels, while the saddle patch is left on to avoid saddle pressure. A hunter clip is used for horses in hard work that are going to sweat heavily.

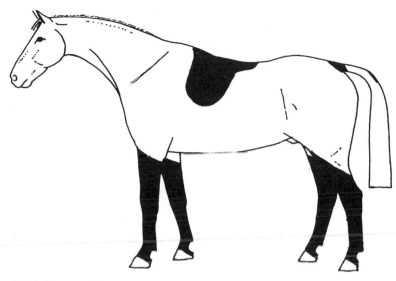

Figure 25.22. Hunter clip.

Blanket clip (Figure 25.23)

With a blanket clip hair is removed from the neck and belly leaving a 'blanket' over the back and quarters. A blanket clip is used for horses that feel the cold or are likely to be standing about, for example riding-school horses. It is also used as a first clip for eventers being fittened during the winter months and is useful for young horses that are unlikely to be working too hard.

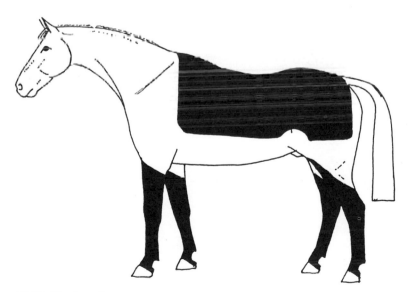

Figure 25.23. Blanket clip.

Trace clip (Figure 25.24)

With the trace clip, hair is removed from the bottom of the neck, top of the legs and the belly. The head is often left unclipped. A trace clip is useful for horses that are turned out during the day in New Zealand rugs and need some protection from the cold.

Chaser clip (Figure 25.25)

A chaser clip is a very high trace clip including the head, so called as it is sometimes used for National Hunt horses as it looks smart but still keeps the back warm.

Dealer clip (Figure 25.26)

With a dealer clip the hair is removed below a line from the stifle, along the bottom of the saddle flap, up the neck and down the side of the face. A dealer clip is a quick clip that makes a horse look presentable, allows to work and yet still leaves plenty of coat for protection.

Before clipping

Make sure that the clippers have been serviced, are in good working order and have sharp blades. Resharpen blades as soon as they become blunt and keep them in pairs in oiled cloth to prevent rusting. Start with a clean horse – a muddy or greasy coat will soon blunt the blades. Having decided which clip to give the horse, it is a good idea to measure lines with string and mark them with chalk. This will ensure that the lines of the blanket and trace clip are even on both sides of the horse. Finally, bandage the tail and put stable plaits in the mane to keep them out of the way.

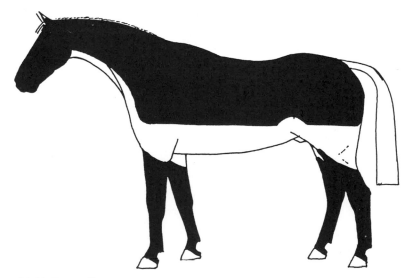

Figure 25.24. Trace clip.

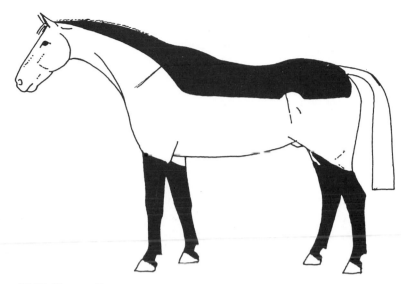

Figure 25.25. Chaser clip.

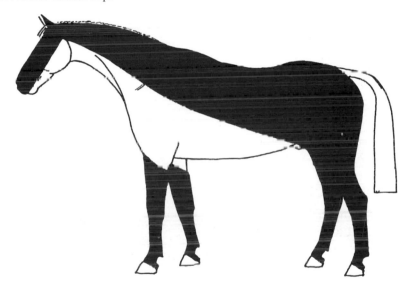

Figure 25.26. Dealer clip.

Clipping equipment

- Clippers and spare blades.
- Oil.
- Soft brush.
- Paraffin.
- Extension lead.
- Circuit breaker.

- Soft rag.
- Rugs and grooming kit.
- Assistant.
- Twitch.
- Dog clippers for head.

The clipping procedure

- The handler should wear suitable clothing and the horse should be clipped in a well-lit box. A box with a non-slip rubber floor is ideal, although some horses are less frightened if clipped in their own stable.
- Assemble the clippers with correct blade tension, oil the clippers and blades, and wipe off excess oil. If the horse has not been clipped before allow it to become accustomed to the smell and sound of the clippers before starting to clip.
- Start clipping in a safe place on the horse, for example the shoulder. This area is flat and not too sensitive. Move the clippers against the direction of hair growth.
- Use long sweeps with firm pressure, moving the skin as necessary in awkward places such as the elbows. An assistant is useful to hold up a front foot so that the skin around the elbow and chest is stretched – this will help avoid nicking the horse.
- During clipping keep the air filters clean and oil the blades regularly, checking that they are not hot.
- As you remove the hair, keep the horse warm by throwing a rug or blanket over it.
- Do not rush, as this leads to mistakes.

After clipping

Once the clip is completed brush the horse off, then wipe over with a damp stable rubber to remove any short hairs left behind. Then rug the horse appropriately. Dismantle, clean and oil the blades and clippers, and store them safely. Wipe clean the cables and leads before putting them away. Collect up the clipped hair in a skip and dispose of it.

Chapter 26
Travelling horses

Travelling is an important aspect of horse care today. Loading, unloading and travelling are hazardous procedures and it is vital to be well prepared and well practised in order to minimise the risk of accidents. Once a horse has had a bad experience, or has travelled badly, it can become very reluctant to load and can panic when on the move.

Clothing for travelling

Horses wear rugs and protective clothing during travelling; what they wear depends on several factors including:

- time of year
- weather
- length of journey
- whether the horse is alone or in company
- how well the horse travels
- type of vehicle.

The equipment needed includes the following (see also Figure 26.1):

- headcollar, rope and poll guard
- sweat rug or thermal travelling rug
- surcingle or roller
- in winter the horse should wear the equivalent of his normal day rug
- travelling boots or bandages with knee boots, hock boots and coronet boots
- tail bandage and tail guard.

Spare rugs should be available in case the rugs get wet or the horse sweats profusely.

Procedure before travelling

Vehicles and trailers must be regularly serviced and checked thoroughly before any journey. Checks should include: the floor, ramp and partitions of the horse space, and tyres of the trailer including tyre pressure, oil, water, fuel, battery and lights.

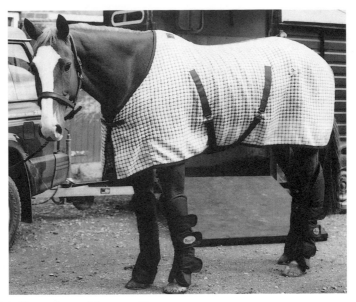

Figure 26.1. Horse dressed for travelling.

Once the trailer has been hitched up check:

- the coupling hitch and safety chain
- indicators, side lights, brake lights and the internal light
- the jockey wheel and cables are clear of the ground.

It is useful to carry insurance and horse registration documents as well as your driver's licence. Up-to-date maps and small first-aid kits for both horses and humans are essential. After travelling, the vehicle should be skipped out, the floor swept and left to dry. It is advisable to do this immediately so that the floor is protected from the rotting effect of urine and wet patches. If the weather is suitable, the floor may be scrubbed and hosed. Remember to lift the rubber matting regularly so that the floor underneath can be cleaned and left to dry out.

Loading a horse into a vehicle

Loading a fractious horse into a vehicle can be dangerous for both the horse and handler, and it is wise to think ahead if you do not know how the horse is going to behave. The procedure is as follows:

- Position the vehicle alongside a wall so that the horse can only escape to one side. Make sure that the gap is very small so that the horse is not tempted to run between the wall and the vehicle.
- Avoid slippery surfaces – concrete and tarmac tend to be slippery. If the horse is going to be awkward it may be better to park on grass.

- Bed down the floor with straw or shavings so that it looks inviting and is less noisy and slippery.
- Swing back and secure the partitions so that the horse is not having to enter a narrow space. It may be better to remove the partitions completely if possible.
- Open the jockey door or the front of front-unload trailers so that it is light inside the vehicle and the horse can see a way out.
- Make sure the ramp is level and firm so that it does not shift under the horse's weight.
- It is very important to have enough experienced help if you suspect that the horse will be difficult; even with well-behaved horses it is useful to have an assistant standing by the side of the ramp. The assistant should not stare at the horse as it approaches – nothing stops a horse going forward more quickly (Figure 26.2).
- The handler standing at the horse's shoulder should lead the horse forward and straight up the ramp (Figure 26.3). It is important not to pull on the horse's head. If the horse stops, pat it, look ahead and walk forward. If it pulls back, do not get into a fight, but move back with the horse until it is happy to move forward.
- Once the horse is inside the vehicle, do not duck under the breast bar, but stand by its shoulder until the back is secured by the assistant. The assistant should stand to one side when lifting the ramp so that if the horse does rush backwards the ramp will not fall on them.

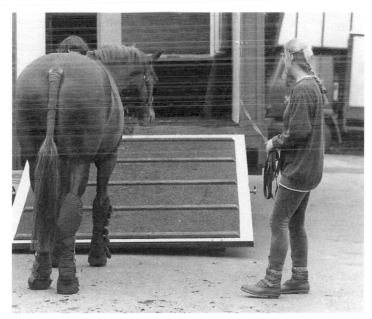

Figure 26.2. Approaching the horsebox.

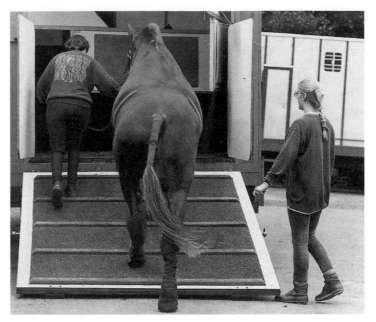

Figure 26.3. Loading into the horsebox.

- Once the ramp has been lifted and secured, tie the horse to a loop of string so that the horse cannot swing round but not so tight that it cannot balance. The string should be breakable, so that if the horse panics and goes down the string will release it.

If you are on your own then the horse should be loaded in exactly the same way, but using a lunge line instead of a lead rope. Once the horse is loaded, the lunge line can be threaded through the tie-ring and the tension on the horse's head maintained as the handler backs down the ramp and lifts it. It is important that the horse does not learn that it can rush back down the ramp, so never load on your own until the horse is reliable.

Coping with a shy loader

Horses can become difficult to load for many reasons including:

- Reluctance to leave the other horses – position the vehicle out of sight and earshot of other horses.
- Fear of the enclosed space or steep ramp.
- Habit – some horses are 'trained' not to load by inexperienced handlers.
- Memories of a bad journey or forceful loading.

Loading difficult horses should not be undertaken lightly; all handlers should be suitably dressed, including gloves, suitable shoes and a hard hat. The equipment needed includes a lunge whip and two lunge lines, food in a bucket, a snaffle bridle for control or a lunge cavesson.

The horse should be led quietly to the ramp and allowed to look where it is going. If the horse has a quiet temperament, first one front leg and then the other can be lifted and placed on the ramp, making much of the horse at each step. If the horse moves back, follow it and start again. This way the horse's confidence can be built up gradually until it is happy to enter the trailer. If a quiet or stubborn horse is not liable to kick, two people can link fingers behind the horse's hindquarters and push up once the front feet are on the ramp.

Alternatively, a lunge line can be buckled to each side of the vehicle, the lines held by two assistants and crossed behind the horse's hindquarters to encourage it forwards. Some horses give in as soon as they realise there is no means of escape, while others can lash out or rear against the lunge lines so care must be taken.

Young horses or horses that are reluctant to leave their companions may load more readily if a companion is loaded first. They can gain confidence from the fact that the other horse is not worried by the ramp or the enclosed space. Once the 'problem' horse is loaded, the companion can be unloaded, but take care that the horse does not panic once its friend has gone. Young horses may benefit from the company of an experienced traveller during their first few journeys.

Transporting horses

Many horses become reluctant to load, especially into trailers, after they have experienced a bad journey or forceful loading. Prevention is better than cure:

- Avoid sudden braking, rapid acceleration and fast cornering.
- Use the gears with brakes to decelerate gently into a corner or to a halt.
- Pull away from a standstill or out of a bend steadily and slowly.
- Pay attention when travelling over a rough or uneven surface.
- Remember that horses can become frightened if they have previously had a bad experience travelling.
- Overhanging branches and uncut hedges along narrow lanes can be very frightening.
- Trailers towed too fast can start to sway and become so unstable that they jacknife or turn over. This is extremely dangerous.

Unloading a horse from a vehicle

The vehicle should be parked in a safe, suitable place with enough room around it. The horse must be untied before the partition, front bar or breeching strap is undone. Many horses can become quite excited in anticipation of being unloaded; they must not be allowed to rush or jump off the ramp (Figure 26.4).

Care of the horse when travelling

The horse should be kept warm in winter and cool in summer, but remember that the vehicle and the number of horses will influence the temperature and the air available. A single horse in a trailer may get cold, even in summer, while a lorry with three or four horses may become very warm even in winter.

There must be adequate fresh air, but no draughts. Many lorries are very poorly ventilated. It is better to put an extra rug on the horse and have more air than a warm stuffy environment.

A non-slip floor which makes minimum noise and hence disturbance to the horse will help the horse travel more calmly as will ensuring that horses have adequate space and that the vehicle has suitable suspension.

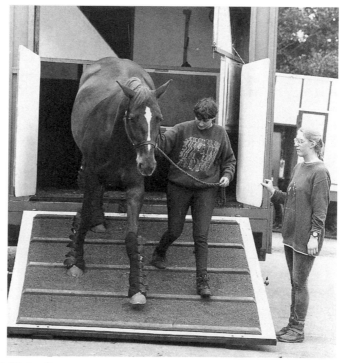

Figure 26.4. Unloading.

Travelling mares and foals, inexperienced travellers and stallions

Some horses have special requirements during travelling. A mare and foal will require about twice as much room as normal; the mare should be tied up while the foal travels loose. The partitions may need to be adapted so that the foal cannot pass under them.

Inexperienced, or very poor, travellers may prefer to travel loose in a large area so that they can find a position that suits them. Studies have shown that travel stress is reduced when horses travel backwards.

Stallions need special partitions to prevent them biting the horse next to them; alternatively they can be muzzled.

Feeding and watering on journeys

One of the major problems horses experience when travelling long distances is dehydration; it is very important to offer the horse water at frequent intervals. If the horse is sweating it is wise to include some electrolytes. Some horses are more fussy about water than they are about food so take some water from home in a couple of containers so that the taste of unfamiliar water does not put the horse off drinking. If the horse refuses to drink try adding a few molasses to the water at home so that you can do the same at your destination and disguise the different taste. Fortunately, most horses will drink when they are thirsty no matter what the water tastes like!

The horse will spend a long time standing still during the journey so to avoid swollen legs or any other metabolic upsets the concentrate ration must be reduced. However, in order to avoid loss of condition, allow the horse plenty of good-quality hay during the journey so that the gut is kept moving and partially full the whole time; this will reduce the risk of colic. Concentrate feeds should be small, easily digested and given at regular intervals.

Chapter 27
The horse at grass

The horse evolved as a nomadic grazer roaming freely over extensive areas to find food and shelter. As the horse grazed it left its droppings behind and moved to a clean area. This is the horse's natural environment. Humans have enclosed horses in smaller, more intensive paddocks where they are more dependent on humans to provide them with their needs.

To spend some time at grass on a daily basis is desirable for all stabled horses and ponies. This is important for psychological health, even for fit racehorses, and many of these now spend time at pasture where the land is available for this purpose.

Some gently ridden horses and ponies spend most of their time at grass. Horses at grass need daily attention.

Requirements of a paddock

Paddock requirements include the following:

• Should be close to the house or stable yard.
• Preferably should be on relatively flat land.
• Should contain well-established meadow grasses with some herbs.
• Trees and hedges should provide natural shelter from the elements or an artificial field shelter should be built (Figure 27.1).

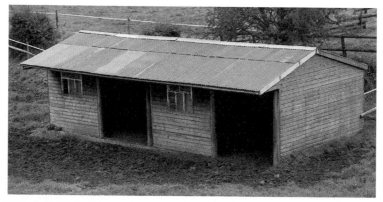

Figure 27.1. A field shelter.

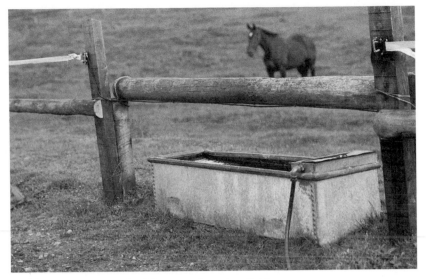

Figure 27.2. A water trough with access from two fields.

- Good quality, safe fencing of the boundaries, easily maintained with no barbed wire.
- Hazardous areas such as ponds should be fenced off.
- Good loam soil base.
- Good drainage to help prevent excessive poaching in winter.
- Good water supply: natural such as an unpolluted running stream with a stone bed or artificial.
- Water troughs should be properly sited and safe (Figure 27.2). Ballcocks should be covered to prevent horses chewing them.

Fencing

Many different types of fencing are appropriate, and it is the responsibility of the owner to make sure fences and gates are safe and secure. If horses are kept in adjoining fields, particularly on studs, then they may benefit from a double line of fencing at least 1.8 m (6 ft) apart.

Commonly used types of safe fencing include:

- hedges
- walls
- post and rail
- stud rails
- high-tensile wire mesh
- plain wire
- electric fencing.

Hedges

Thick, well-trimmed hedges provide a good fence and a degree of shelter. A hedge ideally should be 1.2–1.5 m (4–5 ft) high. Poisonous plants or bushes such as yew should be removed. Any gaps should be filled with another choice of fence, but not barbed wire.

Walls

Stone walls are found in certain parts of the country. If a suitable height and in good condition they may provide good barriers. If too low they may need a rail, two strands of tightened plain wire or a line of electric fencing along the top.

Post and rail

Requires a lot of maintenance and is costly to erect. Wood needs to be creosoted to prevent horses chewing it and to prolong the life of the wood. The fence should be checked daily for broken rails and protruding nails, and repairs undertaken as necessary. Fence posts should be sawn off flush with the fence.

Stud rails

More durable than wood, and more easily maintained. Consist of plastic strips 10 cm (4 in) wide, containing high-tensile wire. These are erected on plastic or wooden posts.

High-tensile wire mesh

Heavy-duty wire mesh topped with a plastic or wooden rail to make it visible to the horse. Small ponies or foals may, however, be able to get their feet through the mesh and injure themselves trying to remove it. Mesh fencing should be inspected daily for tears and holes and repaired.

Plain wire

Must be well erected and strung firmly. Topped with a rail, this is an economical method of fencing. High-tensile steel wire is more expensive than ordinary plain wire, but it lasts longer. It must be erected properly.

Electric fencing

The use of electric fencing is very common. It is inexpensive, easily maintained and portable. It keeps horses away from boundary fences and prevents them playing or fighting over the top. It may also be used for strip fencing for horses and ponies on restricted grazing areas. It is often used to divide up smaller paddocks for temporary reasons such as resting.

The fence runs off a 6-volt battery and consists of iron or plastic-coated posts with insulators at the top.

For permanent fencing, insulators may be directly attached to the wooden fence posts. Visible, fabric strips containing wire are then looped through the insulator rings at either end and attached to the battery. Horses develop a healthy respect for electric fencing and for this reason it is extremely useful for prolonging the life of permanent fencing.

Unsuitable fencing

Horses are liable to injury from unsuitable fencing and some of these injuries may be life threatening as horses get caught up in it. The following should not be used under any circumstances:

- barbed wire
- wire netting
- sheep or pig wire
- iron railings.

Gates

These may be wooden or metal and should be hung so they easily clear the ground when opened. Posts should be set in concrete approximately 1 m (3 ft) into the ground. For security reasons, gates are often now padlocked.

Paddock management

Objectives should include the following:

- To prolong the grazing period over the year by maintaining a vigorous sward of a suitable type.
- Minimise infection from internal parasites such as worms.
- Rotation of smaller paddocks to allow time for maintenance and resting.
- Maintain the pasture free from weeds and poisonous plants.
- Maintain the paddocks keeping them in good order.
- Maintain a dense sward to cover the soil and provide protection to the horses' legs.
- Prevent overgrazing and excessive poaching.

Paddock management is essential to provide horses with nourishment and exercise throughout the year. Many livery yards prevent horses being turned out on pasture whenever it is wet and in some cases all winter. A solution to this common problem is to allow turn out on a rota basis using one or two paddocks or fields through the winter. These should preferably be the ones with better drainage, as they are likely to become poached and lacking in grass. However, horses still benefit from the fresh air and exercise. These poached fields may then be rested from spring, harrowed and rolled.

Stocking rate

This depends on a number of factors and there is no set formula:

- soil quality
- rainfall
- time spent at pasture
- amount of land available
- parasite control
- control of pasture management.

If the pasture were of good quality, then a stocking rate of approximately one horse or two ponies per acre throughout the year would be acceptable. The most significant problem related to stocking rates is the lack of growth of grass through the winter and the abundance factor in the summer.

Pasture management through the year

Spring grass will be expected to contribute to the nutrient intake of horses and ponies. Good pasture should also provide a cushion for feet and legs.

Grass growth fluctuates tremendously during the growing season (spring to late autumn). These fluctuations in grass growth are also dependent on external factors such as temperature, rainfall (or lack of), fertilisation and stocking rates, to name but a few.

Pastures for horses should not be too lush. In spring when young grasses begin to grow quickly, they are very low in fibre (fewer stems and more leaves). Often horses may be seen relentlessly chewing the post and rail fencing (if they can) or chewing trees in their search for long fibre. It is therefore a good idea to leave a small amount of hay out in the field for them to pick at in early spring, as this will contain the long fibre they require.

Harrowing

Assuming pasture has not been hammered over the winter, the first step should be harrowing, to remove the dead and matted grass and moss which clogs up the spring grass that is trying to grow. The dead material also prevents air from circulating. Harrowing will help to break up rough surfaces caused by poaching and to flatten molehills. Any droppings on the pasture should ide-

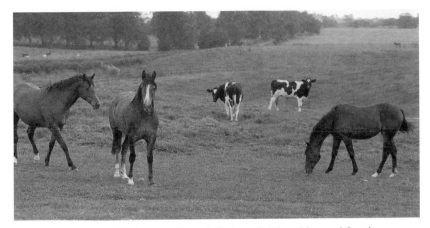

Figure 27.3. Mixed stocking can be financially beneficial and is good for the pasture.

ally be removed prior to harrowing. If not, any worm eggs will be spread widely over the grazing area.

Horses tend to graze paddocks unevenly. They will often select a 'toilet' area for urinating and dunging, and they tend not to graze these areas unless they are very hungry. As a result the grazing areas become shorter (lawns) and the dunging areas become longer (roughs). If the droppings are not being removed on a regular basis, the harrowing should only be carried out on hot dry days! This will kill off worm larvae. If it is damp and warm, they will thrive on the pasture. If droppings are being regularly removed, then harrowing can continue over the season, preferably using the smooth side of a reversible harrow.

Ideally, cattle may be used to graze after horses on a rotational basis. This will help to clean up the paddocks and break the worm life cycle (see Figure 27.3).

Fertilisers

A suitable organic or semi-organic fertiliser should be applied if the acreage available is limited or the pasture is of poor quality, it is, however, not essential. Organic fertilisers release their nutrients slowly and therefore do not result in fast, lush growth. Choice of fertiliser is a personal one and if grass is being grown for hay or haylage then a nitrogen fertiliser should be applied.

Many horse pastures contain high levels of clover, a nitrogen-fixing plant. Bacteria in the roots of clover are able to fix nitrogen from the atmosphere into the soil. High clover pastures for grazing will not need additional nitrogen.

Once the paddocks have been fertilised, they should not be grazed for a couple of weeks. Follow the manufacturer's recommendations. All paddocks that are going to be fertilised should be treated by the beginning of April, even if the soil temperature is still low.

Rolling

The paddock should be rolled either before or after fertilising. If a heavy roller is used after fertilising this will help to incorporate the fertiliser into the soil. Rolling also helps to flatten poached areas and encourages grass plants to tiller (push up new shoots).

If the land is dry enough for a tractor to drive on it without damage, then preparations should begin during March and no later than early April.

Rolling is useful for paddocks that are to be used for hay or haylage as it flattens the soil surface.

Weed control

Good pasture management will help to discourage the growth of weeds, but often this is not enough and further steps should be taken to remove weeds. Topping and selective use of a scythe will help to control them. Docks, thistles and bracken may be spot treated using a knapsack sprayer. Strict regulations now exist with regard to the use of herbicide sprays by untrained people. Unless used by the landowner, the sprayer must hold a certificate of competence after successful completion of a day's training.

For widespread weed invasion, the whole paddock should be sprayed. Consult with the local farmer or seek professional help.

Ragwort needs special attention as it is a poisonous plant (see below).

Clover

Too much clover can be a problem and this may be sprayed with a herbicide containing MCPA (2-methyl-4-chlorophenoxyacetic acid).

Ragwort

The familiar yellow flowers of ragwort are commonly seen growing in horse pastures. Because it is not highly palatable and therefore not a plant that many horses and ponies would choose to eat if pasture was abundant, many horse owners assume that these plants are not causing any harm. However, on sparse pastures or starvation paddocks, ragwort may become tempting to the hungry horse or pony. More importantly, horse and ponies may ingest dried ragwort in hay. Once dried it becomes more palatable to the horse and more difficult for the horse owner to see and remove.

Ragwort is a killer of horses and ponies. Each year hundreds die a slow and painful death due to ragwort poisoning. Ragwort contains dangerous toxins that specifically attack the horse's liver cells, the toxin works cumulatively and with each mouthful of the plant more damage is done. By the time the horse or pony is showing clinical signs as much as three-quarters of the liver may have been destroyed, resulting in terminal liver failure. There is very little that can be done to save these affected horses and ponies.

Horse owners have an absolute responsibility to remove ragwort from their paddocks. It should be dug up and removed and burnt well away from the field. This will help to reduce overall numbers by preventing ragwort seeds being blown onto the pasture and neighbouring fields.

Horse owners should also inform their local authority of areas where ragwort is a specific problem as it is legally a dangerous weed and substantial fines may be, and have been, imposed where the landowners have failed to remove the plant.

Rotating and topping

During the summer, the horses should be rotated around the paddocks with each paddock being given at least 2 weeks' rest. If grass is excessive or a field has been set aside, then this grass may be conserved for winter feeding in the form of hay or haylage. Local farmers should be able to help with this. Rotating with other farm livestock such as cattle or sheep will help to keep the paddocks tidy and will remove parasitic worms from the pasture.

As the summer progresses, the pasture should be mowed to top any new weeds emerging and rejected grasses. This is more important where only horses are kept with no other farm livestock.

Collection of droppings

This is a labour-intensive exercise, but an extremely valuable one. Most importantly this reduces the worm burden of the paddock to a large extent. It prevents the formation of roughs and lawn areas by keeping the grazing sweet. It also improves the appearance of the paddock.

Larger yards and studs use vacuum machines attached to small tractors to remove the droppings.

Pasture improvement

Poor pasture may be improved. For example, a sandy soil may benefit from organic manure and a clay soil from artificial drainage.

Neglected paddocks may be renovated by undertaking the following:

- make good the fencing
- check and install water supplies where necessary
- check drainage and install if necessary
- lime.

Soil acidity

This should be checked every 5 years or so. The local agricultural merchant or garden centre will supply you with a pH testing kit. A pH of less than 7 is acidic. Grass should have a pH of 6.5. Soil that is more acidic will result in good pasture plants failing to thrive and may reduce uptake of important minerals by plants from the soil. Alkaline soil (pH above 7) may benefit from a dressing of farmyard manure, not horse manure. A pH of less than 6 will require treatment with lime or ground chalk. This will add calcium to the soil.

Plant nutrients

Apart from calcium (in soil and lime) other important nutrients to consider are:

- nitrogen (N)
- phosphorus (P_2O_5 – phosphate)
- potassium (K_2O_5 – potash).

Nitrogen is leached out of the soil by rain and so is only used in the growing season. Phosphates and potash are required for plant efficiency. Local agricultural merchants will assist in the assessment of pastures and provide advice regarding these nutrients.

However, too much quick-acting phosphate will upset the horse's calcium: phosphorus balance. Some people are anxious about the use of 'chemical fertilisers' and prefer to use those with an organic base. These are generally slower acting and more expensive, but they provide some minor nutrients which the soil might lack and they may well be free of fluoride which is often found in compound fertilisers. Owners of breeding stock will be anxious that their mares cycle regularly and produce healthy foals every year. They should, therefore, consider soil nutrition as it affects horse nutrition.

Phosphate encourages clover that produces free nitrogen from nodules on its roots. A little clover is desirable in the sward; one plant of wild white clover for each square metre is sufficient. An excess of clover makes the herbage too rich for horses.

The bulk of the sward should come mainly from a late-flowering perennial ryegrass of prostrate growth. A grass called S23 meets this need. Creeping red fescue is productive and gives a good turf; crested dog's-tail also resists treading. In dryer areas, a little smooth-stalked meadow grass may be added to the mixture, and in wetter areas rough-stalked meadow grass is good. Cocksfoot is hard-wearing but grows into clumps. Timothy is persistent, and most horses prefer tall fescue.

The main ingredients in the grass mixture should be presented by two similar varieties. A suitable seed mixture for a hard-wearing, palatable and productive paddock might be as follows:

Species	kg/ha
Perennial ryegrass (two varieties)	18
Creeping red fescue	5
Crested dog's tail	1
Rough- or smooth-stalked meadow grass	2
Cocksfoot, timothy, tall fescue (two of each)	6
Wild white clover	1
	33 (30 lb/acre)

This mixture is mainly for grazing, but an occasional cut of hay may be taken from the sward. It is best not to put herbs into the mixture as they make it harder to use weedkillers (called herbicides!) and for hay to dry out. However, horses like herbs, the deep roots of which bring up minerals from the soil. A compromise can be achieved by hand-sowing a strip of herbs along the fence. These herbs should include chicory, ribwort, yarrow and burnet.

Horse pasture is rarely ploughed up, but the mixture suggested can be used to renovate old pastures as well as to create new ones. If a paddock is thin, renovate by mixing the seed with fertiliser, applying by means of spinner or by hand broadcasting. Seeding must be done in spring or autumn. Chain-harrow before seeding and ring-roll afterwards.

Working horses from grass

Many advantages are claimed for grass-kept horses. It is a natural system, and has much to recommend it. Less straw and hay are used and less time is spent on routine management. The horses need not be ridden because they exercise themselves.

This system has corresponding disadvantages. The horse is often too fat in summer, and in winter the conditions are often wet and muddy. Where a horse is kept at grass, it should be caught up and handled daily if possible. Supplementary feeding will be necessary in winter, and where there is insufficient grass during the summer as well.

It is easier to operate on the 'combined system' where the horse spends part of each day at grass and part in its stable. Thus, in summer the horse, or more particularly the pony, is shut in for part of the day to limit its food intake and also to protect it from flies. In winter the horse may be stabled at night or else shut in well in advance of being ridden so that it can be dried off. This is an ideal method for keeping hunters.

Horses working from grass in winter will usually be given a trace or blanket clip. This makes grooming easier and the horse can gallop about without undue sweating. A clipped horse will need a good New Zealand rug. The best designs have two straps at the front, a well-fitted back and good leg straps so that the rug will stay in place even when the horse rolls.

The unclipped horse can stay out without a rug, but its long coat means that there is the problem of drying its back in wet weather before saddling up. The best method is to put it in the stable with a thatch of straw, lightly covered with a cut-open lightweight sack held in place with a loosely fastened surcingle. After half an hour or so, the worst of the mud may be brushed off. It is undesirable to remove the natural protective grease from an unclipped horse living at grass, and so only a dandy brush should be used. If the back is not cleaned before saddling up, mud will be ground into both the saddle and the horse's back, which could cause sores.

A wet horse must not be left in the stable after riding. If it is to remain stabled, it should be thatched. If the horse is to be turned out, this should be done straightaway so that the horse can roll and keep on the move. A cold, draughty stable and a wet horse will soon lead to a chill.

A variant of the traditional system which, although expensive in initial outlay, offers many advantages of the paddock without the mess, is that of the shelter/stable with a free-draining sand yard attached. The ever-increasing cost of bedding and labour means that this system will become more important.

Whether in field, yard or stable, there is always the problem of how best to feed hay and concentrates. In the field, concentrates may be fed in bowls. Those set in car tyres are good as they tip less easily and have fewer sharp edges. Bowls should be spaced out and it is a good idea to have one more bowl than the number of horses as there will be plenty of swapping when the greedy see off the timid. Hay can be fed on the ground along the fence line to reduce treading. On clay fields, the fence line soon becomes poached. Nets are laborious and a slight hazard, and hay racks tend to be wasteful. Feeding hay in a shed may induce kicking or biting. If available, cheap plastic pods set along the fence are the best answer. Hay is pushed in at one end of a tube, which is like a flute, and the horses pull it out through the holes.

Feed and mineral blocks

Feed or mineral blocks provide useful nutrients for horses and ponies kept at grass particularly where forage (either pasture or hay/haylage) is fed.

Mineral buckets may be placed in the field for horses and ponies with good body condition. Neither feed nor mineral blocks should be used in conjunction with concentrate feeds, unless under veterinary or a qualified nutritionist's supervision. Feed buckets may be made available for horses needing more energy and protein, but with both consumption must be monitored so that intakes are as recommended. If overconsumption occurs they should be removed immediately.

Management routine

When horses are kept solely at grass, a daily visit is essential. The experienced eye will spot small details that may give a clue to more significant events.

Is the horse always standing away from hedges bordering roads because children throw stones at it? Is the good summer weather going to produce a heavy crop of acorns, which will fall and be of sufficient quantity to poison the horse if eaten? Is the coat 'staring', indicating an increased worm burden? These are the sort of questions to ask. Changes are sometimes so slight that only a visit with someone who has not seen the horse for several weeks may draw attention to subtle changes.

The daily check of the horse at grass is usually made entirely by eye. The horse should be looked over for injuries. Particular attention should be paid to the feet. A hand run under the belly, down the legs and over the back may detect something that the eye has missed. This last check may need two people for safety and convenience: it may be carried out weekly. It is a good plan to have a hoof pick and to lift, inspect and pick out the feet at least once a week.

The daily check must include the water supply and the general state of the field, including the grass. By October, for example, grass has less feed value, and hay or concentrates may need to be started or increased.

The field boundary should be walked regularly and any fencing defects noted and made good. Areas by footpaths, public roads or people's gardens all need regular checks for items thrown away, particularly wire, tin, glass or rubber. Like litter collecting, weed removal needs constant attention: poisonous plants such as woody nightshade, foxglove and so on should be uprooted and removed. Ragwort repays pulling up. Docks and thistles do not spread if the field walker carries a sharp billhook or light scythe and constantly tops them.

Horse people have a bad name because of fields that are a mass of mud and weeds, fallen-down jumps, botched-up fencing and tatty buildings. This reputation should be scotched by careful appraisal by the field-owner, and by good husbandry and constant vigilance.

Chapter 28
Lungeing horses

Why lunge?

Lungeing is carried out for many reasons:

- to train the young horse
- to retrain or improve the older horse
- to train the rider
- to exercise the horse
- to warm a horse up prior to ridden work
- for the pleasure of working a horse from the ground.

Some people only lunge mature horses when the roads are too icy to ride or some other reason prevents their normal riding routine. However, lungeing is a pleasant and useful part of the gymnastic preparation of every equine athlete; the hunter, dressage horse, show jumper, eventer, racehorse, carriage horse and so on will all benefit from lungeing if done well. Similarly, it is a pleasing skill in which the lunger gains satisfaction from the quality of the performance. Good lungeing improves a horse's obedience and can be used to build up muscle in the horse as well as developing his rhythm, balance, suppleness and willingness to go forward.

The lungeing equipment

- Bridle: if the horse is being lunged for exercise, a snaffle bridle with the nose-band and reins removed may be used. If the horse is being warmed up prior to work the horse's normal bridle should be used.
- Lungeing cavesson: this has a padded noseband with three metal rings attached at the front. The lunge rein is fitted to the central ring (Figure 28.1).
- Lunge rein, about 10 m (33 ft) long with a large loop at one end and a swivel joint attached to a buckle or clip at the other.
- Side reins.

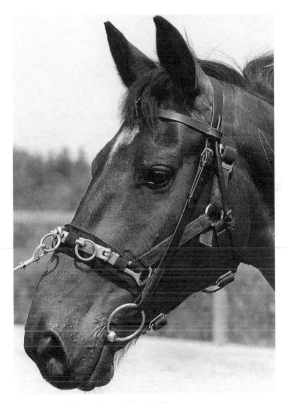

Figure 28.1. Lungeing cavesson and snaffle bridle.

- Saddle or roller adequately padded with a numnah or pad.
- Breastplate: this may be necessary to stop the roller or saddle slipping backwards.
- Brushing boots.
- Lunge whip
- Gloves.

Fitting lungeing equipment

The lungeing cavesson has a thick padded noseband that has to be fastened tightly. To achieve this the cavesson noseband of the bridle must either be removed or lie just below the protruding cheekbones. The lungeing cavesson can then be fastened immediately below the noseband of the bridle. Some lunge cavessons fasten below the bit like a drop noseband. The throatlash of the cavesson, if fitted, should not be tight and, as with a bridle, should allow four fingers to be inserted inside the slack.

Further down the cheekpiece, another strap called the cheek or jowl strap should be pulled tight as it helps to stop the cavesson twisting. Care must be taken with a strong horse in case the cavesson pulls round and the cheek strap moves close to the eye. The lunge cavesson should be set over the bridle but the noseband of the cavesson normally goes under the cheekpieces of the bridle to avoid interference with the action of the bit. However, this is not possible with some Nylon cavessons. If the bridle has reins attached for riding later, the reins should be twisted under the throat and then passed over the head and secured by passing the throatlash through the loop thus formed.

The lunge line should be clipped or buckled to the centre ring on the front of the lunge cavesson. This ring and the lunge line may be fitted with a swivel; one or other is essential to stop the lunge line twisting as it comes off the coils from the lunger's hands. The lunge line should be soft, strong and long; sharp-edged Nylon lines should never be used.

The side reins should be about 2 m (6 ft 6 in) long with a clip at one end and a buckle at the other. The horse should be fitted with a suitable roller with a 'D' ring on each side to which the side reins can be attached. Alternatively, the side reins can be attached to the girth straps on a saddle; this arrangement is normal practice when a horse is being lunged as a warm-up prior to ridden work. The side reins should be passed under the first girth strap in use and secured round the second (Figure 28.2). The stirrups should be run up the leathers and the loop of the leather passed round the tread of the stirrup and then back under itself towards the rear (Figure 28.3).

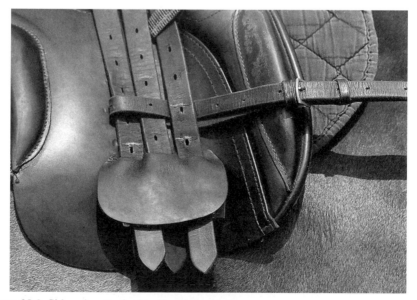

Figure 28.2. Side rein attached to the girth straps.

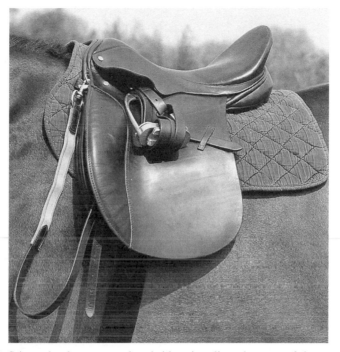

Figure 28.3. Stirrup leathers secured and side reins clipped up out of the way.

Some people like side reins to have elastic in them and some do not; such discussion calls for a long evening and perhaps a drink or two! The side reins should act parallel to the ground, with the horse's head and neck in a posture similar to that when ridden, i.e. the side reins must not be set too low or allowed to slip downwards. The side reins should not be fastened to the bit rings when the horse is first tacked up; they should be clipped to the roller or saddle (Figure 28.3). This arrangement should be adopted until the horse has relaxed on the lunge and again at the end of the lunge work.

For lungeing, the horse must wear brushing boots on all four legs; even with sympathetic and disciplined lungeing on a large circle the horse may knock itself, so protection is essential (Figure 28.4).

Lungers must wear stout footwear in case their toes are trodden on. The footwear should also have a good heel as a smooth under-suface gives poor grip. Properly fitting gloves are essential when lungeing to protect the hands and enhance grip. Those breaking horses on the lunge must wear a hat for obvious reasons; for all others a hat is a matter of preference or exam board protocol (Figure 28.5). Spurs are best not worn when lungeing.

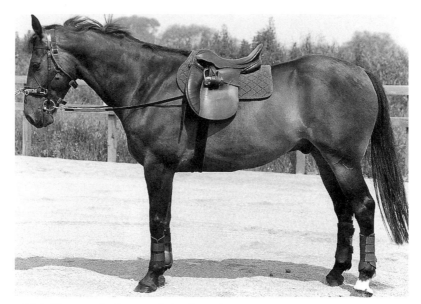

Figure 28.4. Horse tacked up ready for lungeing.

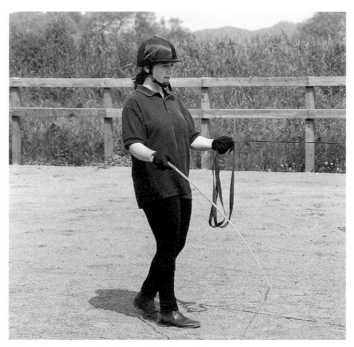

Figure 28.5. Handler correctly dressed for lungeing.

The aids

The main aid to control when lungeing is the voice. Instead of the horse being between the leg and the hand it is between the lunge whip and the rein; the lunge rein is used to keep a light consistent contact with the horse and if the horse becomes strong the tension on the rein is relaxed and retaken consecutively until the horse stops resisting. The horse should be accustomed to the whip.

Lungeing a horse for exercise

The horse is led to the lunge area with the side reins clipped back to the roller. There are two schools of thought about sending the horse forward from the halt. One method is as follows: the horse is stood on the circle facing, for instance, to the left. The lunger has the lunge line leading from his or her left hand to the horse. The spare coils of lunge line may be held in the left hand or, if preferred, in the right. This latter style is better for a frisky horse. The lunge whip is tucked under the left elbow, pointing to the rear. The horse should stand still as the lunger takes a few steps back towards the centre of the circle. Not all horses will stand still, but such discipline and good practice should be instilled in every horse; it is a matter of patient, calm insistence and consistency.

When well clear of the horse the lunge whip can be brought quietly round behind the lunger's back into the right hand to point a metre (a yard) or two to the rear of the horse and towards the ground. The command is 'walk on' but it may be prefixed with either 'and' or the name of the horse; either prefix warns the horse that, whatever else the lunger may have been saying, they are now about to issue a command. The 'and walk on' is enforced by raising the whip to buttock height with a little shake that curls out the thong of the whip so it can be seen by the horse. As the walk proceeds the lunger moves on an inner circle, but by gradually letting out the lunge line makes spiral progress to the centre of the circle. This method establishes the horse on the outer track from the outset.

The second and more common method of sending a horse forward in walk is for the lunger to step just clear of the horse before sending it forward using the whip quietly to encourage the horse to go forwards and outwards. Thus, the horse spirals outwards. The thinking behind this method is twofold: first, it encourages the horse to go away from the lunger rather than the lunger drawing back towards the centre of the circle; second, it does not require the horse to be obedient enough to stand still on the circle – many horses will turn in because they have not been taught good behaviour in this respect. Thus, this method copes with strange horses and those lunged by many different people, as at a riding establishment. With this method of sending the horse out, particular vigilance is required with a fresh or cheeky horse that might plunge forwards and kick out at the lunger.

The walk should be purposeful, long and unhurried with the hind feet over-tracking the print left by the front feet. A walk of this quality may not be achieved in the first few minutes, particularly if the horse has just come from the stable.

Control of the horse is subtle and requires both concentration and anticipation. Lungeing is a great skill and, like riding, there is great pleasure in doing it well. If the lunger stands in the centre of the circle they are in a neutral position with the horse balanced between the whip pointing towards it and the taut lunge line; that is to say, equally between the lunger's two hands (Figure 28.6). If the horse is on the left rein and the lunger wishes to increase the pace, the lunger takes one step to the right. The lunger is now slightly behind the horse and raising the lunge whip a little and clicking the tongue can send the horse forward more purposefully. On the other hand, if the horse is rather too forward, the lunger steps a pace to the left and lowers the whip point towards the ground. Now they are slightly ahead of the horse and with a gentle command of 'steady' can adopt a quieter pace.

Typically, the horse appears to find that the entrance gate to the lunge area has a 'magnetic' effect! Thus, the horse hurries round that part of the circle which heads towards the gate and then dawdles when heading away from the gate. A good lunger will quickly notice such things and by quiet movement will anticipate and counteract them, although this may not be apparent to an

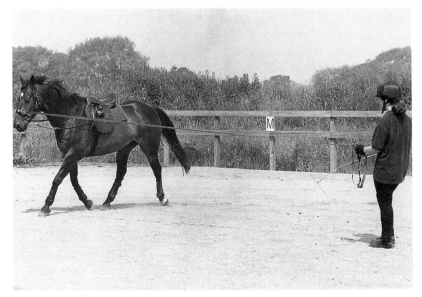

Figure 28.6. Handler in the neutral position.

observer. If the horse pulls outwards, which may happen if the horse is over-fresh or badly trained, then it is helpful to lunge in an enclosed place. This may be the corner of the field or at the end of a school. In severe cases the open side can be enclosed with some jump poles on large oil drums or other temporary fencing. Such provisions should soon become unnecessary as the horse's manners improve.

On the other hand, some horses charge inwards; the procedure is to stand your ground or even advance towards the horse with the lash of the whip looping towards the horse's barrel. If the lunger backs away then the horse has taken control and started to train the lunger. Commonly, the horse will cut corners or fall in on the circle; in this case the whip should be pointed and, if necessary, flicked in the direction of the horse's shoulder. Sometimes a horse behaves like a hooligan and then it is necessary to attach the side reins straight away as clearly the horse is neither going to stretch down or relax, and the side reins will aid control.

When the horse has walked calmly for a few minutes on the left rein (anti-clockwise), it should be sent round on the right rein (clockwise). The procedure is first to halt the horse out on the circle. The horse must not turn in and if it does it should be made to walk on again in the original direction. The command is a low and drawn out 'and whoa' accompanied by gentle vibration on the lung line. If the horse does not halt, shorten the rein and bring it to a standstill. Firmly and consistently repeat this until the horse is obedient to the voice. When the horse is halted, the lunger tucks the whip under his or her elbow, pointing to the rear, and walks towards the horse taking in the coils of line so that it does not hang slack or, worse still, touch the ground. Then, taking the horse on a short line, it is led round or across the circle to face the other way. Proceeding as before, the horse is sent round at a relaxed walk.

The time spent on the lunge will depend on the horse's stage of training, fitness and the type of work on the lunge; some purists like to see a horse walking for 20 minutes before trotting, but at least 5 minutes is a good aim. Having walked well on both reins, the horse can be given the sharp, quick command 'and trot'. If the horse does not respond at once, a touch of the whip will serve as a reminder. A crack of the whip takes only a flick of the wrist and can be useful and effective; however, care must be taken if other horses are close lest they too respond. The point is that the command should be said clearly and sharply, but only once, and the horse must obey instantly. Good lungeing makes the horse a better ride by enhancing obedience.

After the horse has trotted on both reins it can be halted and have the side reins fitted; initially these should be fairly long. The light pressure of the side reins on the bit may tend to shorten the horse's stride and so a little click of the tongue, a flick of the whip plus sideways step to put the lunger a little behind the horse may be used selectively to maintain the quality of the movement. In trot the horse should put its hind feet into the prints left by the forefeet (Figure 28.7). The trot circle should be at least 15 m (16 yards) in diameter.

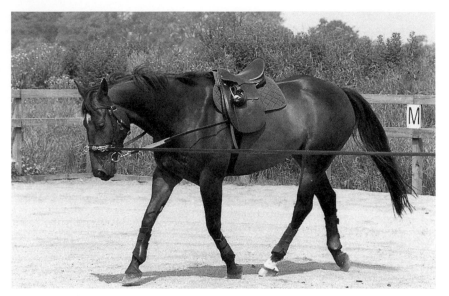

Figure 28.7. A horse working happily on the lunge in trot.

Most lungeing for exercise is carried out at the working trot; this is a purposeful gait, not rushed but with a spring in the step. The side reins are shortened after a while as the horse is asked to accept a contact with the bit. In order to do this it must relax the jaw and flex the neck at the poll. The horse should also engage the hindquarters so that the hind legs step more actively under the body. However, the horse must not drop the contact with the bit by ducking the nose towards the chest so that the face makes a line behind the vertical. From time to time it is a good idea for the trainer or an experienced person to come and watch the lungeing so that bad practices do not creep in. When turning the horse round while it is still wearing side reins, lead the horse forwards in a small half circle; do not turn it on the spot.

Within the trot it is useful sometimes to ask the horse to do a few lengthened strides. The easiest way to achieve this is to select a point of the circle where there is a straight fence on the outside. Then with the lunger running just a few steps parallel to the horse, it can be encouraged to lengthen stride before turning away from the fence back onto the circle. Later it may be possible to produce lengthened strides on the circle, but it is not an essential requirement to be able to do so.

When the horse has worked calmly, yet with good activity at the trot on both reins, it can be asked to canter. Experience will show the best length of side reins in order to allow the horse to move freely forward, yet assist control and produce the round outline of the well-engaged horse (one that is using its hindquarters to propel itself forward actively). Sometimes, particularly in canter, the horse goes faster than intended; in such cases the lunger should never resort to roughness. The lunge line attached to the horse's nose has considerable leverage and so a hefty yank could cause damage to the horse. The procedure if the horse refuses to obey the voice commands of 'steady' or 'trot' is to reduce the length of line fairly swiftly and bring the horse to a halt. Then impose discipline with walk to halt to walk transitions before proceeding to faster paces again.

In the canter it is particularly important that the circle is large enough; 20 m (22 yards) across is ideal so a lunge line of 10 m (11 yards) is required and for a fresh horse it should be longer. If the horse is to be cantered on the lunge, the ground should not be deep or slippery as a poor surface can result in the horse knocking itself, losing confidence or losing the quality of the action. As in all lungeing, it is important that there is always a light, even tension on the lunge line. You should not have a tug-of-war or a slack line. Control of the spare coils of line is a skill needing practice and lack of good line discipline will result in the lunger either tripping over spare line or having line wound round the hand which could result in a nasty accident.

Practice for lungers

Lunge beginners can practice with the line attached to a fence post, letting it out, gathering it in, passing it into the other hand and so on; it is essential that the lunger never fails to have all the line under control and available as necessary. Even in practice, gloves must always be worn so that it is only natural to handle a lunge line when wearing gloves.

Similarly, beginners must practise handling the lunge whip. Typically, the whip is about 2 m (6 ft 6 in) long and the thong with lash an additional 3 m (10 ft). With the thong twisted round the whip it must be carried pointing behind the lunger; it must be brought quietly into the usable position and then tucked out of the way, pointing to the rear again when adjusting the side reins or turning the horse onto the other rein. The whip must not be laid on the ground in case it is trodden on; also, the lunger is in a vulnerable position and not in control when bending to pick it up. In use the whip rarely has to touch the horse, but such a delicate flick needs to be practised.

More advanced work

Trainers schooling horses on the lunge may sometimes shorten the inside side rein, but this is not usual when lungeing horses for exercise. Similarly, trainers may usefully jump horses on the lunge; this is done without side reins and is an advanced skill.

In some cases an ill-disciplined or exuberant horse will go too fast or its hindquarters will keep flying outwards; in such a case a second lunge line is taken from the cavesson, round the hindquarters and so to the lunger's other

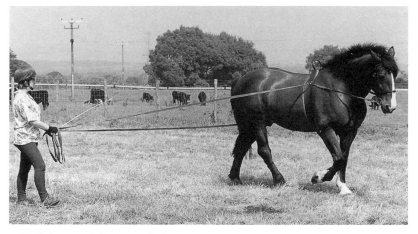

Figure 28.8. Long-reining on a circle.

hand. Great care has to be taken to prevent this line riding up under the horse's tail or slipping to the ground; this too is a form of exercise that is only suitable for those who are more experienced.

In long-reining there is a line to each bit ring and the lines either run through terrets on a roller or pad, or through rings on either side of a roller, and back to the lunger. Long-reining can be carried out using circles (Figure 28.8) or straight lines (Figure 28.9). Unless done with great care and skill the horse may tend to come behind the bit, that is drop the bit by bending the neck too much, tucking the nose into the chest, so that the face makes a line behind the vertical, and not go forwards with sufficient impulsion. Long-reining is a useful and enjoyable advanced skill.

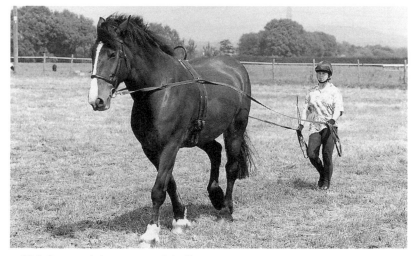

Figure 28.9. Long-reining on a straight line.

Part 6
Horse care in action

Chapter 29
Care of the hunter and sports horse

Getting the horse fit

A fit horse is one that can do the work that is required of it without becoming overtired or overstressed. Getting a horse fit requires a mixture of correct work, feeding and health care. Regardless of the type of horse, the idea of the fitness programme is to improve the horse's ability to tolerate work by gradually increasing its workload and energy intake in a slow, steady progression.

The traditional methods of getting horses fit have developed from getting hunters fit from grass. Traditionally, hunters are brought up from grass at the beginning of August, allowing 3 months to get them hunting fit – equivalent to 1-day-event fitness or 20-mile-distance ride fitness – before the opening meet in November. This 3-month period can be split into three 4-week blocks: preliminary walking and trotting work, development work and fast work.

Bringing up from grass

After the hunting season the hunter will be roughed off and have a complete rest to allow for mental and physical unwinding. The event horse has its break in the winter. The routine for bringing an unfit horse up from grass follows the same basic pattern, although there may be differences from yard to yard:

- *Vaccinations*: if the horse did not have the annual vaccination boosters before the holiday they should be given before starting any work. The horse will need 7 days with no more than light work after vaccination to minimise the risk of any adverse reaction.
- *Teeth*: the vet or horse dentist should check the horse's teeth for sharp edges before the horse comes back into work and again 6 months later.
- *Worming*: a worming programme should be planned, with horses being wormed when they are first brought in, and then every 4–6 weeks.
- *Shoeing*: horses must be shod all round once road work starts; a heavier set of shoes will last longer during this initial fittening period. The horse should be shod every 4–6 weeks.
- *Equipment*: the tack should have been stored in good condition at the end of previous season. Check the stitching and restuff the saddle if necessary.

Hunters can get very fat and soft during their summer break and so a thick numnah and a girth sleeve are a good idea to prevent rubbing and absorb sweat. The numnah and girth sleeve must be washed regularly. Salt water or methylated spirit can be applied to vulnerable areas on the horse to harden up the skin. Many people exercise horses in front boots plus knee boots when on the road; back boots can also be used if the horse's action makes them necessary.

- *Turning out*: the horse will benefit from being turned out for a few hours every day; this will help it unwind and stay sane. The horse has been accustomed to being out for most of the day and if part of the routine is a daily turn-out the horse is unlikely to have too wild a fling and gallop about. In the summer, horses should be protected from flies; otherwise they may become very frustrated and actually start to lose condition. Some people turn the horses out at night, exercise them early in the morning and keep them in during the day to avoid flies. This 'half and half' system is much better both physically and mentally for the horse than suddenly bringing it into work and stabling it full-time.
- *Feeding*: if the horse has not been receiving any concentrate feed, a small feed of a low-energy food such as horse and pony cubes may be fed in the field the week before it is brought up. This will help the horse's digestive system adjust to the feed it will be getting once stabled.
- *Trimming and bathing*: the horse will have its mane, tail, heels and whiskers trimmed, depending on individual preference. If the weather is mild the horse can be washed to help rid the coat of parasites, grease and scurf.
- *Preparation of the stable*: prior to the horse being brought back into work the stable should have been cleared of bedding, well scrubbed and then disinfected. Every so often the walls may need painting or treating with wood preservative. Hay and feed should be ordered and equipment such as buckets, clippers, etc. checked to ensure they are in sound working order.

Preliminary work

The preliminary work exercises the horse slowly for increasing lengths of time to tone up the muscles, tendons and ligaments, and to harden the soft horse's skin. The initial walking and trotting work is very important.

Weeks 1 and 2: walking

The hunter is likely to have spent about 4 months in the field and may be rather fat and very unfit. This means that the work must progress slowly and steadily, starting with 20–30 minutes walking a day, building up to an hour by the end of the first week and 2 hours by the end of the second week. A horse walker can be used to do some of the walking work, or the horse can be led from another horse. Remember that this does not accustom the back muscles to carrying a rider and the girth region stays soft. Ideally, the horse should be walked on the roads for up to 2 hours a day for 4 weeks and never less than 2 weeks – the longer the holiday, the more road work that is needed.

The horse must be carefully checked every day for rubs, galls and injuries. Girths and numnahs must be brushed after use and washed regularly to prevent them irritating the horse's skin.

Weeks 3 and 4: trotting

After at least 2 weeks of walking work, trotting can be introduced; initially the trot should only be for a couple of minutes at a time, building up over the next few weeks to 15 minutes in total.

Development work

The next 4 weeks involve development work – the introduction of canter work so that the heart and lungs become accustomed to exercise. This builds up the horse's stamina while the muscles continue to strengthen and adapt to the work the horse is being given. The ground chosen for the first canter should be flat and not soft or dotted with potholes. The fresh horse may want to buck and gallop so be prepared for this – ask for canter quietly and keep the horse's head up. If the horse is known to be strong make sure that it is in suitable tack.

Canter work should be slow and steady initially and gradually increased so that by the end of the sixth week (mid-September) three or four periods of steady cantering a day can be included in the work. The horse should now be ready to go autumn hunting one or two mornings a week. Initially, the horse should not stay out too long; it is very easy to start early and then stay out until lunchtime and find you have been out for 4 or 5 hours. Although you may not have been galloping and jumping, remember that just carrying a rider for a long time will be tiring to the semi-fit horse.

Fast work

The horse will need clipping as soon as its winter coat has grown adequately.

The hunter is rarely given any fast work during the exercise programme as October hunting usually provides enough cantering and the occasional short gallop (or 'pipe-opener') to prepare the horse for the opening meet. It is wise to school the hunter over cross-country fences once or twice before taking it hunting. It has been 5 or 6 months since the horse last jumped and it is a good idea to remind it about jumping.

During the season

Throughout the hunting season, days of sport will be interspersed with days of exercise. The exercise will vary depending on how hard the horse is working. A Hunt horse may do one or two hard days' hunting a week. This will keep the horse fit and no more than 60–90 minutes walking with a little trotting will be needed on exercise days. Sunday is likely to be a rest day, but rather than stand in its box the horse should be walked out in hand and allowed to graze for 10–15 minutes. This will help reduce the risk of azoturia.

A subscriber's (Hunt member's) horse may only hunt one day a week, that day being considerably less arduous than the Hunt horse's day. The subscriber's horse should have a short walk the day after hunting (usually a Sunday) and possibly a day off midweek when it should be turned out or walked in hand for 10–15 minutes. For the remaining 4 days the horse should have 60–90 minutes of exercise including trotting and cantering. This horse may also benefit from a short gallop the day before hunting to clear its wind and prepare for the next day's galloping.

All horses vary in the amount of exercise they need to keep them in peak condition depending on how much hunting they are doing, their temperament and type. A hunter correctly worked and fed should stay in tiptop condition for the whole of the hunting season.

Roughing off

At the end of the season (March–April) the hunter is usually roughed off and turned out to grass for the long summer's rest. A clipped, corn-fed horse should not suddenly be turned out at this time of the year when the weather is cold, wet and unpredictable; the horse should be gradually 'let down'. Exercise should be reduced and at the same time the concentrate ration should be decreased and the amount of hay increased. As the weather gets warmer the number or weight of rugs should be reduced and the horse turned out for a greater length of time every day. Once the paddocks have dried up sufficiently to allow the horse to stay out all day it can stop being exercised and have its shoes removed. If the feet are likely to crack and spilt it may be necessary to leave the front shoes on. By the end of April or beginning of May, the horse should be able to stay out day and night. A horse roughed off rapidly and turned out too soon tends to lose condition which may take a long time to recover.

During June and July flies can bother the horse, so any field should have adequate shelter. Alternatively, the horse can be brought in during the heat of the day. The horse's feet must be regularly trimmed, it should be wormed every 4–6 weeks and checked daily for injury. The field must also be regularly checked for hazards that may injure the horse.

Feeding

Each horse should be fed as an individual and according to the amount of work done. The hunter has two long days per week and the following points should be considered:

- The horse should be fed to maintain condition over a long season, the use of oil to top up energy supplies is now common.
- Concentrates should be reduced the day before a rest day. Traditionally, hunters had a bran mash on return from hunting, but a warm mash of their

normal feed is more nutritious. They should be turned out on their day off to walk off any stiffness and prevent azoturia.
- Tired horses are better fed smaller quantities of a high-performance feed that contains more concentrated energy.
- Succulents will help the tired horse and soaked beet pulp will help rehydration.

Care of the horse during the season

The day before hunting

It is essential to be properly organised; equipment should be gathered together, cleaned and made ready for the morning. The following list covers the majority of equipment needed for hunting:

- plaiting kit
- grooming kit
- tack – check the stitching for wear and polish bit rings and stirrups if necessary
- brushing boots and over-reach boots if worn
- headcollar and rope
- travelling equipment for the horse
- haynet for the return journey
- sweat rug for the return journey
- full water carrier and bucket
- human first-aid kit
- equine first-aid kit to include a small bowl, scissors, cotton wool, crêpe bandages, gamgee, salt, wound dressings and sprays, and ready-to use poultice

The horse should be thoroughly groomed and have its mane, tail, feet and any white socks washed. If the whiskers and bridle path (parts of the head where the bridle rests) are trimmed they should be tidied up.

The hunting morning

Work backwards from the time of the Meet to calculate the time you should arrive and hence the time you must leave home, start plaiting and doing all the rest of the morning routine tasks and finally the time you must set the alarm clock. The horse must be fed at least an hour before the expected loading up time.

Before leaving, the horse should be groomed, the feet oiled and a tail bandage put on. Any small cuts should be dressed with antiseptic cream to protect them during the day. In countries where mud fever is a problem, the horse's legs and belly are sometimes wiped over with oil to stop mud getting into the pores of the skin.

Hunters often travel tacked up with the headcollar on over the bridle and a rug and roller or surcingle over the saddle. If the journey to the Meet is short, the horse may not wear any protective travelling gear except for a tail bandage. For longer journeys it is preferable for the horse to be adequately protected and tacked up on arrival.

The vehicle should be parked about a mile from the Meet – the hack helps settle the horse. Ensure that all equipment is put safely away and the vehicle locked up before leaving it.

Care after hunting

On a dry day the horse should be walked the last mile back to the vehicle so that it is cool and dry on arrival. However, if it is raining it may be better to keep trotting so that the horse arrives ready to be loaded warm and wet rather than cold and wet.

The bridle can be replaced with a headcollar and the horse either loaded immediately or tied to a string loop on the side of the vehicle. If the vehicle is parked on a busy road, it is wet or the horse excited it is probably better to load immediately. The saddle will have been on for a long time so either the girth can be loosened, the sweat rug and top rug placed on top and the horse travelled home with the saddle on, or the saddle can be removed and the area under the saddle patted briskly to help the circulation in the blood vessels under the saddle to return; sudden removal can cause scalded backs and pressure lumps. The horse can then be rugged up.

The horse can be offered a small drink of water (no more than a quarter of a bucket) and any obvious injuries attended to. Travelling gear can then be put on the horse and it can have another small drink before travelling home with the haynet.

On returning home

The routine followed varies between yards but the following guidelines may prove useful:

- Once the horse has been unloaded it can be taken to the stable, tied up beside a haynet, have the saddle and travelling gear removed, and the rugs thrown back over.
- The horse can be offered water at regular intervals. If it drank a couple of times before being loaded it can have half a bucket of water, followed 15 minutes later by as much as the horse wants to drink. However, if the horse has not drunk all day, it should be restricted to a quarter of a bucket every 15 minutes until the thirst is quenched. Very tired horses may appreciate water that has had the chill taken off it. Dehydrated horses can either be offered electrolytes in the feed or in a separate bucket of water. It is important that the horse drinks, but does not gorge on water, risking colic.
- Meanwhile, the horse can have its feet picked out, shoes checked for soundness and legs checked for injuries such as thorns and cuts. The horse can then

be cleaned. If it is dry the mud can be brushed off and sticky sweat marks sponged off with warm water. If the mud is wet, some people prefer to leave it to dry and to brush it off in the morning while others wash it off immediately either with a hose or sponge and warm water. If the horse is washed it should be towelled dry before being rugged up with dry rugs. Stable bandages will help support tired legs and dry wet ones. The tail should be washed and the plaits taken out. If the horse is very tired, just make it clean enough to be comfortable and leave to rest. Keep offering the horse water until the thirst is quenched.

- The horse can now be left in peace with its haynet and a small feed.
- The tack can be cleaned. Some yards wash the mud off now, leave the tack to dry and soap it the next day, while others clean it completely the same evening.
- The horse may break out in a sweat. Check every 15 minutes for cold, sweaty patches, restless behaviour, disturbed bedding or a reluctance to eat. If the signs are mild keep the horse warm by rubbing its ears until they are warm and walk the horse (if the weather is suitable) until it is dry and comfortable. If the horse does not respond or looks very distressed then veterinary help should be called.
- Before leaving the horse, top up the water buckets. The horse should be checked later in the evening, given more water and hay as well as a late night feed.

The day after hunting

Providing that the horse has eaten up and looks well, it can be fed and given hay as normal. Depending on the routine followed the previous night the horse may be clean or dirty. Any stable bandages should be removed and the legs carefully checked for heat, pain or swelling from cuts, thorns, knocks or strains. The rugs can be thrown back and the saddle and girth area checked for lumps or rubs. The horse can then be unrugged and trotted up in hand to check that it is sound; the horse may seem stiff initially but this should soon wear off. The rugs can then be thrown back over the horse while it is thoroughly cleaned, making sure that awkward areas such as between the hind legs and elbows are attended to. Once the horse is clean it can be exercised. The amount of exercise will depend on how hard the work was the day before; it is likely that 15–30 minutes' walk will be enough. The horse can then be returned to the stable and left in peace to recover from its exertions.

Chapter 30
The competition horse

Competition horses include:

- eventers
- dressage horses (Figure 30.1)
- show jumpers (Figure 30.2)
- endurance
- driving
- polo
- point to point.

Getting the competition horse fit

Bringing the competition or event horse up from grass and then getting it fit varies very little from the programme outlined in Chapter 29. The main differences are that, first, the event horse is being got fit in the winter prior to competing in the summer and, second, the horse needs to follow a more formal fast work plan in order to reach the desired level of fitness.

Bringing the competition horse up from grass

The event horse usually has a rest in the winter and is brought back into work in December or January ready for the first event in March or April. This means that the horse is generally stabled at night and is already being fed concentrates so that unlike the hunter its system does not need to become accustomed to a completely different regime. The horse will also need clipping as soon as it comes into work; a blanket clip keeps the back warm during the preliminary work. The horse can have a hunter clip when it starts to do faster work.

Interval training

Interval training has become popular for training competition horses. It consists of giving a horse a period of canter followed by a brief interval of walk during which the horse is allowed to partially recover before being asked to work again. Interval training increases the horse's capacity for using oxygen to create energy; the point at which the horse runs up an oxygen debt is delayed as much as possible. This results in the horse being able to work for longer before

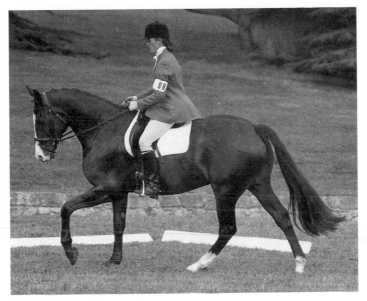

Figure 30.1. The dressage horse.

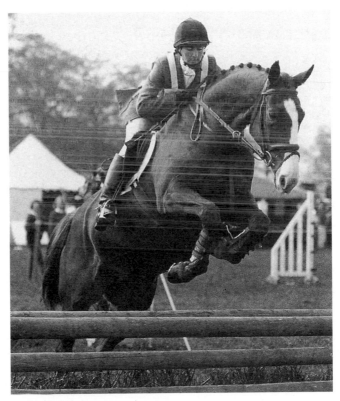

Figure 30.2. The show jumper.

fatigue sets in. The interval training workouts are fitted into the total training programme of the horse.

An essential part of the interval training regime is monitoring the horse's temperature–pulse–respiration (TPR) to gauge the horse's reaction to the work. Interval training cannot cut corners and the following factors must be considered before starting such a programme:

- The horse should be capable of 90 minutes' walk and trot over rolling terrain without distress. The horse conditioned slowly and carefully will stay in peak condition longer than one pushed too fast in the early stages.
- It is essential to keep a notebook with a running record of the horse's response to the workout, allowing the programme to be adjusted accordingly.
- As in any form of training, the rider must be alert to any change in the horse's attitude, appetite, coat, droppings, appearance, muscle tone, etc.

During interval training the horse is cantered at a predetermined speed for a certain time. After this the horse is pulled up and the pulse and/or respiration rates are recorded immediately. The horse is then walked for a set time and rates recorded again. The difference between the two readings is the 'recovery rate' of the horse. This fast then slow work is repeated two or three times.

These workouts are repeated, usually every 4 days, and the pulse and respiration rates recorded at the same points; as the horse gets fitter it will recover faster from the work. Fitness is built up gradually by slowly increasing the total amount of work the horse is asked to do and by increasing the speed and/or length of the workout or using more demanding terrain. If the recovery rate is not good enough after a workout, the work should be adjusted so that the horse is never overstressed.

Points to remember

- Interval training must be monitored by pulse and respiration rate, not by time alone. It is the pulse rate immediately after the workout that shows how much stress the horse has been subjected to, and the recovery rate that shows the level of fitness.
- If the pulse and respiration have not returned to normal within 20 minutes of completing the workout the horse has been overworked and the programme should be adapted accordingly.
- The respiration rate should not exceed the pulse rate; if it does stop work.
- Never complete the day's planned programme if the horse becomes distressed.
- On the other hand, the horse must be stressed enough to stimulate the body systems to become better adapted to exercise. The heart rate must be raised above 100 beats per minute after work.
- The interval training programme should be planned backwards from the proposed date of the competition(s) so that workout days fall appropriately.
- Always warm up and cool down thoroughly before cantering, particularly if the horse has to travel in a lorry or trailer to the work area.

Preliminary work

The preliminary work is no different for the competition horse than for the hunter – they both need plenty of slow work at the beginning of the programme.

Weeks 1 and 2: walking

Not all riders allow their horses to become completely unfit; they may only give their horses a short holiday of 2–4 weeks, after which they are walked two or three times a week for up to an hour each time. This helps to maintain a basic level of fitness and to keep the tendons and bones strong. The risk of girth galls and sore backs is also lessened.

During preliminary work, ideally the horse should be walked on the roads for up to 2 hours a day for 4 weeks and never less than 2 weeks – the longer the holiday the more road work is needed. If the horse has been walked two or three times a week from the field, another 2 weeks on top should suffice once the horse has come in to be stabled. This work strengthens the horse and prepares for the next stage. The walk should never be sloppy; it should be purposeful and with a good rein contact.

Weeks 3 and 4: trotting

After at least 2 weeks' walking work, trotting can be introduced; initially the trot should only be for a couple of minutes at a time, building up over the next couple of weeks to 15 minutes in total. If the trotting is done in an arena sharp turns and small circles must be avoided at this stage. Flat work or lungeing can be incorporated into the routine towards the end of the fourth week; this should be no more than 30 minutes before or after an hour's road work.

It is far better to underfeed than overfeed the horse with concentrates at this stage, but a good amount of hay (or a dust-free equivalent such as haylage) must be fed to prevent the stabled horse becoming bored.

Development work (weeks 5–7)

Development work involves the introduction of canter work and suppling exercises so that the heart and lungs become accustomed to stronger exercise, building up the horse's stamina while the muscles continue to strengthen and adapt to the work the horse is being given.

The initial canter work may be done in a schooling environment where horses often respect their riders more than in an open space. The horse should be cantered for 2–3 minutes at 400 m per minute to start with, bringing the horse back to walk through trot. These little bouts of canter should be built up so that by the end of 2 weeks the horse is cantering for a total of 9–10 minutes split into three or four sessions. The horse should always be walked for 2–5 minutes after each canter.

During week 5 or 6, jumping can be introduced into the programme, starting with pole work, grid work and small jumps in the school. This can be incorporated into the schooling programme so that by the end of the second month the novice horse should have done a small local show jumping class or two.

Discipline work (weeks 8–12)

The third period of the fitness programme is even more specialised; the power and athleticism of the dressage horse (Figure 30.1) and show jumper (Figure 30.2) are developed further, while the racehorse and the event horse are given fast work. Some horses, for example ridden show horses, do not need speed, power or athleticism but should continue to build up body, skin and coat condition and become more highly trained.

Now interval training can start in earnest. Canter work is repeated every fourth day, building the sessions up minute by minute. The day after a canter session should be less stressful with a hack or some gentle schooling. Over the next 2 weeks the sessions are built up so that the horse can do three lots of 5-minute canters at 400 m/minute, with 3 minutes' walking in between.

By now the horse will have been stabled for about 10 weeks. Road work continues each day; it can form a useful warming up and/or cooling down period. Show jumping, cross-country and dressage schooling all continue in a balanced programme.

The final two weeks (weeks 11 and 12)

The first horse trial can be planned for week 12; on a couple of occasions, the last minute of the last canter can be increased to a speed of 500 m/minute.

Table 30.1 shows a sample workout. The heart rate after the third canter should drop below 100 beats per minute after 10 minutes' walking. All horses are individuals and must be treated as such. Tables are merely a guideline and

Table 30.1. Interval training to novice 1-day-event fitness

20 minutes' warm-up	
Canter 1:	5 minutes @ 400 m/minute
	trot 30 seconds
	walk 3 minutes
Canter 2:	4 minutes @ 400 m/minute
	1 minute @ 500 m/minute
	trot 30 seconds to 1 minute
	walk 3 minutes
Canter 3:	4 minutes @ 400 m/minute
	1 minute @ 500 m/minute building
	up to 550 m/minute
	trot 1–2 minutes
	walk at least 20 minutes

do not allow for lost shoes, heavy going or lazy horses. The real skill in training lies in the ability to design programmes for individual horses and to recognise the need to adapt the programme without hindering the horse's progress. The same programme may take up to 2 weeks longer with a different horse.

Roughing off

Once the competition season has finished the horse may be roughed off and turned out to grass for a holiday. The horse's work is cut down or stopped and it is turned out in the field for an increasing amount of time during the day, regardless of the weather. Gradually the number of rugs worn is reduced and the ratio of forage to concentrates increased. The shoes may be removed or left on according to the state of the horse's feet. Hind shoes may be removed if there is danger of horses kicking each other. The horses should have their feet checked regularly while at grass and also should be wormed.

Feeding the competition horse

The competition or event horse has to be fit enough to gallop and jump at speed and yet disciplined enough to perform dressage and show jumping; this has led to many event riders trying to keep their horses happy both mentally and physically by feeding as few concentrates as possible and turning their horses out in the field every day. The 3-day-event horse may have a very rigorous training programme and yet only compete in the run up to the main competition before being turned away, while the lower level horse may compete once a week throughout the long event season. These horses have widely differing feed requirements.

Prior to the event do not be tempted to change the horse's ration. Some people reduce or omit the sugar beet pulp from the feed before the event, while others would only do this on the morning of a cross-country event. If the horse frets away from home, reduce the quantity of concentrate food and use high-energy palatable ingredients such as milk pellets and flaked maize. Generally speaking, however, it is better not to alter the horse's feed too much; you may just cause problems.

A 3-day-event horse should have a concentrate feed no less than 4 hours before the start time of the first phase of the cross-country day. If competing in the afternoon the horse could also be given a small haynet. If the horse has had free access to fresh water there is no reason why the water bucket should be taken away before competing — why should the horse suddenly decide to have a huge drink?

A novice event horse could munch on a haynet while being plaited on the morning of the competition. If the horse is competing early it should not receive any bulk feed while travelling until after the cross-country event. If the horse is competing later it could have a small haynet while travelling. Depending on your competing times, the horse may be able to have concentrate feed between the dressage and the show jumping, providing that there is at least 2 hours' digestion time. The horse should be offered water frequently throughout the day and allowed to wash its mouth out between the show jumping and the cross-country, even if they are very close together.

The fluid and electrolyte balance is very important and the horse must be watched for signs of dehydration. If a pinch of skin on the neck or shoulder lingers after it has been released and the horse has a gaunt tucked-up appearance it may well be dehydrated – this can limit the next day's performance severely. Ensure that the horse drinks and provide electrolytes in the food or water.

Colic can be a problem after severe exertion, and the intestines must be kept moving. Once the horse is cool and the thirst has been quenched it may appreciate a small bran mash, with the normal feed later on. Tired horses are easily overfaced by a large feed, but dividing the normal feed in two and feeding it at intervals may overcome this.

After the competition the horse's appetite will indicate the level of tiredness. Until the horse is eating normally it has not really recovered from the exertions and should be allowed plenty of rest. Hacks and grazing in hand will help the horse relax and recover.

Care of the horse during the competition season

The week before the competition

This is the time for those finishing touches. The mane and tail should be tidied up and the horse clipped if necessary. All tack and equipment must be examined thoroughly and repaired or replaced; any items missing from your check-list must be purchased and ensure that any medications are not out of date. The horse should be shod with stud holes as necessary and the farrier asked to check that the horse's spare set of shoes still fit correctly. The numnahs, boots and rugs, and so on that are being taken to the competition should be clean and in good repair.

The day before the competition

If staying overnight before or after the competition it is essential to be properly organised; clean equipment should be gathered together and packed. The following list gives the general requirements for most situations:

- stable tools, muck skip and muck sack
- shavings or paper bedding
- two haynets
- two water buckets and full water carrier
- feed bowl

- pre-packed concentrate feeds clearly labelled, for example, 'Monday lunch'
- soaked sugar beet pulp if fed
- hay or haylage
- supplements, for example, electrolytes
- grooming kit including extra sponges, towels, sweat scraper and hoof oil
- fly spray
- plaiting kit
- spare set of shoes, studs and stud-fitting kit
- tack cleaning kit
- spare rugs and blankets
- sweat sheets or coolers
- waterproof rugs
- stable bandages and gamgee or wraps
- passport/vaccination certificate
- rule book and details of entry
- equipment for all those going on the trip (food, clothing, toiletries, money, etc.).

Other essential items include:

- tack – depending on the horse and competition
- bandages, brushing boots, over-reach boots plus spares
- spare girth, leathers, irons and reins
- spare headcollar and rope
- hole punch
- lungeing equipment
- travelling equipment for the horse
- human first aid kit
- equine first-aid kit to include a small bowl, scissors, cotton wool, crêpe bandages, gamgee, salt, wound dressings and sprays, ready-to-use poultice and leg coolant.

The horse should be thoroughly groomed; if the weather permits it may be possible to bathe it, and you will need to wash the mane, tail and any white socks. If the whiskers and bridle path are trimmed a last trim will prevent a designer-stubble look.

Packing the vehicle

Equipment should be listed and ticked off as loaded; this will avoid essential items being overlooked. Containers as simple as plastic washing baskets will make loading and unloading easier, but they should not be too large or too heavy as this makes handling tricky. Containers should have an easily read list of contents so that items can be located quickly. Filled water containers and buckets should be packed so that they are easy to get at during the journey for watering the horse.

At the competition

Find out when the class starts or your specific start times so that you know in advance the time your horse is expected to compete. Work backwards from this time to calculate the time you should arrive at the showground and thus the time you must leave home, start plaiting and doing all the rest of the morning routine tasks, and finally the time you must set the alarm clock.

The horse must be fed at least an hour before the expected loading up time. Allow extra time for delays in the journey and about 45–60 minutes to get yourself organised and the horse settled and tacked up before it needs to be ridden. If you have a cross-country course to walk, allow yourself an hour to do this plus 10 minutes to walk the show-jumping course.

Once at the competition ground, park where the ground is as level as possible, and if the weather is warm try to find some shade. If you have help and the horse has had a long journey it should be quietly unloaded and walked in hand; letting the horse graze will help it relax. Meanwhile you can go and declare for the class, pick up your number and find out where everything is. The next step is to brush the horse over; it will have been thoroughly groomed at home and should only need the finishing touches such as hoof oil, quarter marks and the last shaving taking out of the tail. If the competition is on grass the horse may be fitted with studs to give more grip. The type of stud used will depend on the state of the going with pointed studs being used on hard ground and square studs on soft ground. The horse is now ready to be tacked up, mounted and warmed up.

Overnight stays

If staying overnight at a showground or racecourse all the horse's vaccination papers should be up-to-date and ready to show the officials. Before putting the horse into the stable, which may be temporary or permanent, carry out a few checks:

- Clean out contaminated or mouldy bedding.
- Wash out the manger, disinfect and then wash it again.
- Clean out the automatic drinker if present.
- Check that the lights work and are out of reach of the horse.
- Check that glass-covered windows are safe and out of reach of the horse.
- Ensure that there are no sharp edges or projections that may cut the horse.
- The door must be strong with secure latches and bolts.

Once the horse has been unloaded and has had a walk to stretch its legs it can go into the stable for a roll. After being offered a drink, the horse will benefit from a small haynet to munch on so that by the time of offering a feed it is relaxed enough to eat. Even if the horse does not have a late night feed, it should be checked last thing to see that it has settled in this strange environment and is not too warm or too cold.

Care after the competition

After the horse has finished an arduous competition it will have a higher temperature, pulse and respiration rates, and it is important to bring these body systems back to normal as quickly as possible:

- Immediately after the horse has stopped, the rider should dismount and loosen the girth; it is important to keep the horse moving so that the circulating blood cools the muscles. After 5 minutes of walking, the horse can have the tack removed and a cooler or sweat rug put on and walking continued. If the saddle has been on for a long time, it should be left in place for about 10 minutes to allow the circulation in the blood vessels under the saddle to return; sudden removal can cause scalded backs and pressure lumps.
- As soon as the horse stops blowing hard it can have a few sips of water. Until the horse is cool and thirst quenched, it should be given water little and often; as a guide allow five swallows of water for every 50 m walked.
- The pulse and respiration rates of a fit horse that has not been overstressed should return to comfortable levels within 15 minutes and the horse should be checked every 15 minutes thereafter until the values return to normal, which should be within an hour of completing exercise.
- Once the pulse and respiration are within comfortable levels, the horse should be stood in a sheltered place, out of the sun on a hot day and out of the wind on a cool day, and washed down. The lower legs, inside the legs, the head and belly should be sponged.
- During untacking and sponging, the horse must be checked for injury; once it has recovered, these areas can be cleaned and dressed. The horse should also be jogged for a few yards to check for soundness while it is recovering.
- Once the horse has cooled completely it can have a nibble of grass or a small haynet while you attend to the legs. The leg treatment will vary according to personal preference, but after strenuous effort it is a good idea to apply a cold dressing to constrict the blood vessels and soothe any bruising and inflammation that may be present. A clay or cooling gel dressing can be used and applied thickly down the back of the leg from the knee to below the fetlock joint, and then covered in dampened newspaper, tinfoil, clingfilm or plastic with gamgee and a stable bandage applied over the top.
- Although the skin and surface muscles are now cool, the horse may break out in a sweat. Check the horse every 15 minutes for cold, sweaty patches, restless behaviour, disturbed bedding or a reluctance to eat. If the signs are mild keep the horse warm and walk it until it is dry and comfortable. If the horse does not respond or looks very distressed then veterinary help should be called.

Welfare of the competition horse

Whatever type of equestrian sport is being followed it is essential that the competition horse is looked after in the best way possible. The following points are included in a Code of Conduct that has been drawn up by the Federation Equestre Internationale (FEI) in conjunction with the International League for the Protection of Horses (ILPH) and the British Equestrian Federation (BEF).

- In all equestrian sports the welfare of the horse must be considered paramount.
- The well-being of the horse is more important than performance in a competition; horses must not be exploited to satisfy a sponsor or team.
- The pressure to compete must not result in misuse of medication.
- The highest standards of feeding, health and management must be maintained.
- The horse must be travelled with adequate ventilation, feeding, watering and rest periods.
- The horse's rider or driver must be fit and competent.
- No training method should cause pain, injury or distress.

Chapter 31
The leisure horse

A large number of horses are kept by riding schools or private owners as leisure animals. They are not kept to take part in a specific equestrian sport, but provide enjoyment to their riders hacking and taking part in a variety of competitions and club activities. These horses may compete in dressage, hunter trials, show jumping and showing classes, as well as doing the odd day's hunting and the occasional sponsored ride or team chase.

The majority of texts are written for the professional full-time horse person. However, many horse owners are in other full-time work; indeed, they need to work in order to pay the bills associated with keeping a horse! Fitting a horse in around your life and commitments is not easy and must be planned so that neither the horse nor the family are neglected.

The right horse for the job

Selecting the right horse is the first step on the way to a happy partnership. Owning a leisure horse is supposed to be fun; unfortunately, it can turn out to be a nightmare if the horse is unsuitable. The ideal horse is a 'can't go wrong' character; it should be rugged, amenable and a pleasure to own and look after. There are guidelines that will help in choosing the right horse:

- A cob or pony cross is likely to be sensible and easy to feed.
- The horse does not need to be much higher than 15.2 hands. Providing that it is sturdy and has plenty of bone, that is the circumference of the leg below the knee is adequate for the size of horse, it should be able to carry any person's weight. Ability is not related to size and a 15.2 can do anything that a 16.2 can do.
- Smaller horses tend to be more sound and easier to look after. Large often means trouble.
- Avoid Thoroughbreds as they tend to need plenty of work every day and are not suited to being amenable at the weekend having done little all week.
- Avoid buying a young horse unless you have enough time and expertise to train the horse.
- When choosing a horse take a knowledgeable friend with you.
- Before buying the horse have it vetted; the expense is well justified.

Keeping the horse in the stable

The horse is not designed to be kept in a stable; it does not have enough space to move around in, there is very little air space, the air only changes slowly resulting in a stuffy atmosphere and the horse has no real physical contact with other horses. All in all it is a totally artificial lifestyle. However, stabling horses is very convenient for us: we can feed and exercise them, keep them warm and dry, prevent them being kicked or bitten by other horses and keep more animals on a small piece of land. After all, most people cannot afford to buy a paddock but we can afford to rent a stable.

It is important that the stable is an adequate size: for example, 3.5 m^2 (12 ft^2) is a minimum size for a 16 hands horse. Further details regarding the size of stables can be found elsewhere in the book. The stable should also be well ventilated; in most ready-made boxes the window and door are on the same side and as a result the open top half of the door often blocks the window and there is no movement of air through the stable. While the horse must not stand in a draught it is useful to have a window or gap below the eaves on the opposite side from the door to ensure that the air within the box changes regularly, creating a healthy environment. There should also be an exit for air in the ridge of the roof; this allows the warm air to escape from the stable as it rises and effectively 'sucks' air in through the open top half of the door.

Keeping the horse at grass

There are many advantages in keeping the horse at grass: it is a natural system; less straw and hay are used; less time is spent on routine management; and the horse need not be ridden because it will exercise itself. However, there are disadvantages: the horse may become too fat in the summer; it may be wet and muddy in the winter; it still needs to be caught and checked over every day; supplementary feeding will be necessary in the winter and in the summer where there is insufficient grass.

It is easier to operate a 'combined system' where the horse spends part of the day at grass and the rest of the time in the stable. In the summer the horse can be stabled during the day as a protection from flies. In the winter the horse may be stabled at night or brought in well in advance of being ridden to give it time to dry.

A variation of the traditional system of in at night, out by day that, although expensive initially, offers many advantages of the paddock without the mess, is that of the shelter/stable with a free-draining sand yard attached. The horse can be shut in the stable at night and then allowed access to the yard during the day. This way the horse has a little more exercise, plenty of fresh air and a more natural environment.

Horses working from grass in the winter can be given a trace or blanket clip. This makes grooming easier and allows the horse to work without undue sweating. A clipped horse will need a New Zealand rug. An unclipped horse can be turned out without a rug, but the heavy winter coat will take a long time to dry before the horse can be tacked up. The horse will dry quite quickly if put in the stable with a thatch of straw on his back, lightly covered with a cut-open lightweight hessian sack held in place with a loosely-fastened surcingle. After half an hour or so the worst of the mud can be brushed off with a dandy brush. If the horse's girth and saddle area are not free of mud there is a risk that the horse's skin will be rubbed and sore after riding.

After work the wet horse should not be left in the stable. If the horse is to remain stabled, it should be thatched in order to aid drying. If the horse is to be turned out, this should be done straight away so that it can roll and keep on the move.

Keeping the leisure horse fit

The leisure horse is unlikely to undergo a formal fitness programme. The work done will vary according to the rider's ability, facilities and preference, but the horse will rarely by more than half fit, having undergone the equivalent of the preliminary and development stages outlined earlier.

If the horse is going to compete in hunter trials or to go hunting it is important that some faster work is done prior to the event. This faster work may take the form of going round a farm ride, for example, and cantering where possible. This also gives the rider the opportunity to pull their stirrups up and get themselves fit for riding short at the same time. Alternatively, the canter work could be done in the arena – the horse will not be able to go fast but there is no reason why the rider cannot shorten the stirrups, adopt a forward seat and do, say, three 3 minute canters. Both horse and rider may be competent at jumping but unless they are both fit problems are likely to arise towards the end of the course.

Feeding the leisure horse

It must always be borne in mind that the domesticated horse is being given a diet that is quite different from the one it is designed to cope with. In the wild the horse would graze and browse a high-fibre diet for up to 16 hours a day. In an effort to keep the horse slim and athletic we cut down the fibre, reduce the eating time and add highly digestible concentrates to the ration.

It is easy to overestimate the feed requirements of a horse that is working for an hour a day, hacking or doing school work. Just because we have worked hard riding the horse does not mean that the horse has worked equally hard. Many behavioural problems as well as health problems are caused by overfeeding. The golden rules for safe, economical and effective feeding are:

- feed simply
- feed plenty of roughage and as few concentrates as possible
- buy the best quality hay you can afford.

Feeding a low-energy, high-fibre compound feed such as horse and pony cubes along with dust- and mould-free hay should be all that the healthy leisure horse needs. If the horse is inclined to bolt its feed, chaff can be added to slow it down and make it chew the feed more thoroughly. There should be no need to add a supplement or 'a bit of this and a bit of that' to the feed as it will only unbalance the ration that the equine nutritionist has created. In the winter the horse will appreciate carrots in the feed. Horses that are allergic to the dust and fungal spores found in hay may need to have their hay soaked or they can be fed a dust-free alternative such as haylage.

If the horse is turned out onto reasonable grazing in the summer it may only need feed and hay if it is brought in at night. The amount of feed will depend on the quantity and quality of the grazing available. If the horse is inclined to become fat try to turn it out on sparse grazing so that it has to work hard for each mouthful of grass. Keeping the horse in and starving it during the day will only encourage gorging at night.

Caring for the leisure horse after exercise

Although the leisure horse may not work hard in the accepted sense, it will often be hot and tired after exercise. As the horse is only half fit it will find the exercise just as strenuous as the fit horse in an arduous competition.

Selecting a system of management

The important thing with a leisure horse is to set up a system that maximises the pleasure of ownership, whether it is your own stable and paddock or a 'do-it-yourself' livery. Take good local advice to ensure that the system and facilities will meet your needs and provide you and your horse with the greatest enjoyment.

Part 7
Breeding and stud management

Chapter 32
Reproductive, urinary and mammary systems

The survival of a species depends on reproduction: that is the passing of genetic material (genes) from one generation to the next at the time of conception. For reasons of safety, performance and convenience the male horse is most commonly gelded.

Mares are naturally seasonal breeders, that is, they come into season regularly over the summer period which in the northern hemisphere is from spring to autumn.

In some cases, individuals have seasons throughout the year, particularly if they are stabled with plenty of concentrate feed (although this may be a sign that something is wrong).

Thoroughbred breeding

The breeding of Thoroughbreds places additional demands on the mare as an artificial breeding season is used to encourage mares to foal as near as possible to 1 January. All Thoroughbred foals in the northern hemisphere are aged from this date irrespective of their actual date of birth. Foals born nearer to 1 January should be stronger and faster than others born later, for example, in June when they are raced as 2-years olds.

The authorities have determined the breeding season for mares as running from 15 February to 15 July (in the southern hemisphere, the Thoroughbred breeding season runs from 12 August to 15 January).

The natural breeding season of the mare begins around mid-April through to September, with maximum ovarian activity occurring in mid-July. Obviously, a large number of Thoroughbred mares will have difficulty conceiving when their fertility is at its lowest point early in the year.

Inheritance

Genetics is the study of the mechanisms by which the characteristics of the parents are passed on to their offspring. Equine genetics is rather complicated and the description of genetics outlined here has been simplified to provide a suitable introduction to the subject.

There is coded information on the exact make and shape of the parents within an ovum or sperm. This information is contained in chromosomes. Each chromosome resembles a minute string of beads, each bead called a gene and having a special function to perform, such as coat colour. The adult horse has 32 pairs of chromosomes. Each sperm or ovum (the sex cells) produced by an adult horse contains 32 single chromosomes so that when the sperm fertilises the ovum (or egg) the resulting embryo has 32 pairs of chromosomes, half donated by each parent.

Pairs of genes can be described as either homozygous or heterozygous; homozygous means that the genes on the chromosome for a particular characteristic are the same, thus homozygous genes always breed true. Heterozygous means that the genes are different, but in order for the characteristic to be expressed, one gene must be 'dominant' while the other is 'recessive'. Thus, the gene for black coat colour (B) is dominant to the gene for chestnut (b), chestnut is recessive to black. The use of capital letters for dominant genes and lower-case for recessive genes is standard practice, the presence of B stops b from expressing itself. This means that horses containing heterozygous genes will not always breed true; if a heterozygous black horse with the genetic make up (Bb), breeds with another heterozygous black horse there is a 25% chance that the foal will have the genetic make-up (bb). This foal will be chestnut as there are no dominant genes to repress the chestnut colour.

In genetics, the gene that results in horses with pricked ears dominates that giving lop ears; similarly the gene for a dished face dominates that for a Roman nose. The genes also determine the sex of the foal, and the sperm always carries the deciding factor.

Recessive genes may show up if *inbreeding* (breeding between close relations) is practised. Inbreeding can strengthen the genetic make-up provided there is no history of undesirable characteristics. Close inbreeding includes sire to daughter, dam to son, and brother to sister. Animals born with undesirable characteristics should not be used as breeding stock. *Line-breeding* includes grandfather to granddaughter, grandmother to grandson, and cousin to cousin. Line-breeding has less risks but takes longer to establish purity. *Outbreeding* is where there is no relation within the previous five generations.

Mating outside the breed is known as crossing. A true hybrid results from mating with another species, for example, a donkey with a pony. Usually, such hybrids are vigorous but infertile, as is the case with mules. Crossing between different breeds can produce some hybrid vigour. Such vigour was found when horses from the south and cast Mediterranean were crossed with English native improved stock to form the Thoroughbred (see Figures 32.1 and 32.2).

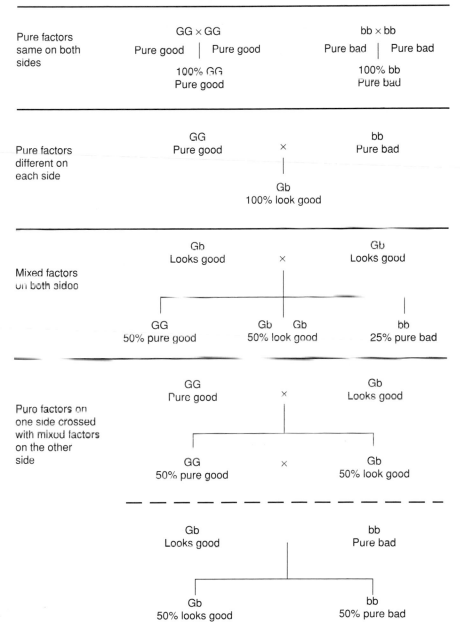

Figure 32.1. Inheritance of a single trait or character.

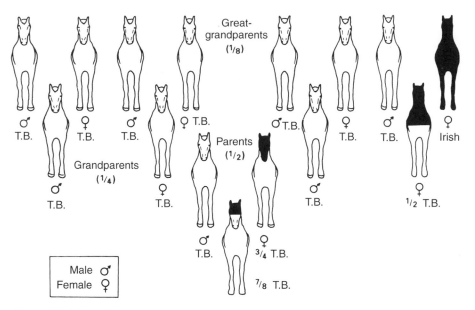

Figure 32.2. Inheritance.

Female reproductive system

The mare's reproductive system (Figure 32.3) produces an egg (ovum) which when united with a sperm will produce an embryo. The system also provides nutrition and protection for the developing embryo. Eggs or ova are produced by the ovaries and at birth these contain the lifetime's egg supply for the mare.

The reproductive system of the mare consists of two ovaries and the genital tract, which is composed of the fallopian tubes, uterus, cervix and vagina. All these are suspended within the body cavity by a sheet of strong connective tissue known as the broad ligament.

The ovaries are attached high in the abdominal cavity just behind the two kidneys. Experts can feel them through the wall of the rectum.

After puberty, mature eggs are released from the ovaries at regular intervals under hormonal control. They are also responsible for the secretion of the female hormone oestrogen.

The uterus of the mare is 'Y' shaped. The highly muscular sac consists of two horns, a body and a neck (cervix). In horses, the embryo develops in the horn of the uterus, whereas in humans the embryo develops in the body.

Mammary system

The mare's udder develops to suckle the foal. The udder consists of the mammary glands in two separate compartments, each leading to a teat. The udder

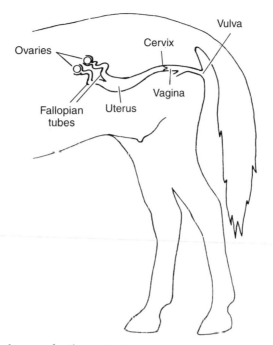

Figure 32.3. Female reproductive system.

and two teats are located between the hind legs for protection. A big mare can produce up to 23 litres (5 gallons) of milk a day.

The mammary glands are well supplied with blood and lymph vessels. The tissues concerned with production are grouped around little sacks called alveoli (similar to those in the lungs), from which run ducts, like the branches of a tree, all joining to go to the trunk. In this case the trunk is the gland cistern. Below this is another gland within the body of the teat (the teat cistern). The teat ends in two small holes, guarded by sphincter muscles, through which the milk is released.

Germs can enter the udder and produce an inflamed condition known as mastitis. The udder then becomes hard and tender to the touch, and swollen lymph ducts will show along the belly. This condition needs veterinary attention.

Oestrous cycle

The oestrous cycle (Figure 32.4) describes alternating periods of sexual activity in the mare. It is controlled by hormones which are initially secreted by the pituitary gland. Mares begin oestrous cycles at puberty, which is usually around $1\frac{1}{2}$ years of age.

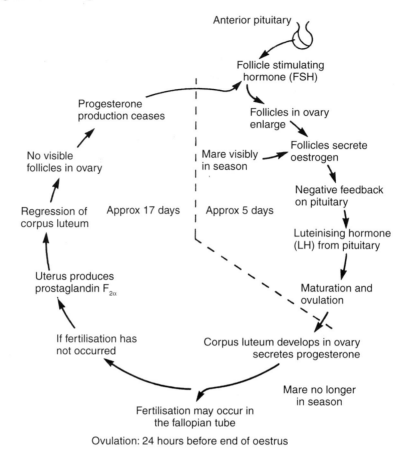

Figure 32.4. Oestrous cycle of the mare.

The oestrous cycle has two phases:

- Oestrus ('heat', 'in season') when the mare is receptive to the stallion and ovulation takes place.
- Dioestrus (between oestrous periods) when the mare is unreceptive.

The cycle typically lasts 21 days in the mare, with oestrus lasting for approximately 5 days and dioestrus for 15–16 days.

Ovulation usually occurs on the last but one or last day of the oestrous period and this is fairly constant, no matter what the length of oestrus is.

Foaling heat

After foaling the mare should come into oestrus some 5–10 days later. This is known as the 'foaling heat' and usually only lasts for 2–4 days. Traditionally, mares have been covered on the ninth day post-foaling, however they often will not be very fertile at this time. The uterus has not had time to return to the normal 'non-pregnant' state and sometimes infection may be present after foaling. Some studs will therefore avoid this time for covering, but in Thoroughbred's where time is of the essence the mares will often be covered.

Behavioural changes

The physical and behavioural changes which occur in the mare throughout each cycle are controlled by chemical messenger substances called hormones.

The oestrous cycle is as follows:

- Pituitary gland produces follicle-stimulating hormone (FSH) that activates the ovaries.
- One ovary forms a follicle which appears as a hard cyst on the surface.
- The ovaries produce oestrogen and the mare comes into season.
- The pituitary gland produces luteinising hormone (LH) which stimulates the egg to mature and be released, i.e. ovulation.
- The hole left by the released egg becomes filled with progesterone secreting cells and becomes the corpus luteum (yellow body).
- Oestrus ends.
- Progesterone, from the corpus luteum, prepares the uterus to receive a fertilised egg.
- If the egg is not fertilised, the uterus produces another hormone, prostaglandin, which kills off the corpus luteum
- Progesterone levels fall.
- The oestrous cycle starts again.

Behavioural signs of oestrus

As oestrus approaches, the mare will often become restless and irritable. She will frequently adopt the urinating posture and ejects urine while repeatedly exposing or 'winking' the clitoris. Mares may be seen doing this to geldings in neighbouring paddocks. When a stallion or teaser is introduced, the mare will tend to exaggerate these postures and she will raise her tail and lean her hindquarters towards the stallion (Figure 32.5). A clear mucous discharge may also be seen. The stallion will often exhibit 'Flehmen' where he rolls up his upper lip and stretches his neck outwards and upwards (Figure 32.6) when the mare is in season. This is in response to pheromones present in the mare's urine. A mare, which is not in oestrus, will react violently towards the stallion's advances and will often kick out. This is the reason why a teaser is often used first to prevent injury to a valuable stallion.

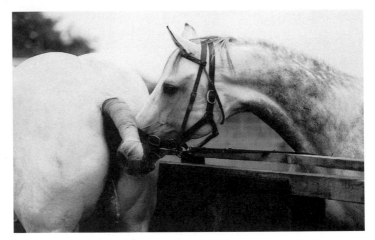

Figure 32.5. Behavioural signs of oestrus in a mare.

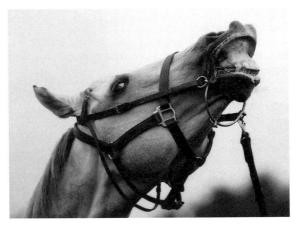

Figure 32.6. A stallion exhibiting Flehmen.

Artificial control of the oestrous cycle

In the management of horses, there are times when some manipulation of the oestrous cycle is required. This is particularly likely in the breeding of Thoroughbred horses. Because of their artificial breeding season, which begins on 15 February in the northern hemisphere, artificial means are used to encourage the mare to come out of the winter anoestrous period and come into season early. These include:

- light – day length
- nutrition
- hormones.

Light – day length

The onset of oestrous activity in the mare is dependent on the hours of daylight. The mare is stimulated into activity as the number of daylight hour's increase. If mares are stabled at the end of December and are subjected to artificial light preferably of increasing duration, then it is possible to advance the onset of normal cyclical activity so that there is oestrus and ovulation.

Nutrition

There is some evidence that improved nutrition may exert a profound effect on ovarian activity. If the mare is kept on a low plane of nutrition or a maintenance ration for a few months prior to the artificial breeding season, then the energy content of the diet is increased, the ovaries should then be stimulated to begin cycling early. The mare should be in good condition.

Hormones

Several different hormones are used to manipulate the oestrous cycle of the mare; these are used to:

* induce oestrus in mares that are in anoestrus
* to prevent oestrus occurring
* to reduce the length of the time between oestrous periods.

The male reproductive system

The reproductive organs of the stallion (Figure 32.7) are designed to create sperm and place it in position within the mare to fertilise the egg.

The reproductive system consists of:

* testes (within the scrotum)
* epididymis
* vas deferens
* accessory glands
* penis.

The functioning of these depends on both hormonal and nervous stimulation. The testicles are carried in a sac known as the scrotum, which is situated between the hind legs of the stallion. This is outside of the body, as the temperature inside the body is too high for sperm development.

In the foetus, the testes develop near the kidneys well inside the body cavity. Approximately 1 month before birth, these testes begin their descent into the scrotum, although they are very small at this stage. Hence, newborn foals normally have both testes in the scrotum at birth or very soon after. The testes have to descend through an opening in the abdominal wall before they reach the

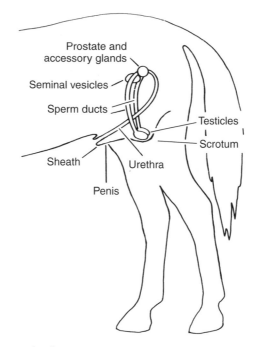

Figure 32.7. Male reproductive system.

scrotum. This is known as the inguinal ring. Sometimes one or both testes fail to descend and remain within the abdominal cavity. These horses are known as rigs (cryptorchids).

By the time the horse is 2 years old, the testes have reached their full size. The growth of the testes is, however, controlled by hormones, which also control sperm production. Once the testes are mature, the male hormone testosterone is produced.

The testes each weigh approximately 300 g (10 oz), the sperm are stored in small coiled tubes joining into one, the epididymis. This is attached to the upper edge of each testis. The epididymis has a tube (the vas deferens) that leads up into the body. The two tubes, one from each testis run side by side as the route taken by sperm before ejaculation. In the abdominal cavity they lead past two seminal vesicles that lie either side of the bladder and which, with neighbouring accessory glands, produce seminal fluid which combines with sperm to form semen.

The penis

This is the male organ of copulation. The internal structure of the penis contains erectile tissue. Erection occurs when the penis becomes engorged with blood when the stallion is sexually stimulated. During erection, the penis of the horse doubles in length and thickness. When erect the stallion is able (with practice) to mount the mare and insert the penis into the mare's vagina. This is called intromission. After some thrusting, semen is ejaculated into the mare and the stallion dismounts.

The end of the glans penis is surrounded by a prominent margin or rose. This enlarges to three times its resting size after ejaculation. The end of the urethra projects through this rose. The free portion of the non-erect penis is covered by the sheath or prepuce, which consists of a double fold of skin, so that two concentric layers surround the penis. This can be quite voluminous and may cause a sucking noise when the horse is trotting.

Sperm

Sperm are produced within the seminiferous tubules in the testes. The process of development of the sperm is known as spermatogenesis. During this process the number of chromosomes halve. The resultant sperm have half the number of chromosomes found in the nucleus of other body cells (e.g. muscle cells, brain cells, etc.), which have 64. The egg also has half the number of chromosomes so that, when fertilisation takes place, the resultant embryo gains half the chromosomes from the mare (egg) and half from the stallion (sperm) The embryo should thus have the full complement of chromosomes.

The whole cycle of sperm development takes approximately 50–60 days in the stallion. The mean daily production of sperm is in the order of 7,000,000,000. The more a stallion is used, i.e. the higher the frequency of ejaculation, the faster the sperm are produced. Each sperm consists of a head, mid-piece and a tail.

The semen (ejaculate) is made up of sperm and seminal fluid produced by the accessory sex glands. The seminal fluid nourishes the sperm on their journey to the egg.

Pregnancy

This refers to the condition of the mare while a foetus is developing within her uterus. The period of pregnancy from fertilisation to birth is known as the gestation period and the average gestation period of the mare is 333–336 days (11 calendar months from the date of last service) there is a range in Thoroughbreds of 310–374 days. In other breeds a range of 322–345 days is normal. The foetus determines when to be born as it approaches full term. The genetic make up and environmental factors such as nutrition of the foetus have a bearing on the length of pregnancy.

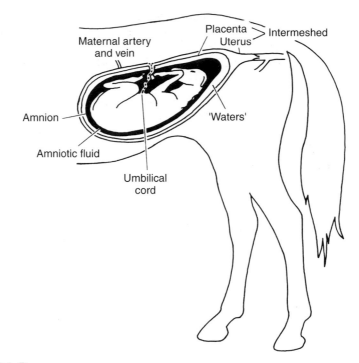

Figure 32.8. Pregnancy.

Pregnancy (Figure 32.8) is the period in which the new embryo develops into an individual being capable of surviving independently from the mother (after birth).

The foetus within the uterus is surrounded by fluids, which cushion and protect against the effects of movement and gravity. The wall of the uterus also allows protection and the foetus cannot lose fluids or heat except through its immediate surroundings, i.e. the mother.

The uterus is a highly muscular organ allowing the foetus to expand as it grows in size. This is very important. First-time pregnancies often result in smaller foals than expected, because the uterus is being stretched for the first time. In subsequent pregnancies, the uterus is able to expand more easily.

The uterus is also kept very effectively closed by the cervix. This prevents the entrance of microorganisms into the uterus, which may harm the developing foetus.

A summary of the development of the foetus is shown in Table 32.1.

Lactation

In the weeks leading up to foaling, the mare's udder (mammary glands) develop and enlarge. These are modified sweat glands. The mare has four

Table 32.1. Summary of foetal development in the horse

Day of pregnancy	Primary development
1	24 hours after conception, the conceptus, i.e. the combination of egg and sperm, start to divide into two cells. This cell division continues into 4, 16, 32, 64, etc. cells
6	The dividing cell bundle arrives in the uterus and at the same time breaks open its outer layer and 'hatches'
18	Foetus now takes on 'C' shape. Gut tube developing and umbilical cord is identifiable
23	All the basic body structures, neural tube (central nervous system and brain), pharynx, gut tube and major muscle blocks are present in a basic form
26	Forelimb bud and eye now evident
40	Nostrils seen, ears forming, all limbs are present, and elbow and stifle joints are discernible
45	External genitalia present
63	Eyelids fused while eye development continues. Sole and frog areas of hoof evident
120	Chin hair and eyelashes growing
180	Tail and mane present
320–355	Birth of a well-developed foal that is capable of walking 20 minutes after birth

glands in two pairs. Each pair of glands exit through a central teat, i.e. there are two teats supplying the four glands.

The mare's mammary glands are situated between the hind legs. Each of the four mammary glands is completely separate from the other, i.e. there is no mixture of milk between the four quarters. It is only in the 2–4 weeks before foaling that milk is produced.

The urinary system

The urinary system (Figure 32.9) is primarily involved in the extraction and removal of waste products from the blood. In particular, it is responsible for the removal of nitrogenous waste and, together with the digestive system, it removes all waste products produced in the body except gaseous carbon dioxide which is removed via the lungs. While removing these waste products, the urinary system is also very closely involved with the water balance of the horse, acid–base and salt balance. These processes are highly complicated and involve the influence of hormones.

The urinary system itself is composed of:

- two kidneys
- two ureters
- bladder
- urethra.

Each day approximately 1000–2000 litres of fluid are delivered to the kidneys of the horse. Since only approximately 5–15 litres of urine are excreted daily, the kidneys must remove most of the substances present in them. If the kidneys did not reabsorb fluid entering them, then horses would lose their entire water and salt content in less than half a day!

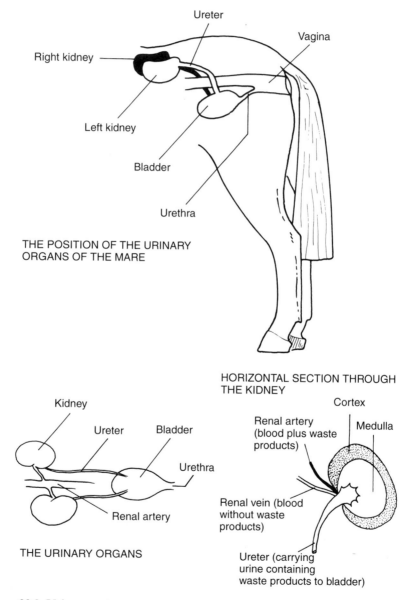

Figure 32.9. Urinary system.

Kidneys

These are a pair. In the horse the kidneys lie on either side of the body, approximately midway between the withers and the croup underneath the spine. The left kidney lies farther back towards the last rib whereas the right kidney lies under the last three ribs. In this position they are well protected from external injury and it is therefore uncommon for them to become bruised.

The kidneys are situated outside the abdominal cavity, but are bound to the upper wall of the abdomen by a layer of peritoneum that prevents the kidneys moving about when the horse moves. There are often large collections of fatty tissue around the kidneys which also help to protect them.

The kidneys are organs that filter plasma from the blood. In other words they are highly efficient sieves, which allow the passage of smaller particles such as plasma through, but not the larger blood cells. From the substances which are filtered through, the kidneys can selectively re-absorb water and other useful constituents, so that they are not wasted.

Most of the domestic animals have bean-shaped kidneys similar to humans, but the horse has two different shaped kidneys, the left one is bean shaped and the right one is heart shaped. In the adult horse each kidney weighs approximately 450 g (1.5 lb) and measures 15–18 cm (6–7 in) in length.

Micturition or urination

This is the term used for the evacuation of urine from the bladder. The urine produced in the kidneys in the collecting tubules is then transferred to the renal pelvis where it enters the ureter and is carried to the bladder. The bladder acts as a storage vessel for urine. Micturition is a reflex activity stimulated by the fullness of the bladder itself.

Horses tend to urinate (stale) at rest when on grass or bedding. Many horses will wait to urinate (if the bladder is not too full) until they are brought into the stable, particularly when the bedding is clean and deep.

Horses adopt a typical posture when urinating, with the hind legs separated, the horse leaning slightly forward. There is contraction of the muscles of the abdominal wall and the tail is raised. Often horses will grunt and groan when urinating. This is normal. Horses produce about 5–15 litres of urine a day (depending on water intake and diet) and will urinate approximately four to six times in that period.

Horse owners should be vigilant in watching their horses urinating habits. Early recognition of abnormal signs will allow prompt veterinary attention if something is wrong.

Possible signs of a problem:

- signs of pain when the horse is urinating
- continual straining
- excessive grunting
- too much or too little urine
- excessive thirst
- absence of thirst
- colour of the urine – should be light-yellow to amber in colour. If it is dark coloured or bloodstained the vet should be called immediately.

Conditions of the urinary system

Diseases of the urinary system are relatively rare in horses. The kidney is an unusual organ in that it can continue to function even when it is quite considerably damaged (up to 70%). Even though this is the case, conditions of the urinary system must always be taken seriously as they can be life threatening.

Cystitis, or inflammation of the bladder, is again relatively rare in horses. The problem may result from passage, e.g. bacteria in the urethra. If the bladder cannot empty itself properly, then infection is more likely to result. Conditions that may cause this are bladder stones or bladder paralysis.

Visible signs include frequent attempts to urinate and severe straining on urinating. Sometimes the condition may be chronic (long lasting) with signs such as urine dribbling and caking of the vulval lips of mares. The urine may be bloodstained.

Treatment depends on the initial cause that must be identified. Antibiotic therapy will be given depending on the organism that has caused the problem. This can be found by culture of urine samples to grow the bacteria. An antibiotic is used which will be excreted at high levels in the urine and therefore kill the bugs in the urinary tract.

Chapter 33
The stallion

Choosing a stallion

The first step in breeding a foal is to choose the stallion that the mare is going to be covered by. The majority of stallions standing at stud are segregated from other horses and cover mares 'in hand', that is both mare and stallion are restrained during the covering procedure. However, many pony stallions run with their mares at grass, covering the mare when his instinct determines, not when a human lets him. While this method is more natural, it is obviously not practical for valuable Thoroughbreds and competition horses.

The Ministry of Agriculture no longer licenses stallions and it is left to the breed societies to make their own arrangements for validating the use of a horse at stud. This validation may involve an inspection to observe conformation, soundness and freedom from hereditary defects.

To breed from a particular breed of stallion it is wise to get in touch with the appropriate breed society. The location of the stud, the breeding record of the stallion, what his progeny look like, what they have done and how much the stud fee is are all-important factors.

When selecting a suitable stallion for a specific mare, it is necessary to consider the following:

- *Value*: the nomination fee should be relative to the mare's value.
- *Conformation*: it is obviously unwise to consider a mating if the mare and the stallion have similar conformation faults.
- *Pedigree*: a considerable amount of data are available to judge the compatibility of bloodlines. Investigation would normally include a study of the sire lines that have been used on members of the same family to analyse the most successful crosses.
- *Performance*: the breeder will carefully consider the performance of the mare and stallion. When breeding racehorses a breeder will normally send a mare to a stallion that has raced over a similar distance.
- *Progeny*: if a sufficient amount of data are available it is helpful to draw a conclusion from the analysis of progeny results.
- *Temperament*: a successful competition horse must have a good temperament.

The final decision may rest on whether the progeny is to be sold or retained to race or compete – if the progeny is to be sold, it is important to consider fashion and market forces.

Decisions concerning the suitability of a mating require considerable experience and understanding of the related factors – there is no fixed formula to gauge the relative importance of each. Thoroughbred horses are not necessarily used solely for the production of racehorses and produce useful stock when mated with non-Thoroughbred mares.

Handling of stallions

While the daily routines for stallions will vary from stud to stud, basic principles need to be observed to maintain their well-being. As with any horse, it is important that stallions receive adequate food and exercise, but these will need to be adjusted according to the season and the horse's workload.

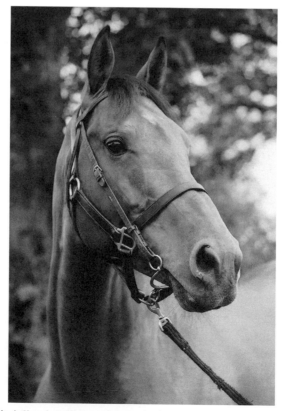

Figure 33.1. A disciplined stallion, safely tacked up.

Maintaining a reasonable level of discipline is essential, but it must be maintained in sympathy with the horse's natural desire to dominate. Access to stallions must be restricted to staff who have sufficient experience and knowledge to work with them safely. Stallions still tend to be naturally aggressive and mishandling will quickly compound any problems.

Exercise

Exercise routines must be established to ensure that a reasonable level of fitness is achieved before the start of the breeding season. Exercise is also required to ensure the mental well-being of the stallion. Lungeing, riding, exercising in-hand and paddock exercise can be considered for inclusion in the routines.

Management

The number of mares that a Thoroughbred stallion will cover is normally limited to between 50 and 60 in any breeding season. Restrictions are made to prevent overuse of the stallion and to protect the value of the resultant progeny. As a general rule, stallions will be limited to three mares per day and about 16 mares per week. Overuse of a stallion will reduce fertility that can take a long time to recover.

As with mares, it will be necessary for stallions to be swabbed according to recommended policy. Swabs are currently taken before the start of each season; they are not normally taken from a stallion during the season unless a problem has been identified.

Covering

When covering it is essential that an experienced handler who is able to maintain complete control leads the stallion. The handler will normally be responsible for guiding the stallion's penis into the mare's vagina and ensuring that ejaculation occurs.

When the horse rears, pressure on his mouth must be limited – harsh handling can cause the stallion to fall over backwards. The stallion normally approaches the near-hind quarter of the mare and is encouraged to mount slowly and carefully. Care must also be taken when the stallion dismounts to prevent spinal and shoulder injuries that can be caused by the mare twisting. The stallion's penis will normally be rinsed with warm water after covering.

Presentation of stallions to clients

The presentation of stallions to prospective clients is also extremely important. Stallions will normally be expected to be well rounded, but not fat, with a well-groomed coat, medium-length mane and trimmed tail. Stallions will normally be viewed from the nearside, but the handler must always remain on the same side as the client. Horses need to be taught to stand and walk properly when being viewed. Clients will often want to watch the horse's action from the front, rear and side. Horses must be encouraged to walk actively and should be turned to the offside.

Teasing

Through the oestrous cycle the behaviour of the mare should alter, especially in the presence of a male horse, and reflect the readiness of her genital tract to conceive and maintain a pregnancy. Significant seasonal and individual variations from the normal cycle can be expected – for instance, early in the season it is not uncommon to encounter prolonged periods of oestrus and dioestrus and lactating mares sometimes become anoestrus after the foal heat. These variations are identified through careful teasing. Routines must be established to ensure the regular teasing of mares, but these will vary from stud to stud. Veterinary examination may also be used to clarify results and these can include blood samples to identify hormone levels, rectal palpation to detect activity in the ovaries, visual examination of the genital tract and endometrial biopsies (microscopic examination of tissue samples from the uterus). The interpretation of teasing and veterinary findings it crucial to the timings of coverings.

Safe teasing practices

Care should be taken to ensure the safely of handlers and horses when teasing and suitable equipment selected to ensure that the mare and the teaser could be restrained. Trying boards can be built to a suitable specification to be safe and strong. Handlers should be given clear instructions regarding:

- protective clothing (gloves, skull cap, footwear)
- suitable equipment to ensure that the mare and the teaser can be restrained
- the correct positioning of the mare and the teaser
- any relevant information about behavioural abnormalities of the horses involved.

Records

Detailed records of teasing must be kept and these should incorporate any individual behavioural characteristics which might be displayed by the mare. Special consideration needs to be given to mares that fail to show normal behaviour at the trying boards – these may include mares that are naturally shy teaser, or mares who have not established a regular oestrous cycle at the start or end of the breeding season.

Chapter 34
The mare

Choosing a mare for breeding

The wrong reason to select a mare for breeding is because she is not fit for anything else. A good reason to select a mare is because she is an outstanding example of quality. It may be that she has proved this quality in competitions, be it in the show ring, the racetrack or elsewhere. Usually it would be wrong to go on breeding from a mare that has difficulty in holding her foetus or in foaling, or from one that is a bad mother. It is also wrong to breed from a mare with poor conformation or a poor temperament.

The oestrous cycle

A mare will normally ovulate every 3 weeks throughout the natural breeding season, which does not entirely correspond with the enforced breeding season of the Thoroughbred industry. In this 3-week period, called the oestrous cycle, the mare will normally be receptive to the male horse (in season or oestrus) for about 5 days and unreceptive (not in season or dioestrus) for about 16 days. The mare will often cease cycling in winter (anoestrus). Anoestrus is a natural response to a poor diet, the cold weather and, the short periods of daylight, which are associated with winter. Mares are often put under lights in January and February to extend artificially the hours of daylight and activate the oestrous cycle.

The teasing/covering procedure was discussed in Chapter 32.

Pregnancy diagnosis

About 16 days after covering it is possible to scan the pregnancy to allow the early diagnoses of a conceptus (Figure 34.1).

Further scans may be performed during the early stages of the pregnancy. In addition to scanning, the veterinary surgeon will normally perform a manual

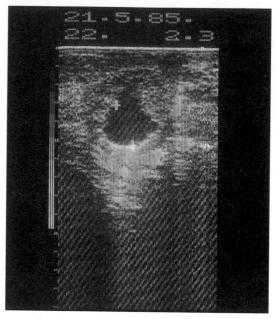

Figure 34.1. A scanner photograph showing a 22-day-old conceptus.

examination of the mare at 6 weeks after mating to confirm the pregnancy. A manual examination is also essential at the end of September for nominations purchased on a no foal–no fee (NFNF) (1 October) agreement.

Alternative methods of pregnancy diagnosis, which may be used include blood and urine tests. While these are less intrusive, they do not offer the accuracy of the rectal examinations.

Maintaining the condition of a pregnant mare

Mares will require feeding and paddock exercise throughout their pregnancy and the farrier, worming and vaccinations according to the stud's policy should pay particular attention to good routine. Teeth should be checked occasionally and rasped as necessary.

Throughout the pregnancy it is desirable that the mare be checked carefully at least twice a day, paying particular attention to any signs of abortion (swollen udder, strange behaviour, discharge from the vulva). If an abortion occurs, it is essential to follow the procedures detailed in the code of practice to ensure that potential problems are not transmitted to other horses and that, whenever possible, the cause of abortion is identified. This should be discussed with the vet.

Exercise is important to mares, although this normally takes the from of free exercise in the paddock. The riding of pregnant mares is not considered harmful in the first months of pregnancy and slow ridden exercise (walking) is unlikely to cause direct harm at any stage of the pregnancy.

Vaccination

Vaccinations must be maintained during pregnancy; influenza (flu), tetanus and equine herpes virus (EHV) vaccinations are recommended. Flu and tetanus injections are sometimes administered late in the pregnancy so that some immunity is transferred to the foal. There are now combined flu and EHV vaccinations that may be used to replace one of the EHV courses. A regular worming routine must be maintained, ensuring that the worming drug used is suitable.

Feeding the broodmare

The pregnant mare

The pregnant mare should be kept healthy and in good condition, not fat. Very overweight mares may have problems foaling, as the foals tend to be large. During winter or summer the mare's ribs should not be seen, but should be detected on touch with no appreciable layer of fat. This will make foaling easier and enhance her chances of conceiving again. If she is in good condition the mare should be fed a low-calorie stud balancer or a good vitamin and mineral supplement. This will maintain her micronutrient intake, without supplying additional calories. In other words, assuming she conceives in April, grass should be adequate in providing calories until September or October depending on the availability of pasture.

As the grass supply wanes hay may be introduced. During the final 3 months of pregnancy the mare's nutrient requirements increase. At the same time the foetus occupies an increasing proportion of her abdomen, thus her capacity for bulk feed may drop. If condition is fine, then maintain the stud balancer and introduce a small amount of stud cubes/mix to prepare the gut for lactation. If she needs more condition, slowly introduce stud cubes/mix and carry on through lactation.

Many native breeds and heavier types will manage very well on good-quality forage and a low calorie stud balancer, through pregnancy and lactation.

It is important that the diet is balanced in calcium and phosphorus as imbalance may lead to a weak foal. In the 24 hours before foaling, the mare should be fed good-quality hay and her stud ration maintained. The mare may go off her feed anyway at this time. Feeding a bran mash after foaling will result in a sudden change of diet and this is not recommended. A small amount of bran may be introduced to the stud diet, which may be mixed with warm water to make it appetising.

The lactating mare

The nutrient requirements of a lactating mare increase dramatically, being equivalent to those of a fit racehorse, particularly in the first 3 months of lactation. The lactating mare needs good-quality hay and high-protein and -energy concentrates, such as stud cubes or stud mix, particularly if she is foaling before the spring grass is available to supplement her diet. As the lactation progresses and the mare has increasing access to grass she should be fed a low-calorie stud balancer, particularly if the mare is pregnant again. If being prepared for the show ring or if grazing is limited, then the stud cubes/mix may be continued but care should be taken not to feed too much cereal/starch at any one feed, no more than 2 kg. The addition of oil helps to provide further calories without overloading the digestive system with starch. Unmolassed beet pulp and alfalfa are both good sources of calcium and readily digestible plant fibre.

Barren and maiden mares

Providing the mare is neither too fat nor too thin, a similar feeding regime to that of the mare in early pregnancy can be followed, ensuring optimum micronutrient nutrition.

Foaling requirements

The facilities that a stud can provide for the foaling of mares will be entirely dependent on the size and nature of the business. However, suggested minimum requirements for a foaling box are as follows:

- good ventilation, but without draughts
- good insulation to prevent condensation and protect water supply
- free draining floor
- adequate lighting and power supply
- free from any obstructions or intrusions
- a sliding or outward opening door
- adequate headroom.

It is essential to have all equipment for foaling clean and available for foaling:

- soap and towel
- tail bandages and head collar
- sterilised surgical scissors
- veterinary gloves
- lubricant

- drawing ropes, only for use by vet or experienced stud groom
- string for tying afterbirth
- antiseptic powder or iodine
- foaling alarm or closed circuit television (CCTV)
- rugs and blankets, including foal rug
- overalls and boots
- disinfectant
- frozen or powdered colostrum, feeding bottle and teat
- kettle
- vet's phone number.

Foaling

A mare will foal approximately 340 days from her last service date, but this can vary from 320 to 365 days. If the mare foals after 325 days of pregnancy, this is as good as full-term and the foal will live. A foal is described as being premature if it is born between 300 and 325 days and the foal may die. As the mare gets nearer to foaling she will get much heavier in weight and slower in her movements, she is less likely to exercise herself and her legs could fill (Figure 34.2).

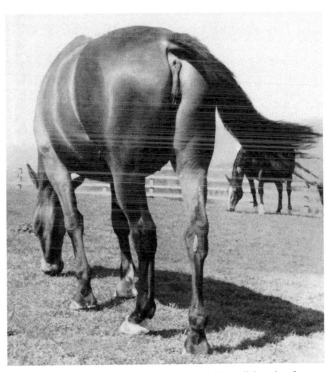

Figure 34.2. Full udder, wax on teats, muscles round the tail-head soft, quarters looking less round, vulva relaxed and moist, and stood apart from the others – this mare did foal that night.

The birth of the foal marks the end of pregnancy; the foal is pushed through the birth canal by contractions of the uterus and abdominal muscles. During the first stage of labour powerful contractions cause a rise in pressure in the fluids surrounding the foetus and these press against the placenta. As the cervix dilates it leaves a weak spot through which the chorio-allantois (placental membranes) bulge until it ruptures, releasing the allantoic fluid. This breaking of the waters marks the end of the first stage. The cervix is now fully dilated and the foal is pushed through the birth canal by contractions of the uterus and abdominal muscles.

Position of the foal

At the start of birth the foal is usually lying on its back with its head, neck and legs flexed. As the contractions begin, the foal extends its forelimbs and head, turning into an upright position with its forelegs and muzzle pressed against the cervix.

Signs of foaling

A mare will normally start to bag-up about 3 weeks before foaling. The udder becomes progressively larger until a waxy discharge of dried milk can be seen on the teats; this often indicates that the mare will foal in the next 24 hours, but it is possible for a mare to foal without waxing-up. Mares may also run milk prior to foaling and that this can result in the loss of vital colostrum. Other signs that might be noted before foaling are changes in behaviour (especially tending to stand away from other mares), elongation of the vulva and relaxing of the pelvic muscles causing dipping of the flank.

Once the mare has waxed up she may foal at any time and should not be left unattended. It is essential that mares are kept under close observation when they are near to foaling, but disturbance must be kept to a minimum. Mares normally foal at night and do not appreciate outside interference.

Stages of foaling

There are three stages of foaling:

- The first stage is from first contractions until breaking of the first waters. This, as in humans, may be a very short time or several hours.
- The second stage is from the breaking of waters until the birth of the foal. If the mare does not foal within approximately half an hour after breaking of waters, the vet should be called.
- The third stage is from the birth of the foal until the expulsion of the after-birth. Mares normally foal late at night and, should the mare not have cleansed by morning, the vet will be required to assist her.

First stage

The first of labour is the movement of the foal lying in its back (head to the rear end of the mare) to the stage where the forelegs and head are at the entrance of the pelvic canal. Some mares will show little sign of the first stage of labour but will normally pace around their box (nesting) and begin to sweat. Most studs will apply a tail bandage and a headcollar when the mare show signs of foaling and mares who have a Caslick's operation will need to be opened by a vet or a senior member of staff. Mares will show a range of signs, including:

- looking at their flanks
- sweating
- showing Flehmen (curled top lip with head and neck outstretched)
- pacing the box and pawing at the ground.

Mares might not show any sign of first-stage labour while others will show prolonged periods of pain interspersed with periods of calm. During first-stage labour, uterine contractions are starting – this continues until the pressure created in the uterus is sufficient to rupture the placenta at the opening cervix. The resultant rush of allantoic fluid (breaking waters) indicates the start of second-stage labour. This must not be confused with the mare urinating.

Second stage

The second stage of foaling commences when the waters break. Normally a rush of fluid will be noticed as the placenta ruptures. The mare will often appear very uncomfortable at this stage and will sometimes lie down and stand up several times. The mare will often stand and lie down repeatedly before finding a satisfactory position to complete the second stage, normally lying down and often with her back against a wall. If all is going well, an opaque whitish-blue bag will appear (the amnion). This has a balloon-like appearance and should contain the foal's first foot. Once the foal's feet appear at the vulva, the presentation of the foal can be checked by carefully placing a gloved hand inside the vagina to feel the front legs and the foal's muzzle. The foal is presented in a diving position, and the foal's second leg and head must be in the correct position. Immediate and expert assistance will be required if the presentation is not correct.

The most difficult stage of the birth process occurs when the foal's shoulders pass through the pelvis (this normally corresponds with time then the foal's poll passes through the vulva). The second leg always follows the first in a manner that will slant the foal's shoulders enabling it to pass more easily through the mare's pelvis. Any problem with posture requires quick action and involves seeking the immediate assistance of a veterinary surgeon or supervisor. In this event, the foal's pasterns should be held firmly and gently pulled down and away from the mare to correspond with contractions.

Second-stage labour will normally will normally last for about 25 minutes, but may last from 10 minutes to 1 hour.

After further contractions from the mare, the foal's head will then be seen covered by the amnion. The amnion will often break naturally while foaling but occasionally may need assistance as a foal can suffocate inside the bag. Once the shoulders are out the mare may rest and should not be disturbed.

After some less violent contractions by the mare, the foal should be born; at this stage the umbilical cord should still be intact, and both mare and foal should be left still and quiet for as long as possible (Figure 34.3).

More often than not the cord will break naturally when either mare or foal moves. At this stage the umbilical stump should be sprayed with purple spray or some other antiseptic product.

If the mare has not moved, the foal should be brought round to the mare's head. It is important at this stage for mare and foal bonding to taken place.

Third stage

Third-stage labour commences when the foal is born and the umbilical cord has ruptured; it involves the expulsion of the placenta (or afterbirth). Once a foal is born, the umbilical cord should be left intact for as long as possible and treated with antiseptic when it breaks. The mare will stand shortly after foaling and will usually expel the afterbirth within about half an hour.

It is advisable to tie up the placenta and amnion while the mare is in third-stage labour. This prevents the danger of the placenta becoming torn and aids the separation and cleansing by applying weight to encourage the separation of the placenta from the uterus. Additional pressure should not be used as this may result in the retention of part of the placenta.

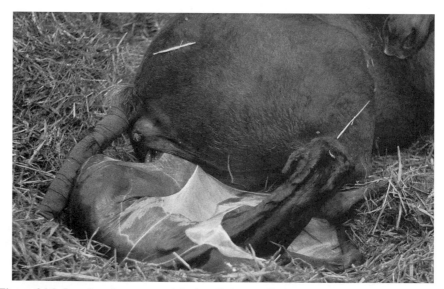

Figure 34.3. Leaving the mare and foal well alone will allow them to bond and settle.

The careful examination of the afterbirth is essential to ensure that it is complete – it is possible for the tip of the non-pregnant horn to tear with a section remaining in the uterus. Placenta retention can have a very serious effect causing widespread infection and laminitis. To examine the afterbirth properly it is necessary to lay it out; two sections will be seen – the white amnion in which the foal lay during pregnancy and the pale red placenta which will almost certainly have turned inside out as the mare cleansed (the attachment side of the placenta will normally be a deep red colour). There should only be one hole in the placenta, close to the point where it attached to the cervix; the hole should be from the body of the placenta opposite the two horns, which must be checked to ensure that they are complete. The severed umbilical cord will run through the amnion to the attachment point, which is normally at the base of the two horns.

Once the mare has foaled the vulva should be checked for tears. If the vulva is torn, it will need stitching by the vet.

Colostrum

For the first month of its life, the foal is unable to manufacture significant levels of antibodies and therefore has a limited natural defence against infections or disease unless it acquires immunity from the mare. Antibodies are not able to cross from the uterine blood to the placental blood, but are transmitted in the mare's first milk, which is know as colostrum. Colostrum contains a high level of antibodies, the gut absorbs these for as little as 12–48 hours, after which the foal will manufacture its own. Failure to absorb sufficient antibodies will leave the foal susceptible to disease; this may occur if the mare runs a significant amount of milk before foaling, or if the foal fails to suckle. The mare may need to be milked and the foal bottle-fed until it has the strength to cope on its own. If the mare was not given a tetanus booster 6 weeks before foaling, then the foal will need the vet to give it protection against tetanus.

Signs of health in the new born foal

Careful observation of the newborn foal is essential to ensure that problems are identified and treated quickly.

Pulse

The normal pulse rate of the newborn foal will be about 60 beats per minute, but rising to 90–100 in the first hour eventually settling back to about 50 per minute. Changes in rate will occur as the foal exercises, but unusual rates in resting foals are always significant. Monitoring the colour of mucous membranes – especially inside the lip and eyelid – can also check circulation.

Temperature

While slight variations do not imply a problem, the normal temperature of a foal will be about 38°C.

Respiration

The normal respiratory rate is 70 breaths per minute at birth, falling to about 40 per minute after 1 hour. A raised respiratory rate in a resting foal could indicate a variety of problems and warrants immediate investigation.

Management of the mare and the newborn foal

Careful consideration needs to begin before mating a mare on the foal heat. Decisions should be based on the age of the mare, the time of the year, any damage caused by trauma during foaling, the degree of involution of the uterus and the results of cervical or endometrial swabs.

The mare's udder must be monitored after foaling as a guide to the foal's health and to ensure that mastitis is detected quickly. Foals that go off suck require prompt attention.

Exercise after foaling is essential for both the mare and the newborn foal. For the mare it assists the uterus shrinking back to its non-pregnant size and the passing of any remaining fluids. For the foal, exercise offers the opportunity to develop balance and strengthen limbs. Growth problems are almost inevitable if the foal is not given adequate exercise.

While there will be variation between the exact policy of different stud farms, it is normal practice to start handling and training the foal within a few days of its birth. Dependent on the season, a foal rug might be used when the foal is exercising and a foal-slip will be used so that the foal can be taught to lead. In wet conditions it is wise to limit the foal's exercise to 1 or 2 hours per day unless a facility is available to offer exercise under cover.

When leading a mare and foal it is normal practice to hold the mare in the left hand and the foal in the right. A second person should be available to follow the foal and ensure that it keeps moving forwards. When the foal gains sufficient confidence, the second person it not required (see Chapter 35).

It is preferable to keep mares with newborn foals away from other horses until a satisfactory level of bonding is achieved (Figure 34.4). It is possible for foals to be swapped if this precaution is not taken.

A degree of protection against flu virus and tetanus in the foal can be gained by vaccinating the mare in the final month of pregnancy, but it is important to discuss a suitable regime with the veterinary surgeon. Worming will normally commence when the foal is about 4 weeks old, but it is important to follow the manufacturer's recommended dosage closely. Foot trimming can be started at about the same time, but the frequency will depend on the rate of growth and any remedial requirements.

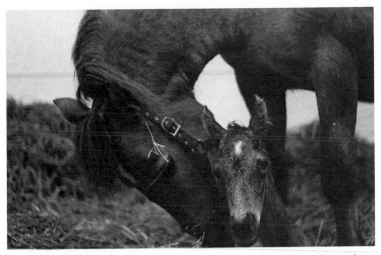

Figure 34.4. Mare–foal bonding is important and best done without distraction.

Foaling complications

When to call the vet

It is important to recognise when to call the vet as prompt action can save mare and/or foal:

- when the waters break and nothing else happens
- when the waters break and one foot only shows, indicating a malpresentation or dystocia
- over-large foal, which gets stuck during foaling
- bleeding from vulva – could be internal haemorrhage
- broken or dislocated pelvis
- recto-vaginal fistula
- bruising and tearing of vulva (stitching and Caslick's operation)
- post-natal laminitis
- mare not cleansed
- prolapse
- colic
- extended labour pains
- presentation of a red bag.

Weaning

The mare should preferably be with other weaned mares with whom she is familiar. The mare should be fed hay with a vitamin and mineral supplement for a couple of days to allow the milk to dry up and avoid complications such as mastitis. Concentrate feed can then be slowly reintroduced.

Chapter 35
Getting the mare in foal

There are several management factors that may help to get the mare in foal, these include swabbing the mare to check for the presence or absence of disease.

Examination of the mare before covering

Before covering

The veterinary surgeon will examine the mare prior to covering and take swabs from the clitoris and inside the cervix to ensure that she is not carrying sexually transmittable diseases or infections that would infect the stallion or prevent her getting in foal.

Swabbing

Swabs are taken for culture and any growth is identified to allow the necessary treatment to be given by the vet. Swabs are normally taken from:

- The clitoris: clitoral swabs can be taken when the mare is not in season and 1 week should be allowed before complete results can be obtained.
- A cervical swab should be taken when the mare first comes into season. This is generally taken as a precaution to find out if the mare has a uterine infection. The cervical swab is taken using a speculum in the mare's vagina so that the swab can be taken from the cervix.
- Bacteria can cause uterine infections. These must be treated by means of irrigation or washing out the mare's uterus by the veterinary surgeon along with antibiotics. She will then be reswabbed the following heat before service may be allowed. Swabbing requirements prior to covering will be dependent on the industry's code of practice, the stud's policy and any significant outbreaks of infection since the policies were written. The Thoroughbred Breeders Association and other breeding authorities produce a code of practice.

For low-risk mares it is recommended that there should be one negative clitoral swab on arrival, plus one cervical swab when in the first oestrus (in-foal mares at foaling oestrus). High-risk mares are ones that have been previously infected or in contact mares plus imported mares other than from France or Ireland.

For stallions and teaser stallions it is recommended that there should be two sets of swabs taken at an interval of not less than 7 days.

All handlers should be made aware of rules of hygiene and the danger of contaminating mares. When handling mares' and stallions' genitalia use tail bandages and disposable gloves. Isolate all aborting mares and have a full investigation. Vulvae discharges to be investigated and the mare isolated.

Once the documentation has been checked, it is normal practice to place a tail bandage on the mare and wash off the perineum around her vulva with warm. Normally, it is not recommended to use detergents or antiseptics/disinfectants as these may disturb the normal protective bacterial flora. It is essential that a visual check be made for discharge when washing off the mare.

Safety equipment in the covering yard

All staff should refer to recommendations regarding safety equipment as issued by their employers. For the handler these might include:

- hard hats
- gloves
- suitable footwear (steel toecaps).

Other safety equipment which might be used to help restrain the mare or stallion and to protect horses and handlers in the covering yard include:

- twitch
- felt boots
- leg strap
- cape or neck protector
- breeding bar
- suitable bridles for mare and stallion.

Clear instructions must be issued to all staff assisting in the covering yard so that each member of the team is fully aware of their responsibilities and familiar with the equipment that will be used. The yard itself should offer a safe environment, including:

- the absence of obstructions or intrusions
- flooring which offers protection and a good footing
- sufficient floor space and headroom
- a dust-free environment.

Once in the yard, the mare will normally be fitted with covering boots (Figure 35.1) that are put on to the hind feet of the mare and designed to soften the blow of a kick. In some cases, a twitch may be applied to the mare's muzzle. A leather cape may be placed on the mare's neck to give protection from the stallion's teeth and a leg strap may be used to hold up a foreleg. The person at the

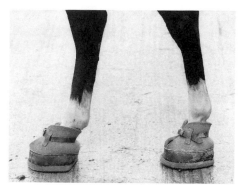

Figure 35.1. Covering boots.

mare's head should stand to the side of the mare out of reach of the stallion's forelegs while he is mounting or covering the mare. On some studs, another member of staff will hold the twitch. Teamwork is essential in the yard and one person present should be responsible for giving instructions.

The stallion will be encouraged to mount from behind (Figure 35.2) and slightly to the near side of the mare. One member of the team will normally be responsible for checking that the stallion has ejaculated. As the stallion dismounts, the mare is normally turned to prevent her from kicking him.

After covering, the mare's tail bandage should be removed and the stallion's penis washed off with warm water. The mare's vulva should be checked for

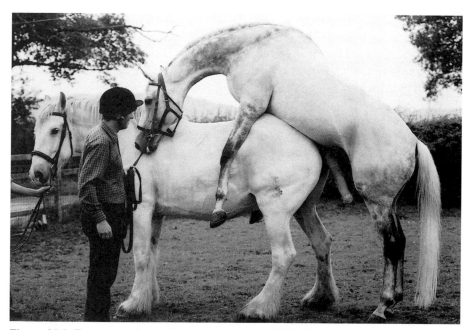

Figure 35.2. Encourage the stallion to mount from behind.

blood and signs of tearing. As with teasing, it is normally better to leave the foal in its stable while the mare is being covered.

It is common practice to walk mares for a few minutes after covering to prevent them straining.

Procedures after covering

It is normal for a teasing programme to be designed to ensure that a second covering is arranged if the mare remains in oestrus and that any return to oestrus after covering can be detected quickly.

Artificial insemination and embryo transfer

Artificial insemination is the technique used to place semen into the mare's reproductive tract using special insemination instruments. This removes the disease risk factor of a natural covering. Artificial insemination is prohibited in the Thoroughbred industry; foals conceived by this method will not be recognised or registered. The industry's concerns relate to possible fraud and the exploitation of 'fashionable' stallions with the resultant significant rise in numbers of their offspring. This would result in reduced value of the offspring. Laboratory equipment and trained personnel are required and this can be expensive. Some non-Thoroughbred studs, particularly those involved with sports horses, are now using artificial insemination to a large extent. Semen must be collected from the stallion using an artificial vagina. The collected semen is evaluated under a microscope and then, if it is normal, will be maintained at 40–44°C for up to 24 hours. If it is to be transported long distances, it may be chilled and placed in a Thermos-type flask. Often the semen sample will be mixed with a preparation known as an extender that contains nutrients and anti-bacterial agents, which will prolong the survival of the sperm.

The use of frozen semen in horses is not as widespread as in cattle due to problems with freezing techniques. Many extenders have been tried, but none have proved to be very successful so far. There is also variation between different stallions and the freezing ability of their sperm using the same extender.

Insemination

Mares are inseminated on day 2–3 of oestrus. Semen is deposited in the uterus by means of a sterile pipette.

Advantages and disadvantages of artificial insemination

Advantages
- Reduces the spread of sexually transmitted disease, such as contagious equine metritis.
- Reduces the risk of injury to mare and stallion.

- Allows stallions with behavioural problems to inseminate mares.
- No transport of mares (with/without foals at foot).
- Mares will not be sent to stud, therefore no keep charges.
- Use stallions further afield as semen may be transported in special containers.

Disadvantages

- Will reduce conception rates if procedure is not carried out correctly.
- Prohibited by many breed societies.
- May lead to errors in respect to parentage as semen may be handled several times before the mare is inseminated.
- May lead to overuse of stallions, thereby limiting genetic variation and increasing inherited faults.

Embryo transfer

Again, this process is well established in sheep and cattle, but is still not widely used in horses. The technique involves the transfer of a fertilised egg from a donor mare into a surrogate mare's uterus. The stallion covers the donor mare and the embryo is flushed out of the uterus 7 or 8 days later. Collection and transfer of embryos can be performed non-surgically with reasonable success. This technique may be used for top-class competition mares allowing them to breed before they retire. This is a great advantage as older mares have more difficulty conceiving.

Recipient mares must be in good health and a similar size to the donor mare.

Chapter 36
The foal and young horse

Handling mares and foals

While the same rules apply to handling mares and foals as to other horses, additional care should be taken. Mares with young foals may be overprotective and show aggression to handlers. Care is needed to ensure that these mares do not injure stable staff or the foal.

Handling the newborn foal

The early handling of foals is the beginning of their training and they must be taught good manners. It is important that this handling should be kind, but firm. Slapping its chest gently and scolding it should discipline a foal that rears or paws. A foal that bites (even in play) should be disciplined. The foal will have to have a foal-slip (small head collar) put on at some point in the first week. The foal-slip is secured with an assistant holding one arm round the chest and the other arm round the quarters. If the foal is hard to catch, the mare can be so placed as to corner it. Right from the start, leading is safer than allowing the foal to run loose. For early leading, a soft web line is placed through the foal-slip and passed back to the left hand. At first, this hand steadies the foal by being placed across its chest. A second loop of similar material is dropped around the foal's quarters and is held on the loins. An assistant should lead the mare and the foal should be kept by the mare's flank. Thus, the mare's leader is in front of the foal, its leader and the mare are on either side of it, and the back strap is behind it. After a week or two, if the mare and foal are coming in at night, the foal will become accustomed to being led and then one person will be able to handle both mare and foal. However, assistance may still be needed at the field gate. The fit of the foal-slip must be checked regularly and adjusted as foals grow quickly.

When foals are 2 months old they may be shown in hand with their mother. For showing it is important that the foal should be polite and lead well. The foal should be accustomed to being stood up in front of the mare and to having the mare stood up in front of it. When being shown, mare and foal will have to be separated to some degree, so that the judge can observe each move without the other masking the picture. All of this handling will help the foal to become accustomed to both humans and discipline. Foals must learn to have their feet picked out as this will prepare them for having their feet trimmed by the farrier.

When leading a mare and foal it is normal practice to hold the mare in the left hand and the foal in the right. A second person should be available to follow the foal and ensure that it keeps moving forwards. When the foal gains sufficient confidence, the second person is not required.

Turning out mares and foals

A rigid procedure is essential when several people are leading mares with foals or young stock. For example, if three mares with foals were led to a paddock, and the first handler, immediately on entering the paddock, were to release his or her mares and foal, the mare might well buck, kick, knock into the foal and then gallop off, thus causing problems for the other leaders, whose charges would want to join in the fun. All studwork involves care, thought, attention to detail and good discipline.

When turning out mares and foals, mares should be turned to face the fence and kept well apart from each other; the gate should be closed before the mares are released. It is better to let the mare go fractionally before the foal to prevent the foal from being trampled or separated from the mare. Caution is needed when introducing a new mare or mare and foal to a group. The group should be given plenty of time to settle after being turned out before the new mares are introduced. The group should be watched carefully until they settle.

When catching young foals in the field it is often necessary to lead the mare to a fence (ideally boarded) so that the foal can be caught between mare and fence, care must be taken not to frighten the foal. It is advisable to have a helper available to assist with catching and to open and close the gate.

Routine healthcare of foals

Vaccination and worming

A degree of protection against flu virus and tetanus in the foal can be gained by vaccinating the mare in the final month of pregnancy, but it is important to discuss a suitable regime with the veterinary surgeon. Vaccination of the foal may take place from about 5 or 6 months, preferably prior to weaning.

Worming will normally commence when the foal is about 6 weeks old, but some studs start as early as 4 weeks. It is important to follow closely the manufacturer's recommended dosage. Foot trimming may be started at about the same time, but the frequency will depend on the rate of growth and any remedial requirements.

Weaning

During the first winter after foaling it is natural for the mare's milk supply to slow down. Foals are weaned so that they become independent of their mother. Weaning of the foal normally takes place at around 6 months of age.

During weaning it is helpful if there are several mares and foals together in the field, which must be well fenced. One of the mares is removed quietly and placed with a companion in a field far removed (out of hearing distance preferably) from the foal. Her foal is left with the friends it knows and soon settles down. A day or so later, another mare may be removed and so on.

Colts and fillies should be separated at this time or a few weeks later.

Feeding youngstock

Foals

Foals have their own food supply in the form of milk. From 2 or 3 months creep feeding will provide additional nutrients to support growth. Creep feeding devices allow the foal to eat, but not the mare. The foal should be fed a 16–18% protein creep feed at a rate of about 1–1.5% of the foal's bodyweight per day [about 0.5 kg (1 lb) of feed per every 1 month of age up to 6 months of age]. Care should be taken to monitor the foal's intake and watch that it is not over- or under-consuming. Foals that have been creep fed are less likely to have a setback at weaning.

Weanlings

The growth-related problem of developmental orthopaedic disease (DOD), which includes epiphysitis, contracted tendons and osteochondrosis, may occur in weanlings and yearlings. It is important that these youngsters receive a balanced and adequate diet, but are not overfed energy during their first winter. DOD is most commonly seen in the overtopped fast-growing foal and there are stud balancers available that supply all the nutrients required for growth without supplying additional calories.

For weanlings that are not overweight, it is useful to feed a reputable stud cube designed for young growing horses along with good quality hay during the winter.

Yearlings

The growth rate will now have started to slow down. Yearlings may be fed 1% of their bodyweight per day of a 14–16% protein concentrate with top-quality hay, depending on their condition. Overtopped yearlings should be fed a low-calorie stud balancer with their forage.

Diseases of foals

Joint-ill

Hot and swollen joints in young foals can be a symptom of joint-ill (infective arthritis or navel ill). The condition is normally associated with an infection acquired through the navel early in life, and is the result of infection carried in the blood and accumulating in the joints. Urgent veterinary attention is essential.

Haemolytic foals

In a small number of cases there is a leaking of foetal blood across the placenta that causes an immune response in the mare. The mare creates antibodies to destroy the foetal cells in her blood stream. If these antibodies are then passed to the foal immediately after foaling via the colostrum, they cause rapid destruction of red cells (haemolysis) in the newborn foal. A swift diagnosis of the problem is essential to save a haemolytic foal. Symptoms include lethargy, jaundiced membranes, and raised respiration and pulse rates if excited or exerted.

Once a mare has produced a haemolytic foal, it is probable that future foals will show the same condition. In these cases it is possible to detect the problem before the foal is born by taking blood samples from the mare. Ensuring that the foal does not drink colostrum from the mare until its intestines are unable to absorb the antibodies can prevent symptoms. The foal should be muzzled at birth and given colostrum from a selected donor mare.

Neonatal maladjustment syndrome

Neonatal maladjustment syndrome (NMS) is a general term for a range of behavioural abnormalities that can occur in newborn foals, often due to a lack of oxygen during birth. Symptoms can involve the suck reflex, balance and sight. Other terms for this condition include dummies, barkers, convulsives or wanderers.

Meconium retention

The faeces, which form in the foal's intestine during the pregnancy, are called meconium. Meconium colic is common and is caused by constipation arising from a failure to pass meconium. The foal may need an enema.

Diarrhoea

It is not unusual for foal's faeces to become loose during the mare's foal heat. It is essential that potential problems are not overlooked at this stage – diarrhoea can be a serious threat to young foals and might be caused by a bacteria or virus. Treatment must be given to prevent foals from becoming dehydrated and it is wise to take action to prevent the scalding of buttocks and hind legs by smearing them with petroleum jelly.

Umbilical hernia

Umbilical hernias are common in foals and are only serious if they become strangulated. Normally correction is performed before this becomes a major risk.

Contracted tendons and limb deformities

Foals will often suffer from slack or contracted tendons and it is essential that management techniques and, when necessary, veterinary assistance are used to prevent problems from getting worse. Angular limb deformities occur with the knee and fetlock deviating from a straight and upright line. Remedial shoeing (or foot trimming) and surgery are used to attempt to correct persistent deviation. Toeing-in and toeing-out can also be associated with this problem. Nutrition needs to be reviewed to check the foal is getting all the required nutrients, oversupply of energy can be harmful.

Deformities

Parrot mouth or over shot jaw is a hereditary deformity in which the upper incisor-teeth overlap the lower incisors. This will makes life difficult for the foal, as it will be unable to bite food and therefore be difficult to keep in good condition. For this reason, in severe cases the foal should be destroyed — especially if upper and lower teeth do not actually touch. If these teeth do touch this is less serious and the foal will be able to lead a normal life.

Chapter 37
Preparation of breeding stock for sale

Thoroughbreds are reared mostly for sale to go into racing. Some Thoroughbreds are bred for flat racing and others for national hunt. National hunt youngstock are more extensively reared and are often out-wintered in groups. They are handled and fed daily. Potentially highly valued competition horse foals are prepared for sale in a similar way to Thoroughbred racehorses.

Preparation for sale by public auction

In order to maximise the chances of receiving a good price for a yearling, the youngster should be presented to the best of the owner's ability. Many yearlings are prepared at the studs where they were bred, others are sent to be prepared by smaller owners to the larger studs (or studs which are renowned for their yearling preparation) for a fee. This can be quite expensive and the cost has to be balanced with the possible increase in the sale price that may be gained with preparation. Many breeders like to prepare their stock themselves.

Yearlings and National Hunt Stores

Care and attention to detail while preparing horses for sale can reap dividends on the day. While pedigree and conformation cannot be changed, a well-presented yearling will draw the eye of prospective purchasers who may give the horse a second look and hopefully create a great deal of interest before bidding begins. On the other hand, a poorly presented yearling will not attract buyers unless the pedigree is outstanding. The yearlings with the best pedigrees and conformation will always attract high prices. Preparation usually begins a minimum of 50 days (usually 100 days) prior to the sale. In fact, many breeders prepare their stock from birth. This slow preparation is much better for the horse. Yearlings need to be prepared physically, mentally and cosmetically.

If the weather is hot, then yearlings will be brought in during the day for work, feeding and rest, and turned out at night when it is cooler and flies are not a problem. Fillies may be turned out together, but colts are usually turned out separately to prevent injuries caused by over-exuberant behaviour.

After yearlings are brought in for preparation they begin a programme of exercise designed to increase muscle and strengthen bone. This exercise may consist of one or several of the following: walking, lungeing, long-reining, horse-walker and treadmill. This exercise programme should be tailored to suit the individual yearling and should not create undue stress on the horse.

Walking

Most yearlings begin preparation by walking which gently conditions the horse and trains it to lead out in hand quietly, as it will have to do at the sale itself. The yearling can also be trained to stand up square in hand for prospective purchasers at the sale.

Lungeing

This should be built up slowly from 2–3 minutes per time and adding 2 minutes per session up to maximum of 12–15 minutes. As the yearling gets fitter some trotting and cantering may be introduced (on both reins). Long-reining may be introduced at this stage.

Treadmill

This should be introduced slowly so as not to frighten the horse. It will provide slow, intense work then faster walking for 3–4 minutes. The yearling should not be expected to work hard.

Horse-walker

An excellent labour-saving device that may also be used to warm up or cool down the horse. The yearling should be placed loose in the walker and not attached by the head.

Presentation

Finally, the yearling must be trained to walk up and present itself to prospective purchasers on the sale days. This will take a lot of practice with many yearlings. Yearlings are usually shown up in either headcollars and chifneys or bridles. Handlers showing off the yearling should be compatible. A tall handler should not present a small yearling and vice versa.

Feeding

Most yearlings receive a high-energy diet to encourage them to put on fat and condition. This must be balanced with all the other nutrients required to maintain their growth.

Feeding an unsaturated oil such as vegetable or corn oil at the rate of two cups per day will help to produce a gleaming coat and will also add calories to the ration. Most yearlings will receive a complete, balanced and formulated ration that has been matched to the forage they consume. Care should be taken with overtopped yearlings that the micronutrient nutrition is correct and that they do not become excessively overweight.

Grooming and bathing

Yearlings should be groomed for a minimum of 30 minutes each day. Their manes are pulled. Most yearlings are rugged up to maintain a short coat (see Chapter 25).

Shoeing

Yearlings have light plates all round.

National Hunt Stores

National Hunt Stores will undergo a more active preparation, as they are older, bigger horses. They will be lunged, long-reined, bitted and some even backed. They will also need to be trained to lead up in hand and stand square in front of prospective purchasers.

Sale day

Most yearlings and the staff looking after them arrive 4 days prior to the sale itself. This gives them time to settle in their new surroundings. Yearlings may be brought out and shown to prospective purchasers many times in the next few days. They should be watched all the time and as normal a routine as possible imposed on them. Staff looking after them should also be smart and well presented, many wear a 'team' jacket as a uniform. On the day of the sale horses will be called to the parade ring about 20 minutes before they are due to be sold.

Yearlings will be walked quietly round as potential purchasers make their final judgements and then taken into the sale ring itself. Bidding takes place in guineas and once the hammer falls, the horse is the responsibility of the purchaser. Many vendors will place a reserve price on the horse and if that price is not reached during the bidding the horse will remain unsold.

Appendix
Equine terminology

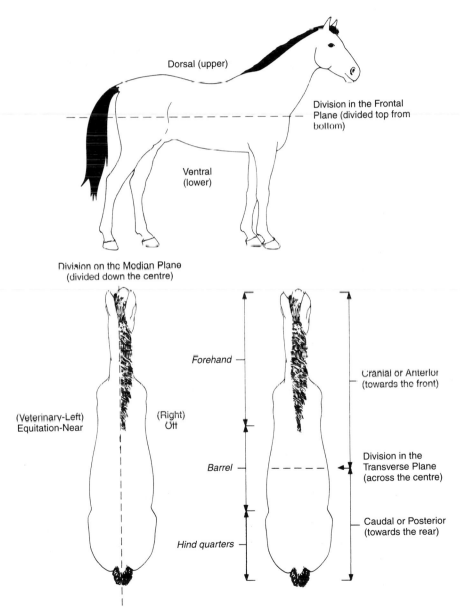

Dorsal (upper)

Division in the Frontal Plane (divided top from bottom)

Ventral (lower)

Division on the Median Plane (divided down the centre)

Forehand

Cranial or Anterior (towards the front)

(Veterinary-Left) Equitation-Near

(Right) Off

Barrel

Division in the Transverse Plane (across the centre)

Caudal or Posterior (towards the rear)

Hind quarters

Equine terminology (*contd.*).

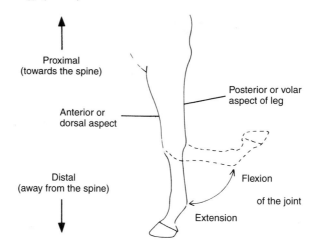

Proximal
(towards the spine)

Anterior or
dorsal aspect

Posterior or volar
aspect of leg

Flexion

of the joint

Distal
(away from the spine)

Extension

Index